Practice in Mental Health–Substance Use

MENTAL HEALTH–SUBSTANCE USE

Practice in Mental Health–Substance Use

Edited by

DAVID B COOPER

Sigma Theta Tau International: The Honor Society of Nursing Award
Outstanding Contribution to Nursing Award
Editor-in-Chief, Mental Health and Substance Use
Author/Writer/Editor

Radcliffe Publishing
London • New York

Radcliffe Publishing Ltd
33–41 Dallington Street
London
EC1V 0BB
United Kingdom

www.radcliffepublishing.com

Electronic catalogue and worldwide online ordering facility.

British Library Cataloguing in Publication Data

A catalogue record for this book is available from the British Library.

ISBN-13: 978 184619 344 6

Typeset by Pindar NZ, Auckland, New Zealand
Printed and bound by Cadmus Communications, USA

Contents

Preface

Approximately six years ago Phil Cooper, then an MSc student, was searching for information on mental health–substance use. At that time, there was one journal and few published papers. This led to the launch of the journal *Mental Health and Substance Use: dual diagnosis*, published by Taylor & Francis International. To launch the journal, and debate the concerns and dilemmas of psychological, physical, social, legal and spiritual professionals, Phil organised a conference for Suffolk Mental Health NHS Trust and Taylor & Francis. The response was excellent. An occurring theme was that more information, knowledge and skills were needed – driven by education and training.

Discussion with international professionals indicated a need for this type of educational information and guidance, in this format, and a proposal was submitted for one book. The single book progressed to become a series of six! The concept is that each book will follow on from the other to build a sound basis – as far as is possible – about the important approaches to mental health–substance use. The aim is to provide a 'how to' series that will be interactive with case studies, reflective study and exercises – you, as individuals and professionals, will decide if this has been achieved.

So, why do we need to know about mental health–substance use? International concerns related to interventions, and the treatment of people experiencing mental health–substance use problems, are frequently reported. These include:

➤ 'the most challenging clinical problem that we face'[1]
➤ 'substance misuse is usual rather than exceptional amongst people with severe mental health problems'[2]
➤ 'Mental health and substance use problems affect every local community throughout America'[3]
➤ 'The existence of psychiatric comorbidities in young people who abuse alcohol is common, especially for conditions such as depression, anxiety, bipolar disorder, conduct disorder and attention-deficit/hyperactivity disorder'[4]
➤ 'Mental and neurological disorders such as depression, schizophrenia, epilepsy and substance abuse . . . cause immense suffering for those affected, amplify people's vulnerability and can lead individuals into a life of poverty'.[5]

There is a need to appreciate that mental health–substance use is now a concern for us all. This series of books will bring together what is known (to some), and what is not (to some). If undertaken correctly, and you, the reader will be the judge – and those individuals you come into contact with daily will be the final judges – each book will build on the other and be of interest for the new, and the not so new, professional.

The desire to provide services that facilitate best practice for mental health–substance use is not new. The political impetus for this approach to succeed now exists. We, the professionals, need to seize on this momentum. We need to bring about the much-needed change for the individual who experiences our interventions and treatment, be that political will because of a perceived financial benefit or, as we would hope, the need to provide therapeutic interventions for the individual. Whatever the motive, now is the time to grasp the initiative.

Before we (the professionals) can practise, research, educate, manage, develop or purchase services, we must commence with knowledge. From that, we begin to understand. We commence using our new-found skills. We progress to developing the ability to examine practice, to put concepts together, to make valid judgements. We achieve this level of expertise though education, training and experience. Sometimes, we can use our own life experiences to enhance our skills. But knowledge must come first, though is often relegated to last! Professionals (from health, social, spiritual and legal backgrounds) – be they students, practitioners, researchers, educators, managers, service developers or purchasers – are all 'professionals' (in the eye of the individual we meet professionally), though each has differing depths of knowledge, skills and expertise.

What we need to remember is that the individual (those we offer care to), family and carers bring their own knowledge, skills and life experiences – some developed from dealing with ill health. The individual experiences the illness, lives with it, manages it – daily. Therefore, to bring the two together, individual and professional, to make interventions and treatment outcome effective, to meet whatever the individual feels is acceptable to his or her needs, requires mutual understanding and respect. The professionals' skills and expertise '*are founded on nothing less than their complete and perfect acceptance of one, by another*'.[6]

David B Cooper
March 2011

REFERENCES

1 Appleby L. *The National Service Framework for Mental Health: five years on*. London: Department of Health; 2004. Available at: www.dh.gov.uk/prod_consum_dh/groups/dh_digitalassets/@dh/@en/documents/digitalasset/dh_4099122.pdf (accessed 29 August 2010).

2 Department of Health. *Mental Health Policy Implementation Guide: dual diagnosis good practice guide*. London: Department of Health; 2002. Available at: www.nmhdu.org.uk/silo/files/mental-health-policy--implementation-guide.pdf (accessed 29 August 2010).

3 Substance Abuse and Mental Health Service Administration. *Results from the 2008 National Survey on Drug Use and Health*. 2008. Available at: www.oas.samhsa.gov/nsduh/2k8nsduh/2k8Results.cfm (accessed 2 August 2010).

4 Australian Government. *Australian Guidelines to Reduce Health Risks from Drinking Alcohol*.

2009. Available at: www.nhmrc.gov.au/publications/synopses/ds10syn.htm (accessed 29 August 2010).

5 World Health Organization. *Mental Health Improvements for Nations Development: the WHO MIND Project.* World Health Organization; 2008. Available at: www.who.int/mental_health/policy/en (accessed 29 August 2010).

6 Thompson F. *Lark Rise to Candleford: a trilogy.* London: Penguin Modern Classics; 2009.

About the Mental Health–Substance Use series

The six books in this series are:
1 *Introduction to Mental Health–Substance Use*
2 *Developing Services in Mental Health–Substance Use*
3 *Responding in Mental Health–Substance Use*
4 *Intervention in Mental Health–Substance Use*
5 *Care in Mental Health–Substance Use*
6 *Practice in Mental Health–Substance Use*

The series is not merely for mental health professionals but also the substance use professionals. It is not a question of 'them' (the substance use professional) teaching 'them' (the mental health professional). It is about sharing knowledge, skills and expertise. We are equal. We learn from each fellow professional, for the benefit of those whose lives we touch. The rationale is that to maintain clinical excellence, we need to be aware of the developments and practices within mental health and substance use. Then, we make informed choices; we take best practice, and apply this to our professional role.[1]

Generically, the series Mental Health–Substance Use concentrates on concerns, dilemmas and concepts specifically interrelated, as a collation of problems that directly or indirectly influence the life and well-being of the individual, family and carers. Such concerns relate not only to the individual but also to the future direction of practice, education, research, service development, interventions and treatment. While presenting a balanced view of what is best practice today, the books aim to challenge concepts and stimulate debate, exploring all aspects of the development in treatment, intervention and care responses, and the adoption of research-led best practice. To achieve this, they draw from a variety of perspectives, facilitating consideration of how professionals meet the challenges now and in the future. To accomplish this we have assembled leading, international professionals to provide insight into current thinking and developments, from a variety of perspectives, related to the many varying and diverse needs of the individual, family and carers experiencing mental health–substance use.

REFERENCE

1 Cooper DB. Editorial: decisions. *Mental Health and Substance Use*. 2010; **3**: 1–3.

About the editor

David B Cooper
Sigma Theta Tau International: The Honor Society of Nursing Award
Outstanding Contribution to Nursing Award
Editor-in-Chief: *Mental Health and Substance Use*
Author/Writer/Editor

The editor welcomes approaches and feedback, positive and/or negative.

David has specialised in mental health and substance use for over 30 years. He has worked as a practitioner, manager, researcher, author, lecturer and consultant. He has served as editor, or editor-in-chief, of several journals, and is currently editor-in-chief of *Mental Health and Substance Use*. He has published widely and is 'credited *with enhancing the understanding and development of community detoxification for people experiencing alcohol withdrawal*' (Nursing Council on Alcohol; Sigma Theta Tau International citations). Seminal work includes *Alcohol Home Detoxification and Assessment* and *Alcohol Use*, both published by Radcliffe Publishing, Oxford.

List of contributors

CHAPTER 2   May Baker
Senior Lecturer – Mental Health Nursing
Faculty of Health and Applied Social Sciences
Liverpool John Moores University
Henry Cotton Building
Liverpool, England

May has worked at Liverpool John Moores University since 2004. She teaches on the pre- and post-registration nursing programme and the MA social work and specialist practitioner course. May's main teaching interests are alcohol and drug awareness, dual diagnosis and motivational interviewing. Previous to teaching she worked for 11 years in acute mental health and as a specialist practitioner in drug services.

David Buckley
Specialist Team Manager
Windsor Clinic Alcohol Service
Mersey Care NHS Trust
University Hospital Aintree
Liverpool, England

David began registered mental health nurse training in 1982 at Winwick Hospital near Warrington. After qualifying he worked briefly as a deputy charge nurse on an acute ward. It was there that David noticed a lack of consistency in the treatment of people experiencing alcohol problems. He took up a staff nurse post at the Windsor Clinic Alcohol Treatment Unit, Rainhill Hospital, and has remained there ever since. David's current role is Specialist Team Manager covering the inpatient unit. David was instrumental in researching and developing a nursing model for specific use with addictions which is in current use at the clinic and has published articles regarding alcohol use through the years. While David's role is managerial he still retains aspects of clinical work in his schedule including assessments, running support groups and contributing to the rehabilitation programmes.

CHAPTER 3   **Dr Zain Sadiq**
Associate Specialist in Psychiatry
Home Treatment Team
South London and Maudsley NHS Foundation Trust
Croydon, England

Zain is a member of the Royal College of Psychiatrists and is the college representative on the Academy of Medical Royal Colleges (AoMRC) SAS Committee. Apart from a busy lead clinical role, Zain is also involved in training and teaching junior doctors and medical and nursing students.

Dr Paul D Morrison
Medical Research Council Clinical Research Training Fellow
Specialist Registrar in Psychiatry
Psychological Medicine
Division of Psychological Medicine and Psychiatry
Institute of Psychiatry
Denmark Hill
London

Paul is a research psychiatrist at the Institute of Psychiatry. He studied in Glasgow and Chicago, before coming to London. At present he is investigating the effects of cannabinoid molecules in humans using electroecephalography (EEG).

CHAPTER 4   **Richard Orr McLeod**
Former Senior Nurse Specialist
Huntercombe Hospital
Four Seasons Healthcare
Roehampton, London

Richard is a former senior nurse and nurse specialist in South West London. He has worked extensively in both inpatient and community settings and has managed prison detox services and forensic dual diagnosis units. His special interests are in dual diagnosis, relapse prevention and post-traumatic stress disorder.

Philip D Cooper
Practice Educator
Education and Workforce Development
Suffolk Mental Health Partnership NHS Trust
St Clements Hospital
Ipswich, Suffolk
England

Phil qualified as a mental health nurse in 2002, and then worked within an acute admissions ward before moving to community mental health. After a brief spell in an assertive outreach team, Phil moved to his current role. Here, Phil was seconded as project manager for the mental health–substance use needs assessment and strategy development project. Phil studied for an Advanced Diploma in Dual Diagnosis before completing an MSc in Dual Diagnosis, in 2007. Phil has authored a number of chapters, and was the founder, and editor, of the international journal *Mental Health and Substance Use: dual diagnosis*; he stepped down from this position in June 2010.

CHAPTER 5   Dr Suzanne Nielsen
Senior Research Fellow/Senior Pharmacist
Clinical Research and Clinical Services
Turning Point Alcohol and Drug Centre
Senior Lecturer (Adjunct), Monash University
Fitzroy, Victoria
Australia

Suzanne is currently the National Institute on Drug Abuse (NIDA) INVEST Clinical Trials Network (CTN) fellow, based at the University of California, Los Angeles (UCLA). She has over 10 years' clinical experience in specialist drug treatment settings with a special research interest in pharmaceutical misuse. Suzanne is on the editorial board of Drug and Alcohol Review and Chair of the Pharmaceutical Misuse Working Group for the Alcohol and other Drugs Council of Australia (ADCA).

Dr Nicole Lee
Associate Professor
National Centre for Education and Training on Addiction (NCETA)
Director, Lee Jenn Health Consultants
Flinders University
Adelaide, South Australia
Australia

Nicole has 20 years' experience in the substance use and mental health fields, including extensive clinical experience. Nicole sits on the council of the Australasian Professional Society on Alcohol and other Drugs (APSAD) and is deputy editor for *Drug and Alcohol Review*. She has previously served as national president of the Australian Association for Cognitive and Behaviour Therapy (AACBT) and on the board of the Alcohol and other Drugs Council of Australia (ADCA). Nicole is well known internationally for her work in addiction treatment, especially in co-occurring substance use and mental health disorders and treatment of methamphetamine use problems. She is currently part of a team developing Australia's National Pharmaceuticals Strategy, and has published extensively in substance abuse and mental health treatment, including peer-reviewed literature, book chapters and training and clinical guidelines.

CHAPTER 6   David Jones
Director
Quit Now Ltd

Walsall, West Midlands
England

Dave has worked as a clinician, manager and lecturer in the addictions for the last 15 years. He is the director of Quit Now Limited, a company that offers treatment, training and consultancy related to smoking cessation (www.quitnow-walsall.co.uk). Dave has worked as a lecturer at the universities of Wolverhampton and Nottingham, and been an honorary tutor in dual diagnosis at the Institute of Psychiatry, Kings College, London.

CHAPTER 7   Professor David J Kavanagh
Research Chair
Institute of Health and Biomedical Innovation and
School of Psychology and Counselling
Queensland University of Technology
Queensland, Australia

David was educated at Sydney and Stanford Universities, and has an extensive record of research funding and publication on substance misuse and its comorbidity with mental disorders, and currently leads the OnTrack research group, which is developing and testing online interventions in this area. Since 2008, he has been the co-chair of a committee that plans strategic initiatives on comorbidity for state government health services in Queensland, and has previously served on several national committees on substance misuse, comorbidity and service development.

Dr Dawn Proctor
Postdoctoral Research Fellow and Clinical Psychologist
Institute of Health and Biomedical Innovation and
School of Psychology and Counselling
Queensland University of Technology
Queensland, Australia

Dawn was previously a senior clinician within the Queensland alcohol and drug detoxification unit. She completed her doctoral training at the University of Manchester, specialising in metacognitive therapy for anxiety disorders. Dawn is currently involved in the development of online interventions for a range of mental health concerns and in exploring the application of metacognitive techniques for dual diagnosis.

CHAPTER 8   Francesca Miller
EMDR and Body Work Therapist
Clinical Nurse Specialist Alcohol
Chorley, Lancashire
England

Fran qualified as a mental health nurse in the late 70s and worked for 15 years in acute and forensic mental health services. She left the health service in 1994 to take a job as an alcohol counsellor in the voluntary sector. Concerned about the lack of innovation and research into the aetiology and treatment of addiction, Fran trained in a number of psychological and complementary therapies in an attempt to answer her own questions about the recurring themes and presentations she was noticing in her work. Fran returned to the health service in 2000, and her chapter is a synthesis of her experience as a nurse, counsellor, trainer, clinical supervisor, EMDR and body work therapist, amid the emerging and exciting findings of the neuropsychology movement.

CHAPTER 9 Dr Walter Busuttil
Medical Director and Consultant Psychiatrist
Combat Stress
Leatherhead, Surrey
England

Walter served in the RAF for 16 years. He helped set up mental health rehabilitation services for combat veterans returning from the first Gulf War. He was part of the clinical team that rehabilitated the released British Beirut hostages. Walter has published and lectured internationally about treatment and rehabilitation of chronic and complex presentations of post-traumatic stress disorder and has helped to set up services for its treatment nationally. He is the current chair of the UK Trauma Group.

CHAPTER 10 Dr Arthur G O'Malley
Consultant Infant, Child and Adolescent Psychiatry
Specialist in Trauma Focused Psychotherapy
Specialist in Perinatal and Infant Mental Health
5 Boroughs Partnership NHS Foundation Trust
Runcorn, Cheshire
England

Art is an accredited EMDR practitioner and a member of the UK and Ireland EMDR association. He is a member of the European conference organising committee for the London Conference and the Child and Adolescent Committee. Art has presented at the AGMs, and at the European conferences in Paris and London. He has presented widely in the fields of trauma, the developing brain, attachment disorders, personality disorders, emotional dysregulation in ADHD and ASD diagnosis and management. Art has an interest in infant and maternal mental health and set up a joint parent–infant mental health clinic. This is designed for parents of infants where there are significant difficulties in the parent–infant relationship. The trauma-focused approach includes EMDR, sensorimotor psychotherapy, mindfulness and trauma-focused CBT. The infant mental health is addressed using the Watch Wait and Wonder dyadic psychotherapy approach (WWW). Art actively supervises therapists towards accreditation as both practitioners and consultants. He recently completed MacArthur Story Stem Battery training (MSSB) under the guidance of Professor Jonathan Hill, which he plans to use to evaluate the clinical effectiveness of the combined clinic which incorporates trauma-focused therapies and Watch Wait and Wonder psychotherapy.

CHAPTER 11   Marilyn White-Campbell
Geriatric Addiction Specialist
Manager, Geriatric Mental Health Outreach Geriatric Addiction Specialist
Long Term Care
Community Outreach Program in Addiction (COPA)
Toronto, Ontario
Canada

Marilyn has worked with older adults with substance use and mental health issues with the COPA programme – one of Canada's first addiction treatment programmes for seniors – for over 24 years. She is considered a pioneer in the field of addictions/ concurrent disorders and older adults. Marilyn is co-author (with Kate Graham *et al.*) of *Addictions Treatment for Older Adults: evaluation of an innovative client-centered approach*. Marilyn is on the International Advisory Board of *Mental Health and Substance Use: dual diagnosis*. She has presented nationally and internationally on the Canadian Model for Treatment of Older Adults with Substance Misuse.

CHAPTER 12   Dr Christina KME Sonneborn
Psychiatrist and Head of Service
Forensic Youth Service, GGzE
AX Eindhoven, The Netherlands
Dual Diagnosis Programme
Novadic-Kentron
AE Vught, The Netherlands

Christina completed her general medical training in Germany and undertook her psychiatric training in the UK. She subsequently trained as a psychotherapist in Belgium where she lives with her Belgian husband and three children. She has been working as a consultant psychiatrist in the Netherlands since 1998, combining her appointment as a psychiatrist/psychotherapist at a forensic inpatient service for young adults (16–24 years) with leading an integrated dual diagnosis service for patients with complex mental health and substance use problems.

CHAPTER 13   Dr Lorne M Korman
Scientist, British Columbia Mental Health and Addiction Service
Research Director, British Youth Columbia Concurrent Disorders Network
Clinical Associate Professor of Psychiatry
Department of Psychiatry
University of British Columbia
Vancouver, British Columbia
Canada

Lorne is a registered psychologist. He has authored publications on DBT and the treatment of borderline personality disorder, anger and addictions, gambling, and on emotion in psychotherapy. Recently, Lorne helped establish a DBT programme in British Columbia for individuals who are deaf. He has been featured in the APA training video *Working with Anger*, and is currently the principal investigator on a trial of a DBT adaptation for young adults with anger and addiction problems.

Dr Kyle Burns
Psychiatrist
Deaf, Hard of Hearing and Deaf-Blind Well-Being Program
Vancouver Coastal Health
Burnaby, British Columbia
Canada

Kyle is currently a consulting psychiatrist to the Deaf Well-Being Program, a mental health programme for individuals who are deaf or hard of hearing. He has been part of developing the first dialectical behaviour therapy team for deaf and hard of hearing individuals in Canada. Kyle also works with the Vancouver Inner City Youth Mental Health Program and founded a DBT team that works with disenfranchised youth and young adults in inner-city Vancouver.

CHAPTER 14   David Marteau
Section Head – Substance Misuse
Offender Health
Wellington House
London

Dave has worked in the substance misuse field for 25 years. He is currently the substance misuse policy lead for offenders (England). He is the author of a book and several chapters on the nature and treatment of problematic substance misuse.

CHAPTER 15   Rami T Jumnoodoo
Project Lead Relapse Prevention
Brent Rehabilitation and Supporting Services
Central and North West London NHS Foundation Trust
Bushey, Hertfordshire
England

Rami qualified as a general nurse and then a registered mental nurse. He has a first-class degree in psychiatric nursing and a Masters in Mental Health Interventions. Rami is experienced in many fields of psychiatry and psychology. He has been commended for awards for his current role and post. Rami has developed several accredited programmes on relapse prevention in mental health. He recently won the CSIP Positive Practice and the Human Resources and Nursing Times awards. His work is achieving international recognition.

Dr Patrick Coyne
Nurse Consultant
Manager of Addiction and Offender Care, Education and Training
Addiction and Offender Care
Soho Centre for Health and Care
London

Patrick qualified in 1986, and has held a number of posts in adult mental health, elderly care, and substance misuse. He commenced his senior position as a consultant research advisor before taking a post in substance misuse and mental health. Patrick has a number of publications and has presented work both nationally and internationally on nursing, health promotion, substance misuse and workforce development. Patrick developed the clinical nurse specialist post in HIV and substance misuse service during the 1990s, and has undertaken private consultancy. Patrick provides consultancy support for the sustainable development of the Relapse Prevention in Brent Mental Health Services Initiative (RPBrent) and beyond for the past 12 years.

CHAPTER 16   Sharon H Hsu
Graduate Student
Addictive Behaviors Research Centre
Department of Psychology
University of Washington
Seattle, WA
USA

Sharon is a doctoral candidate in clinical psychology and has received the Ruth L Kirschstein National Research Service Award, funded by the National Institute on Alcoholism and Alcohol Abuse. This award will support her to conduct dissertation and related training goals. Sharon earned her bachelor's degree in psychology with completion of the honours programme from the University of California, San Diego. Her research interests include understanding how culture may shape factors associated with addictive behaviours among ethnic minorities and how such empirical evidence can be used to enhance existing evidence-based treatment.

Professor G Alan Marlatt
Director, Addictive Behaviors Research Centre
Department of Psychology
University of Washington
Seattle, WA
USA

Alan's major focus has been the field of addictive behaviours. In addition to over 200 journal articles and book chapters, he has published several books including *Harm Reduction* (1998). He has received continuous funding for his research from agencies such as the National Institute on Alcohol Abuse and Alcoholism, the National Institute on Drug Abuse (NIDA), and the Robert Wood Johnson Foundation. Most recently, Alan received the Distinguished Scientific Contributions to Clinical Psychology Award by the American Psychological Association. Alan currently serves as the principal investigator on a NIDA-funded grant examining the efficacy of Mindfulness-Based Relapse Prevention.

Alan sadly passed away in March 2011, just as this book was being sent to press.

CHAPTER 17   Dr John R Ashcroft

Speciality Grade Psychiatrist
Hope House
Blackpool Substance Misuse Service
Blackpool, Lancashire
England

John is an Associate specialist psychiatrist in substance misuse. He studied at Imperial college of Science Technology and Medicine in London and achieved undergraduate degrees of BSc (Hons) in Neurosciences and Medicine (MBBS). He is a Member of the Royal College of Psychiatrists. In 2008, John was awarded a postgraduate diploma in clinical neuropsychiatry with merit by the University of Birmingham. He has recently been invited to become an advisory board member of the journal *Mental Health and Substance Use* published by Taylor and Francis International. He has special interests in clinical neuropsychiatry and dual diagnosis.

USEFUL CONTACTS   Jo Cooper

Former Macmillan Clinical Nurse Specialist in Palliative Care
Horsham, West Sussex
England

Jo spent 16 years in specialist palliative care, initially working in a hospice inpatient unit, then 12 years as a Macmillan Clinical Nurse Specialist (CNS). She gained a Diploma in Oncology at Addenbrooke's Hospital, Cambridge, and a BSc (Hons) in Palliative Nursing at The Royal Marsden, London, and an Award in Specialist Practice. Jo edited *Stepping into Palliative Care* (Radcliffe Medical Press, 2000) and the second edition of *Stepping into Palliative Care*, Books 1 and 2 (Radcliffe Publishing, 2006). Jo has been involved in teaching and education for many years. Her specialist subjects include management of complex pain and symptoms, terminal agitation, communication at the end of life, therapeutic relationships, and breaking bad news.

Terminology

Whenever possible, the following terminology has been applied. However, in certain instances, when referencing a study and/or specific work(s), when an author has made a specific request, or for the purpose of additional clarity, it has been necessary to deviate from this applied 'norm'.

MENTAL HEALTH–SUBSTANCE USE

Considerable thought has gone in to the use of terminology within these texts. Each country appears to have its own terms for the person experiencing mental health and substance use problems – terms that includes words such as dual diagnosis, coexisting, co-occurring, and so on. We talk about the same thing but use differing professional jargon. The decision was set at the outset to use one term that encompasses mental health *and* substance use problems: *mental health–substance use*. One scholar suggested that such a term implies that both can exist separately, while they can also be linked.[1]

SUBSTANCE USE

Another challenge was how to term 'substance use'. There are a number of ways: abuse, misuse, dependence, addiction. The decision is that within these texts we use the term *substance use* to encompass all (unless specific need for clarity at a given point). It is imperative the professional recognises that while we may see another person's 'substance use' as misuse or abuse, the individual experiencing it may not deem it to be anything other than 'use'. Throughout, we need to be aware that we are working alongside unique individuals. Therefore, we should be able to meet the individual where he/she is.

ALCOHOL, PRESCRIBED DRUGS, ILLICIT DRUGS, TOBACCO OR SUBSTANCES

Throughout this book *substance* includes alcohol, prescribed drugs, illicit drugs and tobacco, unless specific need for clarity at a given point.

PROBLEM(S), CONCERNS AND DILEMMAS OR DISORDERS

The terms *problem(s)*, *concerns and dilemmas* and *disorders* can be used interchangeably, as stated by the author's preference. However, where possible, the term 'problem(s)' or 'concerns and dilemmas' had been adopted as the preferred choice.

INDIVIDUAL, PERSON, PEOPLE

There seems to be a need to label the individual – as a form of recognition! Sometimes the label becomes more than the person! 'Alan is schizophrenic' – thus it is Alan, rather than an illness that Alan lives with. We refer to patients, clients, service users, customers, consumers, and so on. Yet, we feel affronted when we are addressed as anything other than what we are – individuals! We need to be mindful that every person we see during our professional day is an individual – unique. Symptoms are in many ways similar (e.g. delusions, hallucinations), some need interventions and treatments are similar (e.g. specific drugs, psychotherapy techniques), but people are not. Alan may experience an illness labelled schizophrenia, and so may John, Beth and Mary, and you or I. However, each will have his/her own unique experiences – and life. None will be the same. To keep this constantly in the mind of the reader, throughout the book series we shall refer to the *individual*, *person* or *people* – just like us, but different to us by their uniqueness.

PROFESSIONAL

We are all professionals, whether students, nurses, doctors, social workers, researchers, clinicians, educationalists, managers, service developers, religious ministers – and so on. However, the level of expertise may vary from one professional to another. We are also individuals. There is a need to distinguish between the person with a mental health–substance use problem and the person interacting professionally (at whatever level) with that individual. To acknowledge and to differentiate between those who experience – in this context – and those who intervene, we have adopted the term *professional*. It is indicative that we have had, or are receiving, education and training related specifically to help us (the professionals) meet the needs of the individual. We may or may not have experienced mental health–substance use problems but we have some knowledge that may help the individual – an expertise to be shared. We have a specific knowledge that, hopefully, we wish to use to offer effective intervention and treatment to another human being. It is the need to make a clear differential, for the reader, that forces the use of 'professional' over 'individual' to describe our role – our input into another person's life.

REFERENCE

1 Barker P. Personal communication; 2009.

Cautionary note

Wisdom and compassion should become the dominating influence that guide our thoughts, our words, and our actions.[1]

Never presume that what you say is understood. It is essential to check understanding, and what is expected of the individual and/or family, with each person. Each person needs to know what he/she can expect from you, and other professionals involved in his/her care, at each meeting. Jargon is a professional language that excludes the individual and family. Never use it in conversation with the individual, unless requested to do so; it is easily misunderstood.

Remember, we all, as individuals, deal with life differently. It does not matter how many years we have spent studying human behaviour, listening and treating the individual and family. We may have spent many hours exploring with the individual his/her anxieties, fears, doubts, concerns and dilemmas, and the illness experience. Yet, we do not know what that person really feels, how he/she sees life and ill health. We may have lived similar lives, experienced the same illness but the individual will always be unique, each different from us, each independent of our thoughts, feelings, words, deeds and symptoms, each with an individual experience.

REFERENCE

1 Matthieu Ricard. As cited in: Föllmi D, Föllmi O. *Buddhist Offerings 365 Days*. London: Thames and Hudson; 2003.

Acknowledgements

I am grateful to all the contributors for having the faith in me to produce a valued text and I thank them for their support and encouragement. I hope that faith proves correct. Thank you to those who have commented along the way, and whose patience has been outstanding. Thank you to Jo Cooper, who has been actively involved with this project throughout – supporting, encouraging, listening and participating in many practical ways. Jo is my rock who looks after me during my physical health problems, and I am eternally grateful.

Many people have helped me along my career path and life – too many to name individually. Most do not even know what impact they have had on me. Some, however, require specific mention. These include Larry Purnell, a friend and confidant who has taught me never to presume – while we are all individuals with individual needs, we deserve equality in all that we meet in life. Thanks to Martin Plant (who sadly died in March 2010), and Moira Plant, who always encouraged and offered genuine support. Phil and Poppy Barker, who have taught me that it is OK to express how I feel about humanity – about people, and that there is another way through the entrenched systems in health and social care. Keith Yoxhall, without whose guidance back in the 1980s I would never have survived my 'Colchester work experience' and the dark times of institutionalisation, or had the privilege to work alongside the few professionals fighting against the 'big door'. He taught me that there was a need for education and training, and that this should be ongoing – also that the person in hospital or community experiencing our care sees us as 'professional' – we should make sure we act that way. Thank you to Phil Cooper, who brought the concept of this book series to me via a conference to launch the journal *Mental Health and Substance Use: dual diagnosis*, of which he was editor. It was then I realised that despite all the talk over too many years of my professional life, there was still much to be done for people experiencing mental health–substance use problems. Phil is a good debater, friend and reliable resource for me – thank you.

To Gillian Nineham of Radcliffe Publishing, my sincere thanks. Gillian had faith in this project from the outset and in my ability to deliver. Her patience is immeasurable and, for that, I am grateful. Thank you to Michael Hawkes and Jessica Morofke for putting up with my too numerous questions! Thank you to Jamie Etherington, Editorial Development Manager, and Dan Allen of the book marketing department, both competent people who make my work look good. Thanks also to Mia Yardley, Natalie Mason, Camille Lowe and the production team at Pindar,

New Zealand, for bringing this book to publication, and the many others who are nameless to me as I write but without whom these books would never come to print; each has his/her stamp on any successes of this book.

My sincere thanks to all of you named, and unnamed, my friends and colleagues along my sometimes broken career path: those who have touched my life in a positive way – and a few, a negative way (for we can learn from the negative to ensure we do better for others).

A final heartfelt statement: any errors, omissions, inaccuracies or deficiencies within these pages are my sole responsibility.

Dedication

This book is dedicated to the people who have made the most important and meaningful impact in my life – personal and professional. All have made a positive difference, whose love and non-judgemental attitudes know no bounds.

Jo Cooper (née Harvey) – her wisdom and compassion outstretches mine, and her love makes my life complete and meaningful.

Joyce Cooper (née Wolstenholme) – a 'lassie from Lancashire' with spirit, care, love and motherliness.

In the fondest memory of

➤ Emily Ada Harvey (née Bliss: 1907–58): a lady I never met but whose qualities I have witnessed in her daughter and to whom I am eternally grateful for the precious gift of life she gave to me.

➤ Albert Edwin Harvey (1903–86): A 'gentle man' whose standards I respected and would love to equal. I hold them fondly and dearly.

➤ Rose Hannah Harriet Harvey (née Hart: 1909–93): The 'mother-in-law' who never lived up to the stereotypical image, and a lovely stepmother to Jo – and me.

➤ Charles Dennis Cooper (1925–2002): A 'gentle man' whose sound judgement I would love to emulate. His kindness of heart and ability to bring calm during my adulthood made me feel supported and loved.

Finally

To our children (Phil, Marc and Caroline), their partners (Sarah, Vicky and John), and our grandchildren (Ella Maisy, Megan Louise, Daisy Mae, Daniel John Charlie and Noah Jacob), thank you for the pleasure and love you bring to our lives.

CHAPTER 1

Setting the scene

David B Cooper

Listening itself is an art. When we listen with a still and concentrated mind, it's possible to actually be responsive to what the words are saying. Sometimes deep insights come in a flash, unexpectedly.[1]

INTRODUCTION

The difficulties encountered by people who experience mental health–substance use problems are not new. The individual using substances presenting to the mental health professional can often encounter annoyance and suspicion. Likewise, the person experiencing mental health problems presenting to the substance use services can encounter hostility and hopelessness. 'We cannot do anything for the substance use problem until the mental health problem is dealt with!' The referral to the mental health team is returned: 'We cannot do anything for this person until the substance use problem is dealt with!' Thus, the individual is in the middle of two professional worlds and neither is willing to move, and yet, both professional worlds are involved in 'caring' for the individual.

For many years, it has been acknowledged that the two parts of the caring system need to work as one. However, this desire has not developed into practice. Over recent years, this impetus has changed. There is now a drive towards meeting the needs of the individual experiencing mental health–substance use problems, pooling expertise from both sides. Moreover, there is an international political will to bring about change, often driven forward by a small group of dedicated professionals at practice level.

Some healthcare environments have merely paid lip service, ensuring the correct terminology is included within the policy and procedure documentation, while at the same time doing nothing, or little, to bring about the changes needed at the practice level to meet the needs of the individual. Others have grasped the drive forward and have spearheaded developments at local and national level within their country to meet such needs. It appears that the latter are now succeeding. There is a concerted international effort to improve the services provided for the individual, and a determination to pool knowledge and expertise. In addition, there is the ability of these professional groups to link into government policy and bring about the political will to support such change. However, this cannot happen overnight. There are major attitudinal changes needed – not least at management and practice level. One consultant commented that to work together with mental health–substance use problems would be too costly. Furthermore, the consultant believed it would create 'too much work'! Consequently, there is a long way to go – but a driving force to succeed exists.

Obtaining in-depth and knowledgeable text is difficult in new areas of change. One needs to be motivated to trawl a broad spectrum of work to develop a sound grounding – the background detail that is needed to build good professional practice. This is a big request of the hard-worked and pressured professional. There are a few excellent mental health–substance use books available. However, this series of six books is groundbreaking, in that each presents a much needed text that will introduce the first, but vital, step to the interventions and treatments available for the individual experiencing mental health–substance use concerns and dilemmas.

These books are educational. However, they will make no one an expert! In mental health–substance use, there is a need to initiate, and maintain, education and training. There are key principles and factors we need to bring out and explore. Some we will use – others we will adapt – while others we will reject. Each book is complete. Conversely, each aims to build on the preceding book. However, books do not hold all the answers. Nothing does. What is hoped is that the professional will participate in, and collaborate with, each book, progressing through each to the other. Along the way, hopefully, the professional will enhance existing knowledge or develop new concepts to benefit the individual.

The books offer a first step, relevant to the needs of professionals – at practice level or senior service development – in a clear, concise and understandable format. Each book has made full use of boxes, graphs, tables, figures, interactive exercises, self-assessment tools and case studies – where appropriate – to examine and demonstrate the effect mental health–substance use can have on the individual, family, carers and society as a whole.

A deliberate attempt has been made to avoid jargon, and where terminology is used, to offer a clear explanation and understanding. The terminology used in this book is fully explained at the beginning of the book, before the reader commences with the chapters. By placing it there the reader will be able to reference it quickly, if needed. Specific gender is used, as the author feels appropriate. However, unless stated, the use of the male/female gender is interchangeable.

> *Patience and perseverance have magical effects before which difficulties disappear and obstacles vanish.*[2]

BOOK 6: PRACTICE IN MENTAL HEALTH–SUBSTANCE USE

The professional's role is to see where the individual is in his/her life, to support and steer that individual to a level of stability that is acceptable to him/her. You may not be able to 'fix it', but you can encourage acceptance and bring hope. To achieve this we must use the best evidence-based practice and ensure quality in that practice.

For the individual and family it is important that we achieve an intervention that is right – what works for one person may not work for another. Matching the intervention to the person leads to a more effective outcome. The individual, working with others experiencing similar problems and experiences, in a supportive environment, should not be overlooked as an effective intervention.

We listen to the individual and take action to work alongside the move towards his/her goals. Sometimes, one way does not work, and an alternative is tried. However, the good professional never gives up on the individual and family members – no one 'deserves it'. The door should always be open; accepting of the individual and family members at whatever point she/he enters our care (*see* Book 1, Chapter 7).

To achieve this, we need an understanding of what is available to aid the individual and family member to achieve his/her own goals: where he/she wants to be – what is acceptable to him/her – not what is acceptable to us! To do this, we need the basics – then we develop that knowledge to practise and utilise skills.

As mentioned in the Preface, the ability to learn and gain new knowledge is the way forward. As professionals, we must start with knowledge, and from there we can begin to understand. We commence using our new-found skills, progressing to develop the ability to examine practice, to put concepts together and to make valid judgements.[3] This knowledge is gained through education, training and experience, sometimes enhanced by our own life experiences.

However, we must always remember that those we offer care to, and their family members, bring their own knowledge, skills and life experiences, some developed from dealing with ill health. Therefore, in order to turn our clinical practice to effective outcomes for the individual and family, we must demonstrate a mutual understanding and respect of that expertise.

We need to appreciate and understand the concerns and dilemmas that face the person. We have to adapt our practice to respond to those individual needs. It is important to remember that each person is unique. Yes, there may be similarities in symptoms, and specific needs addressed for sexuality, spirituality and age, etc. However, we must accept and acknowledge that each person will have variations and specific needs that have to be considered when offering appropriate practices, and when interacting with the individual. Moreover, we must be aware of the needs of the family and carers who have their own specific requirements.

To get to this level of skill we need a grounding – a sound knowledge of the theories behind the practices – how they work, who may benefit, and the principles behind the interventions. This must be research led and be fluid in that we take on board the updates and modifications to the intervention as knowledge and skills progress. These are the philosophies from which effective practice and interventions are offered. Taking all we have understood and learned from the previous books in the series, this book offers some practical examples of interventions offered by the professional in specific circumstances to the individual and family. To provide effective care there is a need for a 'starting point' of intervention – then an understanding of the types of interventions that may improve the quality of life for the person and family. Thus, Book 6 provides the basis of best practice when offering effective interventions and treatment.

Chapters 2–6 look at practice in relation to alcohol, cannabis, stimulants, prescription drug and tobacco use in relation to mental health. David Kavanagh and

Dawn Procter (Chapter 7) explore the impact of substance use in schizophrenia and offer some evidence-based practice examples through case studies, etc. that will enhance interventions for the individual and family.

Fran Miller (Chapter 8) looks at how eye movement desensitisation and reprocessing (EMDR) offers a way forward as an effective intervention for mental health–substance use problems. EMDR is a continuing theme when Walter Busuttil from Combat Stress examines current practice with post-traumatic stress disorder and substance use (Chapter 9), and Art O'Malley looks at practice in relation to attention deficit hyperactivity disorder and substance use in children (Chapter 10).

We acknowledge that all practice intervention cannot be the same; in Chapters 11 and 12 the authors look specifically at the complex needs of the older adult (Chapter 11) and the young adult (Chapter 12), both requiring changes in intervention to meet these needs. In Chapter 13, Lorne Korman and Kyle Burns examine how dialectical behaviour therapy can be helpful when working alongside the young adult and how this is best achieved at a practice level.

When the individual is within the judicial system the process of effective intervention produces some specific areas for consideration. Such intervention is not as easy as we would like to believe in terms of facilities, skills, low staffing levels and expertise. In Chapter 14, Dave Marteau offers some guidance on how such concerns and dilemmas might be approached, and what could be the way forward for effective practice interventions.

SELF-ASSESSMENT EXERCISE 1.1

Time: 7 days
- Before reading Chapters 15 and 16 think of something you really like to eat or drink on a regular basis. Your preferred drink can be tea, coffee, alcoholic or soft drink or you may prefer chocolate.
- Set a day to commence and then stop using your chosen substance (no tea or coffee or so on). Only choose one substance.
- Note how you feel before starting and then complete a daily diary for the next seven days.
- Have you experienced craving? If so, in what form did this take? What was the worst time of day? What did you do to overcome this craving?
- Did you relapse? If so, what triggered the relapse? Was there anything you would do differently to avoid relapse? Did you recommence your previous usage? Was this usage more excessive than previously?
- Did you recommence the trial? If not, why not?

In Chapter 15, Rami Jumnoodoo and Patrick Coyne open up our thinking in relation to relapse prevention in mental health – pivotal in any effective therapeutic intervention involving the individual and family – and how they have developed their approach from current practice in the substance use field. Sharon Hsu and Alan Marlatt (Chapter 16) develop the debate when considering relapse prevention within mental health and substance use. Here the authors draw on their pioneering research and experience to demonstrate how effective relapse prevention can make a real difference in successful treatment outcome for the individual and family.

John Ashcroft (Chapter 17) brings Book 6 to a close with a reminder that what we think we see (i.e. someone under the influence of substances) may not be what is actually impacting on the individual, and that we constantly need an open mind. We should not exclude thorough physical assessment at any time. Brain injury can and does mimic the effect of substance use on the individual's behaviour and that leads to ineffective practices and interventions or even death if we fail to properly assess for physical, psychological and substance use consequences in the person presenting for treatment.

> *When it is obvious that the goals cannot be reached, don't adjust the goals, adjust the action steps.*[1]

CONCLUSION

This is the final book in the series of six textbooks aimed at improving the quality of care, intervention and treatment of people experiencing mental health–substance use problems. It is important to remember that there is a constant theme throughout the series – the need for properly funded education and training. Just as important, there is constant reinforcement of why we need to know about mental health–substance use. These books are aimed at the professional, educator, service developer, manager and student, for we all need to be aware of the unique needs of the individual and family. Moreover, we need this knowledge, skills base, and high level of competence, if our practice is to be effective.

It is hoped that these books are helpful and informative. One would hope that we feel sufficiently stimulated to further develop our knowledge and skills, having extended and developed this grounding in mental health–substance use. We can build upon our knowledge using the 'To Learn More' sections as a guide to further study. As one enters each new area of knowledge, so our understanding improves – of what is needed, and what is not – and how we can apply this knowledge and theory through to practice and service development. With that comes the ability to use an open, non-judgemental and accepting approach to the problems identified by the individual and family presenting for intervention, treatment, advice or guidance.

As our knowledge and understanding constantly change, the challenge we face is to remain open and accessible to new evidence-based knowledge, information and practices that will help each of us provide appropriate therapeutic interventions:

➤ at the appropriate level of expertise
➤ at the appropriate time
➤ at the appropriate level of understanding of the individual, and her/his presenting concerns and dilemmas
➤ at the appropriate cost.

We cannot afford to assume we know all there is to know about each individual and/or family member we meet – all individuals are not the same and one size does not fit all. If these books encourage us to be wise and flexible in our service development, intervention, treatment, care and practice, and to respond effectively and efficiently using research-led knowledge, practice and skills, then we, the authors contributing to this series of books on mental health–substance use, have achieved our aim. If these books help you appreciate some of the problems encountered by the individual, family, and carers, they have achieved their aim. Together, we can bring about much needed changes for the individual and family experiencing mental health–substance use problems. Now is the time for our collective action to bring about this much needed, essential, long overdue change to practice for those experiencing mental health–substance use.

> *Compassion can be roughly defined in terms of a state of mind that is non-violent, non-harming and non-aggressive. It is a mental attitude based on the wish for others to be free of their suffering and is associated with the sense of commitment, responsibility and respect towards others.*[5]

REFERENCES

1 Joseph Goldstein. As cited in: Föllmi D, Föllmi O. *Buddhist Offerings 365 Days.* London: Thames and Hudson; 2003.

2 John Quincy Adams, 6th US President. Available at: http://thinkexist.com/quotation/patience_and_perseverance_have_a_magical_effect/150955.html (accessed 19 November 2010).

3 Bloom BS, Hastings T, Madaus G. *Handbook of Formative and Summative Evaluation.* New York: McGraw-Hill Book Company; 1971.

4 Confucius 551–479 BC. Available at: http://thinkexist.com/quotation/when_it_is_obvious_that_the_goals_cannot_be/202375.html (accessed 19 November 2010).

5 The 14th Dalai Lama. As cited in: Föllmi D, Föllmi O. *Buddhist Offerings 365 Days.* London: Thames and Hudson; 2003.

CHAPTER 2

Alcohol and mental health

May Baker and Dave Buckley

PRE-READING EXERCISE 2.1 (ANSWERS ON P. 21)

Time: 20 minutes
1   Can you remember how many alcohol units you have drunk in the last two weeks?
2   Can you list two common and two serious mental health problems?
3   Can you identify any link between alcohol use and mental health problems?

- Once you have read the chapter repeat this exercise and compare your answers.
- What have you learned from this exercise?

INTRODUCTION

This chapter examines the relationship between mental health and alcohol use within the practice area. It will ask the reader to look at problems and issues in case scenarios. Reflection and critical thinking will aid exploration of the points of concern and interest.

LEARNING OBJECTIVE

Identify the link between mental health problems and alcohol consumption.

ALCOHOL

Alcohol could be seen as the nation's favourite drug, albeit a legal one. In England alone 90% of people drink alcohol.[1] Alcohol is a social lubricant and is widely accepted within British society, crossing cultural, social and generational barriers. However, in the last three decades patterns of use have changed.[2] More people are drinking at home, and there is binge drinking and consuming beyond the recommended limits set by the UK Department of Health.[2]

Women are more likely to have problems associated with alcohol in relation to disease, with serious implications for the foetus in pregnancy.[2]

If we combine alcohol use with someone experiencing a mental health problem such as anxiety, depression or schizophrenia, potential problems could lie ahead. It is important to be realistic about this and professionals should be aware that drinking within sensible limits can be enjoyed even if someone is experiencing mental health problems. However, this would depend on the amounts consumed and the nature of the problem.

MENTAL HEALTH PROBLEMS

Mental health problems are common throughout the world.[3] The prevalence of mental health problems in the general population in the UK is 10%–25%.[3] Living with and experiencing mental health problems can be disabling for the person, cause great anguish and frustration and may lead a person to the brink of despair and desperation. The stigma attached to someone experiencing mental health problems can sometimes be just as debilitating as the label of mental illness.

Mental health problems can be separated into two distinct groups:[3] common and serious mental health problems (*see* Table 2.1). Common mental health problems are sometimes described as 'less serious conditions'. This interpretation can be misleading as any psychological problem can be debilitating for the person, no matter how it is categorised.

TABLE 2.1

Common mental health problems	Serious mental health problems
• Anxiety	• Schizophrenia
• Depression	• Bipolar disorder
• Obsessive compulsive disorder	• Depression and psychosis
• Phobias	
• Panic disorder	

Statistics for mental health–substance use problems have identified an increase in people seeking help, advice and treatment.[4] There is a chance that alcohol can interfere with the efficacy of prescribed medication.[5]

Some antidepressants are less efficient when taken with alcohol and some medications increase the sedative effect.

It is estimated that heavy drinking is linked to 65% of suicides.[6] Excessive alcohol use is strongly associated with vulnerable groups, such as the homeless and offenders,[7] and is implicated in violence, criminality and child neglect.

SELF-ASSESSMENT EXERCISE 2.1

> **Time: 10 minutes**
> - When should the professional advise the individual to totally abstain from alcohol consumption?
> - Are there any times when drinking can help a person cope with mental distress?

PSYCHOLOGICAL PROBLEMS ASSOCIATED WITH HEAVY OR BINGE DRINKING

Psychological problems associated with heavy or binge drinking include:
- irritability/poor concentration
- depression
- anxiety
- panic attacks
- sleep problems
- paranoia
- memory loss.

We can conclude that consuming alcohol while experiencing mental health problems can be problematic for the person, the family and the professional. Some people think that using alcohol helps them to cope, and they may find it difficult to associate their drinking with any deterioration in their mental state. However, we have to accept that people will use alcohol to excess and need to acknowledge and work with people who wish to continue harmful drinking behaviour in a non-confrontational and non-judgemental manner.

Important questions to be asked

Some important questions to be addressed during screening and assessment include the following.
- How much alcohol are you drinking?
- How often are you drinking alcohol?
- Does this link to your mental health problem?
- How does this link to your mental health problem?
- How does this impact on your life?

LEARNING OBJECTIVE

To understand the process of identification, assessment, planning and evaluating alcohol and mental health problems within a person-centred framework.

PERSON-CENTRED PRACTICE

Person-centred working is paramount. A person-centred approach is essential to empower and recognise the person in her/his own right. The individual should be allowed to voice his/her concerns and opinions and should be actively encouraged to state what is important to her/him (*see* Book 4, Chapter 2). Whether this is family, carer involvement or the person's own views, the individual should be listened to and treated respectfully.[8] This helps the professional to focus on the person and not the condition. People are complex with highly multifaceted lives. They have physical, psychological, social and spiritual needs; some factors being more important than others. Therefore, the professional should be aware of the support systems that a person may need in order work alongside them through their problems.

REFLECTIVE PRACTICE EXERCISE 2.1

Time: 20 minutes
- Think of an issue in your work where you practised a person-centred approach.
- How did you recognise it?

IDENTIFYING ALCOHOL-RELATED PROBLEMS IN PRACTICE

How do we identify if the individual's drinking is affecting their mental health? First, we have to know what sensible limits are for men and women and how these are calculated (*see* Table 2.2). Second, we should screen for alcohol use (*see* Book 4, Chapter 8; Book 5, Chapter 8). This helps to identify people who are at risk through drinking. Some alcohol screening tools provide a framework for harm minimisation, and thus help avoid the consequences of harmful drinking, while others identify chronic use, binge drinking or accidents associated with alcohol use. *See* Box 2.1 for some alcohol screening tools.

BOX 2.1 Screening tools

- CAGE[9]
- AUDIT[10]
- PAT[11]
- GAIN-Short Screener (GAIN-SS)[12]
- Psychiatric Diagnostic Screening Questionnaire (PDSQ)[13]

Professionals working within mental health services should always ask about alcohol use and complete a risk assessment.[14] Conversely, professionals working in the field of alcohol/substance use should ensure that they ask questions about any mental health problems experienced by the individual. This may be in the form of taking a history, sharing of information via referral or a third party, such as family, or if the person informs you they are experiencing mental health problems. Professionals should also be aware of congruence. Do you see the same picture that the individual sees? Does it add up?

TABLE 2.2

UK Formula for Calculating Alcohol Units	UK Sensible Guidelines for drinking[15]
$$\frac{\text{Alcohol by Volume} \times \text{mL}}{1000}$$ **8g of ethanol =** **a standard drink (UK) =** **1 unit =** • 25 mL spirits at 40% volume • ½ pint of lager at 3.5% volume • 100 mL wine at 10% volume.	Women 2–3 units daily (14 units weekly) Men 3–4 units daily (21 units weekly) • Weekly units should not be consumed all at once. • 2 days' abstinence is recommended. • Binge drinking for women is >6 units and for men >8 units in any one session.
US Sensible Guidelines for drinking[16]	**Australian Sensible Guidelines for drinking[17]**
13.7 g of ethanol = **a standard drink (US)** • 1.5 ounces of 80-proof spirits • 12 ounces of beer • 5 ounces of wine. Women: 1 standard drink daily Men: 2 standard drinks daily • Weekly units should not be consumed all at once.	**10 g of ethanol =** **a standard drink (Australia) = 1 unit** • 30 mL nip (spirits) at 40% volume • 375 mL bottle (beer) at 3.5% volume • 100 mL wine at 13% volume. Women: 2 standard drinks (2 units) daily Men: 4 standard drinks (4 units) daily • Weekly units should not be consumed all at once. • 1–2 days' abstinence is recommended.

SELF-ASSESSMENT EXERCISE 2.2

> **Time: 30 minutes**
> - Access the internet and search for screening tools that may be useful to your professional practice.
> - Check these out using self-assessment.
> - How easy/difficult are they for you to use?
> - How easy/difficult are they for the individual to use?

WHAT DO YOU SEE?

Ideally, the individual should present for assessment sober. If a person is intoxicated, it is very difficult to carry out an assessment of their needs. *See* Box 2.2 for signs of intoxication.

There may be reasons for you to be concerned about the individual's physical health and decide that clinical investigations are needed. These may include:

➤ taking a blood sample to measure markers that could indicate excessive/dependent alcohol use

➤ using a breathalyser to measure blood alcohol concentration; this can measure

tolerance, which increases when more alcohol is needed to gain the same effect
➤ arranging a medical examination to identify physical problems associated with alcohol use.

BOX 2.2 Signs of intoxication

- Unsteady on feet
- Slurred speech
- Smell of alcohol
- Disinhibited behaviour
- Delayed reflexes
- Accidents

Physical features that can help us to identify dependence include:
➤ the smell of alcohol on the person's breath
➤ a slight tremor or shake of the hands
➤ bloodshot eyes
➤ small vascular breaks in the skin around the nose, cheeks or chest (spider naevi – *see* www.google.co.uk/images?hl=en&rlz=1G1TSEACENGB355&q=spider-naevi&um=1&ie=UTF8&source=univ&ei=JMbOTJ2ME5SSjAecg43YBw&sa=X&oi=image_result_group&ct=title&resnum=2&ved=0CC8QsAQwAQ)
➤ ascites (swelling of the abdomen)
➤ overweight or underweight/malnutrition.

There are also long-term physical problems associated with heavy dependent drinking (*see* Box 2.3). If dependence is identified, the person would need to go through a process of detoxification. This is a carefully managed procedure using a reducing dose of a given medication that is managed until withdrawal symptoms have gone. It is not a treatment for alcohol-related problems as this is ongoing, following through detoxification and beyond. Physical dependence on alcohol means that when it is taken away the person experiences withdrawal symptoms. These symptoms range from sweating, sickness and shaking to more serious conditions such as delirium tremens (DTs) and seizures.

KEY POINT 2.3

Alcohol withdrawal can be complicated and potentially life threatening.

The individual may present with no obvious physical signs but can still have problematic alcohol use. Therefore, it is important to recognise this and treat each person individually.

BOX 2.3 Long-term physical problems

- Diabetes
- Neuropathy
- Raised blood pressure
- Cancer of mouth, larynx
- Cancer of liver
- Pancreatitis
- Foetal harm
- Wernicke-Korsakoff psychosis
- Cirrhosis of the liver

WHAT IS THE PERSON SAYING?

We also have to take into account the person's story:

➤ What does the individual have to say about his/her drinking behaviour?
➤ Does she/he think it is a problem – for her/him or the family?
➤ Is it causing problems at work?
➤ Is the story corroborated by family or friends?
➤ What is the story of the family or friends?
➤ Does the individual feel supported?
➤ Does the individual feel coerced into seeking help?

There are many social problems associated with heavy or binge drinking and this may lead to mental health problems such as anxiety, depression or suicidal thoughts. The professional should recognise this and be aware that sometimes the person does not always think he/she has a mental health problem but may mask the symptoms or deny they exist.

SOCIAL PROBLEMS ASSOCIATED WITH HEAVY OR BINGE DRINKING

Social problems associated with heavy or binge drinking may include:

➤ lack of pleasure in activities
➤ relationship difficulties
➤ debt problems
➤ work problems
➤ legal problems.

Case study 2.1: James

James (57), a businessman, has been referred by his general practitioner who is concerned about his alcohol consumption affecting his health. He has been diagnosed with high blood pressure and has been prescribed medication which is made less effective by alcohol use.

At assessment, James is accompanied by his wife Mary. James is well dressed and articulate but vague at times and frequently turns to Mary for verification of events.

James smells of alcohol but denies drinking for two days. His explanation of his drinking habits and his activities differs from Mary's account, although James does not argue when she contradicts him but looks puzzled rather than upset. Mary states that James is actually drinking less overall than he used to.

Mary reports that over the last few months James has become increasingly forgetful and frequently makes things up. James has been a heavy drinker for many years, though up until recently this does not seem to have affected him adversely and he still manages to run his business with support from his staff.

SELF-ASSESSMENT EXERCISE 2.3

Time: 20 minutes

After reading James' case study:
- What are your initial thoughts on how James is presenting at assessment?
- Is there a possible alternative explanation?
- Does James actually have a drinking problem? Justify your answer.
- How would you proceed with assessment?
- How would you support Mary?

ASSESSMENT

Undertaking an assessment (*see* Book 5, Chapter 9) can be fraught with many problems for the professional. Therefore, using a systematic approach will help. Having a good knowledge base around alcohol and mental health problems will assist when trying to obtain a comprehensive picture. This also means the professional needs to have the ability to communicate effectively, taking into account the diversity of the person. This could include language and cultural differences (*see* Book 4, Chapters 4 and 5; Book 5, Chapter 5). One of the most important skills needed is that of communication; not only with the person and family but alongside other professionals (*see* Book 2, Chapters 11 and 12). The professional has a responsibility to the individual and family; therefore, an assessment of risk should be completed especially in relation to safeguarding children and vulnerable adults (*see* Book 1, Chapters 4, 6–8 and 12; Book 3, Chapters 2–7; Book 5, Chapters 4 and 7).[18] This is a statutory responsibility for all professionals but this does not have to compromise your relationship with the individual. Confidentiality is vital when building a trusting relationship and the individual should feel that what they say to you is treated with respect and kept in confidence. However, on occasions confidentiality may be breached. If this happens it should always be on a need-to-know basis, usually with other professionals who can assist and advise on the matter of concern (*see* Book 1, Chapter 12). The individual should be guided and supported to confide this information personally to the correct agency.

SELF-ASSESSMENT EXERCISE 2.4

Time: 5 minutes
- How would you explain confidentiality to James?

MOTIVATION

People present differently and they will have various tolerance levels and a variety of mental health problems. Some will be seeking help for the first time while others may have had problems lasting many years. Trying to identify how motivated the person is to change at that particular time can ease the transition and help the individual set appropriate goals. Prochaska and DiClemente[19] describe six stages of behaviour change:

➤ pre-contemplation – not recognising the problem
➤ contemplation – recognition
➤ action – doing something about it
➤ making changes – attempting behaviour change
➤ maintaining change – maintaining change
➤ relapse – returning to the behaviour.

SELF-ASSESSMENT EXERCISE 2.5

Time: 20 minutes
Think how you would:
- calculate consumption
- assess tolerance
- assess mental health problems
- decide whether any clinical investigations are needed
- assess readiness to change
- decide whether detoxification is needed.

Case study 2.2: Maggie

Maggie (27) self-referred for assessment. She arrives for her appointment with her four-year-old daughter Abigail, who appears happy, well and cared for. Maggie smells strongly of alcohol and appears to be slightly intoxicated.

Maggie is not currently registered with a general practitioner. She moved to the area two years ago and has no relatives or friends locally except for her partner. On assessment, Maggie discloses domestic violence issues and says she is fearful of her partner but realises she needs him as he supplies her with heroin. Maggie has been smoking this for the past year as she says it helps her to forget her problems.

Maggie mentions that she had previously seen a psychiatrist, as she was depressed. She was given 'tablets' but they did not help. She has not been in contact with any services since moving to the area. Maggie decided to ask for help with her drinking as she is unable to cope and does not know where to turn to. Maggie does not want to contact drug services as they may take Abigail from her.

SELF-ASSESSMENT EXERCISE 2.6

Time: 20 minutes
Thinking back to Maggie's case study:
- How would you discuss confidentiality with Maggie?
- How would you develop trust in the initial stages of the relationship?
- How would you prioritise?
- Take the top three issues – describe how you would go about addressing these further.

MAKING A PLAN

Once the assessment has been completed and you have a clear picture of what the actual problems are it is time to talk about taking the next step.

This could be potentially difficult for you if at this stage the picture is still not clear. You may struggle to make sense of all the information and you may be unsure of what to do next. If this happens, think about the value of a second opinion or how you would liaise with colleagues in order to help the process.

Planning goals can also be difficult for the person as they will have to consider a host of other factors such as their family, job and friends. They will also need to be offered the support from you as a facilitator and will need encouragement and empathy. It is of equal importance to remember that the family may also need support from you and/or other agencies.

One way to stay focused on the goal is to use the acronym SMART.[20]

The person's aims and goals should be:
➤ **S**pecific
➤ **M**easurable
➤ **A**chievable
➤ **R**ealistic
➤ **T**ime framed.

Therefore, setting an achievable goal will also determine which interventions the person wishes to adopt. Setting realistic goals will encourage self-esteem, self-worth and a feeling of achievement when these goals are realised. Setting the person up to fail will bring about mistrust and a sense of worthlessness or even guilt.

PLANNING GOALS

In order to set goals you need to know which interventions are needed. Offering choices will certainly help. However, guidance from you will most likely be needed. A menu of interventions should be offered as the more choice a person has the more likely they will find one that suits their needs (some are listed below). What is important is that the correct option is chosen to suit the person's needs at that particular time, including:

➤ medication management for detoxification/maintenance (*see* Chapter 5; Book 5, Chapter 13)
➤ psychotherapeutic intervention – counselling, cognitive behavioural therapy, Motivational Interviewing (*see* Chapter 13; Book 4, Chapters 9–15; Book 5, Chapters 11 and 12)
➤ group work.

The person you have assessed will now have to decide what path he/she may wish to take.

You will need to be knowledgeable and have a good working relationship with identifiable agencies and, if necessary, liaise with them on the individual's behalf.

SELF-ASSESSMENT EXERCISE 2.7

Time: 15 minutes
- How could you develop a good working relationship with relevant agencies?
- What barriers could inhibit this?

Case study 2.3: Carol

Carol (47) is being treated for depression by her general practitioner with an antidepressant called dothiepin. She lives with her 20-year-old daughter Susan and has struggled to leave the house since her acrimonious divorce several years before. Carol drinks a bottle of vodka three or four times a week. At her appointment Carol has a low blood alcohol of 20 mgs%. Carol's account of her drinking is confirmed by Susan.

Carol complains of being unable to sleep and goes wandering at night, though she will sleep for several hours in the day. During her sleepless hours she feels hopeless and feels like ending it all. Carol has a history of taking overdoses, though not for several years.

Carol appears agitated and weepy, and though she has obviously made an effort to appear presentable, looks somewhat dishevelled.

SELF-ASSESSMENT EXERCISE 2.8

Time: 30 minutes
Thinking back to Carol's case study:
- What is the most important issue?
- What questions would you ask to ascertain the relevant information?
- How would you deal with this crisis?
- What agencies would you involve?

INDECISION

Sometimes the individual can be in denial about their drinking or they find it difficult to see how their alcohol use is affecting their life. This may be due to an exacerbation of the symptoms of the mental health problems. Their partner, family or friends may have coerced them to seek help, or the individual simply may not have made up her/his mind what to do next. Whatever the reason, indecision can block the path forward, so it is important to recognise this early and address it.

Case study 2.4: Gakere

Gakere (38) has recently moved to the area. He reports drinking a couple of cans of lager in the morning, afternoon and evening. At assessment, he has a blood alcohol of 210 mgs% and appears quite sober.

   Gakere was admitted to a mental health hospital for a few weeks last year when he lived in another city. At the time he felt paranoid and suspicious; he thought that his friends were out to get him. Gakere did not like the hospital as the nurses were 'trying to poison' him. Gakere gives very little detail on this event and is extremely anxious about giving you information. He reports suffering from panic attacks and says his general practitioner prescribes him an antidepressant called citalopram, which he says is ineffective. Gakere is very wary of people trying to help him and has only agreed to see you because his landlady has persuaded him as she thinks he needs help for his drinking problem.

Calculating consumption

When the professional asks Gakere for more details it emerges that 'a couple of cans of lager' amount to eight 500 mL cans of lager (9%) per day.

SELF-ASSESSMENT EXERCISE 2.9

Time: 10 minutes
Thinking back to Gakere's case study:
- What may lead you to believe that Gakere has a high alcohol tolerance?

Factors to consider
- Why might the antidepressant be ineffective in treating Gakere's panic attacks?
- Why would Gakere appear uncomfortable in your presence?
- How would you deal with this?
- How would you explain to Gakere that his drinking could be making his problems worse?
- Would you recommend that Gakere reduces his alcohol or detoxifies?
- How would you persuade Gakere to let you refer him to other services?
- Which services would you refer Gakere to?

HOW ARE ACHIEVEMENTS MEASURED?

The nature of mental health–alcohol use problems are complex. Thus, when evaluating progress, you should always support self-efficacy and encourage any achievement no matter how small. To say how effective the process has been depends on what the person sought initially. It could mean abstinence or minimising the harm from alcohol. Sometimes it can help if people can visualise their goals and successes (*see* Figure 2.1).

KEY POINT 2.4

Professionals must ensure that the individual receives the correct advice and, if appropriate, referral for intervention and treatment.

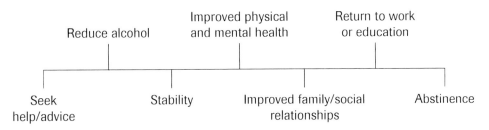

FIGURE 2.1 A linear continuum

It is important to have discussed relapse prevention, ideally at the planning stage (*see* Chapters 15 and 16; Book 4, Chapter 13). This will ensure that the person is aware that relapse is sometimes a normal part of the process of recovery. The individual should not be shocked and despondent if he/she relapses but should see this as a learning opportunity from which to progress to her/his chosen goals. The professional should use their skills to help the individual prevent a longer relapse by trying to minimise any damage quickly. This may depend on the relationship you have with the individual, and how involved they have been in their care planning. If there appears to be little progress made, it is vital to encourage the individual to remain involved. It may just take longer than anticipated.

CONCLUSION

This chapter discussed the link between alcohol and mental health problems. It used case studies to help identify how to:

➤ assess
➤ plan
➤ implement
➤ evaluate

. . . care for people seeking help with mental health–alcohol use problems. The focus was to enable the reader to utilise their existing skills, and to learn new ones to enhance this process. It is not possible to cover all aspects associated with mental health–alcohol use problems here. However, the reader should now be aware of the complexity of alcohol use when someone experiences mental health problems. In order to progress, as professionals we should remain open to new ways of thinking and practice. However, we have to recognise that it is the individual and not the problem that always comes first.

REFERENCES

1 Department of Health. *Safe. Sensible. Social: the next steps in the National Alcohol Strategy*. London: Department of Health; 2007. Available at: www.dh.gov.uk/prod_consum_dh/groups/dh_digitalassets/documents/digitalasset/dh_082203.pdf (accessed 1 November 2010).

2 Alcohol Concern. Available at: www.alcoholconcern.org.uk/publications/factsheets-and-booklets (accessed 30 November 2010).

3 Department of Health. *Care Services Improvement partnership. National Institute for Mental Health in England: designing primary care mental health services, Guidebook*. London: Department of Health; 2006.

4 Institute of Alcohol Studies. *Alcohol and Mental Health Factsheet*. 2007. Available at: www.ias.org.uk/resources/factsheets/mentalhealth.pdf (accessed 1 November 2010).

5 British National Formulary. Available at: www.bnf.org/bnf/extra/current/450003.htm#guideprescribing (accessed 1 November 2010).

6 World Health Organization. *Alcohol and Mental Health (Briefing)*. European Ministerial Conference on Mental Health; 12–15 January 2005: Helsinki, Finland.

7 Alcohol Concern. *Alcohol and Mental Health Factsheet Summary*, July 2007. Available at: www.alcoholconcern.org.uk/publications/factsheets-and-booklets/alcohol-and-mental-health-factsheet (accessed 1 November 2010).

8 Videbeck SL. *Mental Health Nursing*. 1st ed. London: Lippincott Williams and Wilkins; 2009. pp. 28–9.

9 Ewing JA. Detecting alcoholism: the CAGE Questionnaire. *Journal of the American Medical Association*. 1984; **252**: 1905–7.

10 Babor TF, Higgins-Biddle JC, Saunders JB, *et al*. *The Alcohol Use Disorders Identification Test*. 2nd ed. Genève: World Health Organization; 2001. Available at: http://whqlibdoc.who.int/hq/2001/who_msd_msb_01.6a.pdf (accessed 1 November 2010).

11 Smith SG, Touquet R, Wright S and Das Gupta N. Detection of alcohol misusing patients in A&E department: the Paddington Alcohol Test (PAT). *Journal of Accident & Emergency Medicine*. 1996; **13**: 308–12.

12 Dennis ML, Chan YF, Funk RR. Development and validation of the GAIN Short Screener (GSS) for internalizing, externalizing and substance use disorders and crime/violence problems among adolescents and adults. *American Journal on Addictions*. 2006; **15**: 80–91.

13 Zimmerman M, Mattia JI. The psychiatric diagnostic screening questionnaire: development, reliability and validity. *Comprehensive Psychiatry*. 2001; **42**: 175–89.

14 Department of Health. *Refocusing the Care Programme Approach: policy and positive practice guidance*. London: Department of Health; 2008. Available at: www.nmhdu.org.uk/silo/files/dh-2008-refocusing-the-care-programme-approach-policy-and-positive-practice-guidance.pdf (accessed 1 November 2010).

15 Kipping G. The person who misuses drugs or alcohol. In: Norman I, Ryrie I, editors. *The Art and Science of Mental Health Nursing*. Maidenhead: Open University Press; 2004. pp. 486–7.

16 United Stated Department of Agriculture and United States Department of Health and Human Services. *Dietary Guidelines for Americans.* Chapter 9 – Alcoholic Beverages, Washington, DC: US Government Printing Office; 2005. pp. 43–6. Available at: www. health.gov/DIETARYGUIDELINES/dga2005/document/html/chapter9.htm (accessed 4 November 2010).

17 Stockley C. Australian Alcohol Guidelines health risks and benefits. The Australian Wine Research Institute, 2001. Available at: www.aim-digest.com/gateway/pages/guide/articles/ Aus_guide.htm (accessed 4 November 2010).

18 Department for Children, Schools and Families. *Every Child Matters: HM Government information sharing guidance.* June 2009. Available at: www.dcsf.gov.uk/everychildmatters/ resources-and-practice/IG00340/ (accessed 1 November 2010).

19 Prochaska JO and DiClemente CC. Toward a comprehensive model of change. In: Miller WR, Heather N, editors. *Treating Addictive Behaviors: processes of change.* New York: Plenum Press; 1986.

20 Norman I, Ryrie I, editors. Assessment and care planning. In: Norman I, Ryrie I. *The Art and Science of Mental Health Nursing.* Maidenhead: Open University Press; 2004. p. 203.

TO LEARN MORE

- Department of Health. *Mental Health Policy Implementation Guide: dual diagnosis good practice guide.* 2002. Available at: www.dh.gov.uk/en/Publicationsandstatistics/Publications/ PublicationsPolicyAndGuidance/DH_4009058
- Department of Health. *Best Practice in Managing Risk: principles and evidence for best practice in the assessment and management of risk to self and others in mental health services.* 2007. Available at: http://webarchive.nationalarchives.gov.uk/+/www.dh.gov.uk/en/ Publicationsandstatistics/Publications/PublicationsPolicyAndGuidance/DH_076511
- Edwards G, Marshall EJ, Cook CC. *The Treatment of Drinking Problems.* 4th ed. Cambridge: Cambridge University Press; 2003.
- Alcohol Concern – available at: www.alcoholconcern.org.uk/
- Drink Aware – available at: www.drinkaware.co.uk/
- National Treatment Agency – available at: www.nta.nhs.uk/
- Mental Health Foundation – available at: www.mentalhealth.org.uk/campaigns/alcohol/
- Mental Health and Higher Education – available at: www.mhhe.heacademy.ac.uk/
- MIND – available at: www.mind.org.uk/about
- Sainsbury Centre for Mental Health – available at: www.scmh.org.uk/

ANSWERS TO PRE-READING EXERCISE 2.1

1 This is easier to do if you start from today and work back each day at a time. Remember to include afternoon and weekend drinking both at home and outside (i.e. public house/restaurant).

2 Anxiety and depression are normally described as common mental health problems whereas schizophrenia and bipolar are normally described as serious mental health problems.

3 Suicide or attempted suicide increases significantly if the person has a history of heavy drinking. Anxiety and depression are strongly associated with alcohol dependence. Excessive use of alcohol can lead to an exacerbation of the symptoms of schizophrenia.

CHAPTER 3

Cannabis and mental health

Zain Sadiq and Paul D Morrison

OBJECTIVES

After reading this chapter, you should have:
- ➤ an understanding of the short- and long-term sequelae of cannabis use, particularly on mental health
- ➤ an overview of the legislation in the UK regarding cannabis use
- ➤ more confidence in taking a good substance use history
- ➤ a better understanding of the growing evidence base about cannabis use and mental illness
- ➤ knowledge of the different interventions available for people who use cannabis and their effectiveness.

INTRODUCTION

There is increasing evidence about the detrimental effects of cannabis use. Mental health professionals often encounter individuals who run into problems with this drug. It can be challenging to establish whether there is a severe underlying mental disorder in a person abusing cannabis, particularly one who is psychotic. Treatment of psychotic illness–cannabis use disorder presents a significant challenge for professionals.

Here we have formulated an evolving clinical scenario typical of everyday practice, which serves well for discussion in small groups. In this clinical case, the management which ensues is not offered as an 'ideal' template, or as some sort of standard to be followed. Indeed shortcomings are evident at several points, although this only becomes clear with the benefit of hindsight. Thus, professionals are encouraged to consider where they would have come to an alternative judgement and where their management of the case would have differed. The case is discussed in more detail towards the end of the chapter.

There is also a set of multiple-choice questions. We recommend that you answer them before starting the chapter and then take them again after completion, thereby comparing your pre-/post-test scores.

MULTIPLE CHOICE QUESTIONNAIRE 3.1 (ANSWERS ON P. 38)

Time: 10 minutes

1 According to the United Nations Office of Drugs and Crime, which of the following are true?
a Worldwide, 10% of adults use cannabis each year
b Worldwide, 4% of adults use cannabis each year
c Use of cannabis has decreased since the mid-1990s
d Worldwide, amphetamine use is higher than cannabis use
e Cannabis use is more prevalent in males

2 Which of the following are true?
a In the Western world, ~1% of cannabis users become daily users
b The age at first use has fallen in Western countries
c Driving under the influence of cannabis has been shown to be safe
d Cannabis is not addictive
e Cannabis does not impair educational attainment

3 Which of the following are true?
a In the UK, cannabis has been reclassified as a class B drug
b In the West, compared to 10 years ago, more people are seeking help for cannabis dependency
c A cannabis withdrawal syndrome does not exist
d Statistically, people who use cannabis are more likely to go on to use other illegal drugs
e Cannabis is an effective treatment for depression

4 Which of the following are true?
a Cannabis is a risk factor for the development of schizophrenia
b The main psychoactive ingredient in cannabis is cannabidiol
c There is no dose-response relationship between cannabis and the risk of developing schizophrenia
d Schizotypal personality traits confer vulnerability for THC-induced psychoses
e People with schizophrenia tend to use stronger forms of cannabis

5 Cannabis use can be associated with the following (choose as many as applicable):
a Paranoid delusions
b Auditory hallucinations
c Ideas of reference
d Improved memory
e Increased levels of motivation

6 With regards to cannabis and mental health problems, which of the following may be true?
a People with schizophrenia obtain symptom relief from THC
b Very few people with schizophrenia have a cannabis use disorder (CUD)
c People with schizophrenia feel more relaxed following THC
d Exposure to cannabis *in utero* is associated with severe developmental delay
e Cannabis is associated with symptom relapse in people with schizophrenia

7 **Which of the following are true?**

  a In the UK, the concentration of THC in street preparations has risen

  b Skunk is a less potent variety of cannabis

  c Skunk now dominates the UK cannabis market

  d Skunk contains no cannabidiol (CBD)

  e Most UK skunk is imported

8 **In terms of pharmacological treatment for cannabis use disorders, which of the following are true?**

  a Nefazodone is highly effective in promoting abstinence

  b Bupropion reduces the severity of cannabis dependence

  c Oral THC reduces the severity of cannabis withdrawal

  d When a primary mental disorder has been diagnosed in addition to the substance use disorder, this should be treated according to the standard practice for that disorder

  e The evidence base for the pharmacological treatment of cannabis dependence is now robust, and guidelines should be developed as a priority

9 **When it comes to psychological treatments for cannabis use disorders, which of the following are true?**

  a Confrontational techniques are the most effective

  b The FRAMES approach utilises best practice for the delivery of substance use-related brief counselling interventions

  c Studies are in agreement that cognitive behavioural therapy is better than motivational interviewing

  d Motivational interviewing is not person-centred and the person's views are not important at all

  e There is a robust evidence base showing that cannabis users with schizophrenia derive clear (and cost-effective) benefits from cognitive behavioural therapy

Case study 3.1: Mike – part i

Mike (19) presents to the Accident and Emergency department with his parents at 3 a.m. They state that he has been acting 'bizarrely' for the last two weeks but things 'have reached crisis point'. As the on-call member of the psychiatric liaison team you are asked to assess Mike. He appears generally settled but conveys that he is somewhat displeased at having been brought to hospital. His parents are 'anxious' to give some background history.

They state that Mike is their only child and lives with them in their family home. Both parents are high school teachers. They state that Mike left school with top grades but dropped out of university last year and for the last six months has been working at a local supermarket, while 'he was supposed to be thinking' about reapplying for a different course. They describe him as a 'polite and kind-hearted boy, by nature'. Previously, he had a few 'good', close college friends, and some long-term school friends and their shared interest was computing. They state that he never got into any trouble, but they have been concerned recently about the company he has been keeping. He has been leaving the house and not returning until the early hours. Apparently, he has told them that he smokes 'weed'. They say this was a huge shock, especially since he always tended to be 'anti-drugs', although in retrospect 'it all made sense'. Now there are major household shouting matches about weed and his late nights. They can smell the cannabis from his room. Although 'an issue', this is preferable to his 'disappearing off' at nights. His mother adds that he has started smoking cigarettes as well, and remarks, 'Even his appearance has gone to pot'.

There is no previous history of mental illness and no family history of functional psychiatric illness, although his maternal grandfather suffered from alcoholism. He is physically well and not on any prescribed medication.

Mike's parents feel that things had become more serious about two weeks ago, when he suddenly decided to stop going into work. He told them that some of his colleagues were plotting against him and were constantly talking about him behind his back. He claimed that his employers had hired detectives to follow him everywhere because they wanted to accuse him of stealing cigarettes from the store. Things seem to have intensified over the last few days. His parents state that he has been even more irritable and that he was unable to sit in their company as usual. They had heard him muttering to himself in his room. Yesterday he was apparently extremely agitated and was obsessed with the electricity sockets and light bulbs. They feel that they cannot manage him at home.

SELF-ASSESSMENT EXERCISE 3.1

Time: 10 minutes
- How would you proceed?
- What would you wish to clarify about the drug use?

Case study 3.2: Mike – part ii

You interview Mike alone. He is predominantly amenable, calm and coherent. He feels comfortable to tell you the following.
- He has been smoking cannabis for 'about a year or two'.
- He denies other drugs, and drinks alcohol very rarely ('two or three bottles of lager at most'). He has started buying cigarettes recently and smokes about 10 per day.
- He previously smoked 'the odd joint'. In the last six months, he has only been able to obtain skunk (high-potency cannabis). He states that he now smokes about 'two or three' joints per day. He feels he can control this, although on closer questioning, he states that he has never had any periods of abstinence.

- He feels that the cannabis relaxes him and makes him 'more chilled'.
- He states that he smokes skunk with his friends or sometimes alone, in his room at the computer. He sometimes feels 'weird' when smoking with friends, and seems to get 'a bigger hit' than the others.

In terms of his odd behaviour, Mike does not understand why his parents are so worried. He says he cannot recall behaving in the ways that they have described to you. He acknowledges feeling that people are 'playing' with his mind but refuses to cooperate further with your line of questioning. He feels his parents are still angry about his dropping out of university.

SELF-ASSESSMENT EXERCISE 3.2

Time: 20 minutes
- What more would you like to find out about the psychiatric symptoms?
- What is your differential diagnosis so far? State reasons for and against each category.
- List the diagnostic criteria for cannabis dependence.
- Does Mike fulfil these criteria?
- What is your management plan?

Case study 3.3: Mike – part iii

Mike is admitted informally to a general psychiatric ward. He is commenced on 10 mg of olanzapine (oral) and 1 mg of clonazepam (tds). A urine drug screen is done and is positive for cannabis. At the busy ward-round, three days later, Mike denies any psychiatric symptoms and feels that it was 'all down to stress', although he agrees that he may have been overdoing the weed. The decision is made to discharge him. A follow-up appointment with community psychiatric services is arranged. In the corridor, after the ward-round, his parents recognise you. They express some concern that he may go back to his old habits. The advice is to contact the family general practitioner in the event of a crisis, and to encourage him to attend his psychiatric outpatient's appointment.

Case study 3.4: Mike – part iv

Two months later, Mike is brought to the Psychiatric Intensive Care Unit (PICU) after being picked up by police under UK Section 136 of the Mental Health Act.[1] A neighbour alerted police to his bizarre behaviour. It transpires that Mike (barefooted and dressed in his boxer shorts and a hooded top) was 'hanging around' the local shops. He was making 'strange' gestures with his hands and shouting. At interview, Mike is over-aroused and suspicious. He believes that you can read his mind and is actively responding to 'voices' from the electricity sockets. His parents arrive and are keen to talk to you alone. Mike gives his consent. They explain that things were settled for three weeks, although he had not wanted to return to the supermarket. The old pattern re-emerged; as before, he was expressing 'psychotic ideas' and hearing voices. He refused to see the general practitioner and did not attend any psychiatric appointments. Things reached a head in an altercation with the local Asian grocery store owner after he threatened to beat the man up, apparently because he felt he was 'disrespecting' him. His self-care had deteriorated.

Mike describes to you how certain ethnicities are involved in a conspiracy against him. He expresses ideas about being followed by people whom he feels are employed by a secret organisation which orchestrates terrorist activities all around the world. He does not know why this occurs but he holds these beliefs with 100% conviction. He also feels that this organisation has the means to control people's minds directly via the electricity grid.

SELF-ASSESSMENT EXERCISE 3.3

Time: 5 minutes
What is the most likely diagnosis?

Case study 3.5: Mike – part v

Mike is admitted to PICU under Section 2 of the UK Mental Health Act.[2] He is initially treated with intramuscular (IM) haloperidol and lorazepam. Twenty-four-hours later, he begins to accept oral medication and is commenced on olanzapine 10 mg per day. A urine drug screen is positive for cannabis and cocaine. He admits to having had some skunk a few days before but cannot understand the positive cocaine result. All blood tests and physical examination are normal. Mike continues to harbour psychotic symptoms but is transferred to an open ward two weeks later as he is no longer agitated. The olanzapine is increased to 20 mg per day during the third week of treatment. His section is rescinded and by about eight weeks, Mike is almost asymptomatic. He is discharged back home under the care of the Home Treatment Team (HTT). Mike engages well with the team and allows them to supervise his medication daily. However, he resumes using cannabis. In the street (four weeks later), Mike punches an Asian man, whom he believes to be an 'operative agent'.

SELF-ASSESSMENT EXERCISE 3.4

> **Time:**
> - What should the management plan be now?
> - What is the most likely diagnosis?
> - Is this different from your previous diagnosis?

CANNABIS: CAUSE FOR CONCERN?

Cannabis use, especially among the young, has generated increasing concern in recent years.[3]

> **KEY POINTS 3.1**
>
> Worldwide, cannabis is the most commonly used illicit drug.

Rates of use are higher in the Western world, and higher in males. For some reason, use of cannabis is particularly high in people diagnosed as suffering from schizophrenia. People presenting with their first episode of psychosis have double the rates of cannabis use compared to their peers.[4-6] Overall, about one in every four people with schizophrenia has a comorbid cannabis use disorder.[7] There are indications that people experiencing schizophrenia have a preference for more potent varieties of cannabis which are high in delta-9-tetrahydrocannabinol.[8] Cannabis was formerly believed to be a relatively benign recreational drug in comparison to stimulants and opiates. However, a growing body of evidence now indicates that cannabis is not without adverse or undesired effects. High levels of cannabis use are related to:

➤ poorer educational outcomes
➤ lower income
➤ greater welfare dependence
➤ unemployment
➤ lower relationship satisfaction
➤ lower life satisfaction.[9]

Cannabis use is also associated with subtle cognitive impairment, which appears to persist after discontinuation of the drug.[10] Most of the attention, certainly in the media and in government, has focused on the link between cannabis use and psychotic illnesses such as schizophrenia. This has been one of the main drivers for the reclassification of the legal status of cannabis in the UK (*see* Box 3.1).

BOX 3.1 The UK 2009 legal status of cannabis

The UK Government reversed their earlier (Class C) decision and reclassified cannabis as a Class B drug in January 2009. The maximum penalties are:
- For possession: five-year prison sentence or an unlimited fine, or both
- For dealing/supplying: 14-year prison sentence or an unlimited fine, or both

CANNABIS AND THE BRAIN

The major psychoactive properties of cannabis are attributable to the molecule Δ^9-tetrahydrocannabinol (THC), one of over 60 plant-derived cannabinoids. There are also cannabis-like substances produced naturally by the brain itself – the endocannabinoids. THC elicits psychological effects via stimulation of a receptor called the cannabinoid 1 receptor (CB1).[11] All drugs of addiction (including cannabis) activate the release of dopamine in deep regions of the brain.[12] It was initially hypothesised that the ability of cannabis to elicit psychosis stemmed from the release of dopamine. The addictive properties of cannabis were also ascribed to increased dopamine release. However, the picture is more complex. It now appears that the endocannabinoid system itself is much more central than was previously thought. Indeed there is evidence that the addictive properties of a range of drugs depend on the endocannabinoid system. Drugs blocking endocannabinoid signalling show a remarkable ability to reduce the addictiveness of a range of substances including alcohol, nicotine, opiates and cocaine.[13] So far, this work has not yet translated beyond an experimental setting. However, this approach is promising for the development of new interventions against a wide range of addictions. The ability of THC (and stimulants – *see* Chapter 4) to induce transient psychotic thinking is also believed to depend upon perturbations of natural endocannabinoid signalling.[14] Of the other plant-derived cannabinoids (or phytocannabinoids), cannabidiol (CBD) has aroused interest. Ironically, and in stark contrast to THC, cannabidiol might even be an effective remedy for schizophrenic psychosis.[15] Newer forms of street cannabis, termed 'skunk' or sinsemilla, are notable in that they contain no CBD, but high (and still rising) concentrations of THC.[16] Understandably, the widespread use of sinsemilla among young people in the West has become a major public health concern.

CANNABIS DEPENDENCE

It was widely held that, in contrast to alcohol, nicotine, stimulants and opiates, cannabis had no propensity for addiction. This is not the case. Animal studies have clearly shown that THC carries the signature of being an addictive compound.[13]

KEY POINT 3.2

It is estimated that about 10% of cannabis users meet diagnostic guidelines for addiction.[17]

Increasing numbers of people in North America, Australia and Europe have been seeking help for CUDs.[18] On average, those seeking help will have made more than six serious attempts to stop or reduce their cannabis use.[18] Proponents of cannabis legalisation have often pointed to the lack of any significant cannabis withdrawal syndrome as evidence of non-addictiveness. However, a pronounced cannabis withdrawal reaction can be triggered by CB1 receptor blockers, in animals and in humans.[3] Normally, the slow clearance of cannabis from the body can mask any major withdrawal symptoms. However, many individuals report withdrawal symptoms including:
➤ irritability
➤ anxiety
➤ muscle pains
➤ chills
➤ stomach upset
➤ anorexia
➤ sleeping difficulties.[19]

CANNABIS AND PSYCHOSIS

Since the 19th century, there have been descriptions of acute schizophrenia-like psychotic symptoms in healthy subjects who have taken cannabis. This has been confirmed in modern studies using purified preparations of THC.[20,21] Studies have shown that in people who go on to develop schizophrenia, those who use cannabis develop their illness some five years earlier.[22] Furthermore, patients who use cannabis have more psychotic symptoms, more frequent and earlier relapses, and have more episodes of inpatient treatment.[23–25] Patients who use cannabis are less likely to comply with psychiatric medication.[26]

Whether cannabis could actually 'cause' schizophrenia was controversial but numerous epidemiological studies are in agreement that early onset cannabis use is a risk factor for schizophrenia (relative risk x ~2).[27,28] Furthermore, in people who had used cannabis on more than 50 occasions the relative risk increased by x 6.[29] A recent Danish study showed that among people presenting to psychiatric services for treatment of acute cannabis psychosis, 50% went on to be given a diagnosis of schizophrenia in the next year.[30] Recent studies have argued against reverse causality; in which psychotic symptoms precede cannabis *self-medication*.[31]

Experimental studies have shown that, in schizophrenic patients, purified THC does not aid anxiety or side-effects from neuroleptic drugs.[32] Cannabis is certainly neither necessary nor sufficient for schizophrenia and additional components acting in combination are required. The age when the drug is first used appears to be an important factor. In a longitudinal study, use by the age of 18 doubled, whereas use by the age of 15 quadrupled, the odds of subsequent schizophrenia in adulthood, suggesting that cannabis may be affecting adolescent neural/mental development.[33]

Between 1970 and 2002, cannabis use in British teenagers increased 18-fold. Hickman and colleagues[34] predicted that by 2010, a substantial increase in both the incidence and prevalence of schizophrenia would be apparent.[34] Under a conservative model, in which heavy use carries a two-fold risk, they calculated that cannabis would be responsible for 10% of new schizophrenia cases, which rises to

25% if light use *also* carries risk. There is already some evidence to support such predictions from studies in South London by Jane Boydell and colleagues. During the period 1965 to 1999, there was a rapid increase in the proportion of first-episode schizophrenic cases using cannabis in the 12-months prior to diagnosis, which significantly exceeded a far less dramatic increase observed in a control group of non-schizophrenic patients.[35] Over the same period, the incidence of schizophrenia in South London has doubled.[36]

One remaining mystery is why people experiencing schizophrenia use cannabis more avidly than the rest of the population. Furthermore, what motivates a person with schizophrenia to persist in taking cannabis when the outcome can be so immediately detrimental? One possibility is that those people who develop schizophrenia are also more prone to cannabis dependence (and dependence to other substances). But, to date, there have been few studies testing this hypothesis directly.

THE TREATMENT OF CANNABIS USE DISORDER

The successful treatment of cannabis use disorders (CUDs) is challenging, whether occurring as part of a coexisting major mental illness or not. Compared to the management of nicotine, alcohol and opiates, there is a scant evidence base for the treatment of CUDs,[18] but recent work has been encouraging.

Psychotherapies/behavioural interventions

There have been several trials of the efficacy of various supportive psychotherapies.[18,37] Stephens and colleagues[38] showed that two sessions of individualised assessment and intervention (IAI – which comprised elements of cognitive behavioural therapy [CBT]) and motivational enhancement therapy [MET] – *see* Book 4, Chapters 7 and 10; Book 5, Chapters 11 and 12), was as effective as 14 relapse prevention/social support (RSPG – *see* Chapters 15 and 16; Book 4, Chapter 13) sessions in reducing cannabis use at four months, and both psychotherapies performed better than a control group.[38] Motivational enhancement therapy utilises a non-confrontational, non-judgemental clinical style to enhance an individual's awareness of their drug use and its impact on their life. The aim is to enhance their motivation for change and guide them towards commitment and action.[18] In a study of 229 outpatients, Copeland and colleagues[18] found that subjects randomised to one session of CBT or six sessions of CBT were equally likely to achieve abstinence at one month and both active groups outperformed controls.[18] However, the treatment effect was short-lived in that the likelihood of maintained abstinence was the same between actively treated groups and controls. In a trial of 450 cannabis dependent subjects, nine sessions of CBT/MET/case management was superior to two sessions of CBT, which was itself superior to a control condition, in promoting abstinence at four months.[39] Maintained superiority of the longer intervention over the shorter intervention was reported, although the robustness of this finding has been questioned.[37] Two studies investigated whether contingency management (cash transferable vouchers) promoted abstinence from cannabis. In the first study, four sessions of MET were as efficacious as 14 sessions of MET plus behavioural skills training, but the addition of voucher incentives augmented the efficacy of the 14-session intervention.[40] Subsequently, this group found that a voucher-based intervention was successful up until the point that vouchers were discontinued, but that the combination of 14 sessions of CBT and vouchers promoted longer term abstinence.[41] These findings were replicated in a study by Kadden and co-workers, where the psychotherapy component consisted of MET+CBT.[42]

Pharmacotherapies

The utility of various pharmacotherapies for cannabis withdrawal and cannabis dependence has been explored. However, to date, the studies involve a small number of participants. Unsurprisingly, oral formulations of THC can reduce the symptoms of cannabis withdrawal.[40] In a laboratory-based study, lofexidine did not reduce cannabis withdrawal symptoms, but improved sleep and decreased relapse, while the combination of oral THC and lofexidine produced a robust symptomatic improvement.[43] Preliminary randomised-controlled trials (RCTs) for cannabis dependence (valproate, nefazodone, bupropion) have been disappointing.[37]

MENTAL HEALTH–CANNABIS USE DISORDERS

> **KEY POINT 3.3**
>
> The management of a cannabis use disorder is more challenging in people suffering from schizophrenia.

Evidence indicates that cannabis usually worsens a pre-existing psychotic disorder. Many professionals will be familiar with individuals who, following a period of successful inpatient treatment, resume cannabis use (stopping their psychiatric medication) and require further intensive treatment. It is also common to encounter individuals who believe that cannabis (as opposed to psychiatric medicines) helps their underlying symptoms, despite evidence to the contrary in the form of readmission to hospital.

Hjorthoj and colleagues[45] have undertaken a systematic review of the literature on the treatment of CUDs in people with schizophrenia.[45] They conclude that the evidence at present is insufficient and that, in terms of outcome, many studies have failed to 'tease out' cannabis from other substances as a whole. The size and rigour of many studies has been found wanting. Similar to the findings above (in non-mental health–substance use individuals), contingency management in the form of vouchers promoted abstinence, but only during the active phase of treatment with no long-term maintained effect. Supportive psychotherapies (MET and CBT) were *ineffective* in most studies where cannabis use was measured as a separate outcome, but effective in studies that grouped substances together as a whole.[45]

To date there have been no randomised controlled trials of medications aimed at cannabis use/dependence in people with schizophrenia.[45] However, there are reports that antipsychotics (quetiapine and clozapine) can reduce cannabis use and craving.[46,47] Definitive placebo-controlled trials – of this class of molecule, for this outcome, in people experiencing schizophrenia – are unfeasible, given the obvious ethical concerns of replacing an anti-psychotic with placebo. The findings above and future open-labelled studies will probably constitute the best available evidence for professionals.

It is evident that more research is needed, to clarify which of the currently available interventions (psychosocial/pharmacological) is best for CUDs, whether complicated by severe mental illness or not. Nordstrom and colleagues[37] conclude that a number of supportive psychotherapies are effective (in uncomplicated CUDs), but with the exception of vouchers, no particular brand of psychotherapy is superior. Furthermore, long-term treatment appears to be no more effective than shorter therapies.[37] Copeland and Swift[18] reach the same conclusion regarding the efficacy of brief psychosocial interventions – and argue that, given the increasing demand for the treatment of CUDs, there remains a strong need for the development of more effective interventions, aimed not just at treatment, but at early-detection and prevention.[18] Hjorthoj and colleagues[45] recommend that future studies should test combinations of psychosocial and pharmacological interventions, and incorporate elements of contingency management.[45] The evidence suggests that contingency management (in the form of cash redeemable vouchers) is effective, in cannabis-dependent individuals, whether mentally ill or not. Copeland and Swift[18] point out that contingency management has not always been viewed as a practical strategy by many professionals, but the weight of the evidence is hard to ignore.

There is little doubt that people experiencing schizophrenia should be encouraged to comply with neuroleptic medication and remain engaged in treatment (whether they use cannabis or not), given what is known about relapse following discontinuation. However, it is encouraging that neuroleptics may also help decrease cannabis use. Although most people will not be oblivious to the furore surrounding cannabis and schizophrenia, it can be a worthwhile exercise sharing recent findings from the literature.

KEY POINT 3.4

Most people (whether schizophrenic or not) are surprised by just how detrimental cannabis use can be in major mental illness.

Finally, there remains a need for a paradigm shift and the development of new pharmacotherapies. Ironically, the endocannabinoid system itself appears to be a promising target for broad-spectrum anti-addictive compounds. The prototype molecule rimonabant (a CB1 antagonist) showed broad-spectrum efficacy in preclinical studies. Initially, it was introduced for obesity, but was later suspended due to concern over depressive side-effects.[3] Newer compounds with similar mechanisms are now under investigation. A major challenge will be developing CB1-targeting drugs devoid of serious psychiatric side-effects. Preliminary results with CBD have been encouraging, but much more work is needed to investigate whether this molecule has 'real' therapeutic utility, in psychosis and in dependence. Surprisingly, perhaps, the main barriers to progress are not necessarily technical or pharmacological. Instead, current-day researchers are encumbered by (ever-increasing) bureaucratic requirements, which stifle the development of promising new treatments. That this has happened, so that the champions of micro-management have triumphed over clinicians, is tragic for the art of drug discovery in medicine. In addition, unless the balance can be redressed, it does not bode well for future individuals experiencing mental health–cannabis use disorders.

CASE DISCUSSION
Case studies: Mike – parts i–iii

Mike is suffering from a psychotic episode. The most likely factor is his use of high-potency cannabis (skunk). The clinical features of schizophrenic psychosis and cannabis psychosis can be identical. Thus, it is impossible to rule out the possibility that this is the first manifestation of a schizophrenic psychosis. His functioning may have deteriorated long before this crisis. Particularly, why did he stop university? Was he experiencing positive symptoms (suspiciousness, delusional thinking and disturbed perception) at that point? Alternatively, did his motivation, drive and level of interest suffer? The features of the so-called cannabis-amotivation syndrome mimic the negative symptoms of schizophrenia. It is interesting that he reports get-ting 'a stronger hit' from cannabis than his friends. Personality and genetic variables are thought to underlie why some people are more vulnerable than others. It could be argued that he is started on olanzapine with too much haste. The evidence sug-gests that current antipsychotics do not protect against cannabis psychosis. Thus, an as required benzodiazepine as a sole treatment may have been preferable. One danger is that the apparent benefits of olanzapine (and hence the justification to continue it) are in fact more attributable to 'washout' of THC from his system. That said, it can be argued that he is discharged without adequate arrangements for follow-up. Moreover, the concerns of his parents are not addressed fully (*see* Book 3, Chapter 2; Book 5, Chapter 4). Could Mike have been seen, while on the ward, by a community-based key-worker, who would then have been able to begin establishing a therapeutic relationship (*see* Book 4, Chapter 2)? Notably, he shows some insight at the ward round prior to discharge and accepts cannabis may have played a role. The key tasks for the key-worker would have been:
➤ continued monitoring of Mike's mental state
➤ building the therapeutic relationship so that Mike's cannabis use can be addressed, making use of supportive psychotherapy
➤ ensuring there are lines of communication available should things go wrong.

Case studies: Mike – parts iv–v

Mike falls through the net, returns to drug use and becomes psychotic again. The suspicion is that cannabis has uncovered a schizophrenic illness. However, has he been experimenting with cocaine (crack)? Again, the symptom profile cannot dif-ferentiate drugs from endogenous illness. For precise diagnostics, what is needed is a period of abstinence from cannabis. It is wise to be clear about the intended purpose of antipsychotics. Are they being prescribed for symptom management (to reduce positive psychotic symptoms, or as a sedative) or are they being prescribed for the prophylaxis of relapse in schizophrenia?

Mike is vulnerable and the intensity of his symptoms has increased. There is also a sense that his delusions are crystallising. With each relapse, he becomes less insightful and less amenable for a psychological approach. His presentation mimics that of a person experiencing an endogenous psychosis. Notably, however, he makes a relatively swift recovery. Whether this is due to cannabis washout or an effect of treatment is unknown. The continued prescribing of neuroleptic medication needs careful consideration on an individual basis. The judgement will be informed by the balance between desired effects and side-effects. In any case, is he compliant? Following reorientation back to reality, the aims remain the same:

➤ continued monitoring of his mental state
➤ building the therapeutic relationship so that supportive psychotherapies can be utilised to tackle his use of cannabis
➤ revisiting the contingency arrangements.

CONCLUSION

We have used a case study approach to help identify the problems associated with mental health–cannabis use disorders. We have looked at the challenging issues for the individual, family and professional. The case study built around Mike demonstrates the conflict that arises with and between the individual and the family.

More research is needed to determine whether people experiencing schizophrenia are more prone to cannabis use dependence – but this appears to be the case. For instance, it is known that the rates of cannabis use are higher in people who are diagnosed as suffering from schizophrenia. Furthermore, in the study by Di Forti and colleagues,[8] people experiencing their first psychotic breakdown were six times more likely than their matched peers to have a preference for stronger forms of cannabis.

Why do people with mental illness persist in using cannabis and why do they appear to prefer the most potent forms? At present, no clear-cut answers emerge. It is clear that the endogenous cannabinoid system is involved in reward/reinforcement/addiction, as well as the process of psychosis. This is also the case for the neuromodulator, dopamine. The next few years are likely to confirm the importance of cannabinoids in the process of addiction, and for some a cannabinoid hypothesis may come to rival the more long-standing dopamine hypothesis. But this is to misunderstand the neurobiology. The cannabinoid and dopamine systems are intimately linked throughout the reward pathways, thus both systems are important. Teasing out the detail will rely on modern molecular neuroscience, for example conditional gene knockout technology, *in vivo* voltammetry and electrophysiology. The prospect is that as we learn more about the neurological underpinnings of addiction, we will also learn more about the process of psychosis.

REFERENCES

1 Mental Health Act 2007 – Section 136. Available at: www.dh.gov.uk/en/Publications andstatistics/Publications/PublicationsPolicyAndGuidance/DH_084351 (accessed 2 November 2010).

2 Mental Health Act 2008 – Section 2. Available at: www.dh.gov.uk/prod_consum_dh/ groups/dh_digitalassets/@dh/@en/documents/digitalasset/dh_097244.pdf (accessed 2 November 2010).

3 Murray RM, Morrison PD, Henquet C, *et al.* Cannabis, the mind and society: the hash realities. *Nature Reviews.* 2007; **8**: 885–95.

4 Barnett JH, Werners U, Secher SM, *et al.* Substance use in a population-based clinic sample of people with first-episode psychosis. *British Journal of Psychiatry.* 2007; **190**: 515–20.

5 Hambrecht M, Hafner H. Cannabis, vulnerability, and the onset of schizophrenia: an epidemiological perspective. *The Australian and New Zealand Journal of Psychiatry.* 2000; **34**: 468–75.

6 Van Mastrigt S, Addington J, Addington D. Substance misuse at presentation to an early psychosis program. *Social Psychiatry and Psychiatric Epidemiology.* 2004; **39**: 69–72.

7 Koskinen J, Lohonen J, Koponen H, *et al.* Rate of cannabis use disorders in clinical samples of patients with schizophrenia: a meta-analysis. *Schizophrenia Bulletin.* 2010; **36**(6): 1115–30.

8 Di Forti M, Morgan C, Dazzan P, *et al.* High-potency cannabis and risk of psychosis. *British Journal of Psychiatry.* 2009; **195**: 488–91.

9 Fergusson DM, Boden JM. Cannabis use and later life outcomes. *Addiction.* 2008; **103**: 969–76, discussion 77–8.

10 Solowij N, Stephens RS, Roffman RA, *et al.* Cognitive functioning of long-term heavy cannabis users seeking treatment. *Journal of the American Medical Association.* 2002; **287**: 1123–31.

11 Iversen L. Cannabis and the brain. *Brain.* 2003; **126**: 1252–70.

12 Hyman SE, Malenka RC. Addiction and the brain: the neurobiology of compulsion and its persistence. *Nature Reviews.* 2001; **2**: 695–703.

13 Gardner EL. Endocannabinoid signaling system and brain reward: emphasis on dopamine. *Pharmacology, Biochemistry, and Behavior.* 2005; **81**: 263–84.

14 Morrison PD, Murray RM. From real-world events to psychosis: the emerging neuropharmacology of delusions. *Schizophrenia Bulletin.* 2009; **35**: 668–74.

15 Zuardi AW, Crippa JA, Hallak JE, *et al.* Cannabidiol, a cannabis sativa constituent, as an antipsychotic drug. *Brazilian Journal of Medical and Biological Research = Revista brasileira de pesquisas medicas e biologicas/Sociedade Brasileira de Biofisica.* 2006; **39**: 421–9.

16 Potter DJ, Clark P, Brown MB. Potency of delta 9-THC and other cannabinoids in cannabis in England in 2005: implications for psychoactivity and pharmacology. *Journal of Forensic Sciences.* 2008; **53**: 90–4.

17 Hall W, Degenhardt L. Prevalence and correlates of cannabis use in developed and developing countries. *Current Opinion in Psychiatry.* 2007; **20**: 393–7.

18 Copeland J, Swift W. Cannabis use disorder: epidemiology and management. *International Review of Psychiatry.* 2009; **21**: 96–103.

19 Haney M, Ward AS, Comer SD, *et al.* Abstinence symptoms following smoked marijuana in humans. *Psychopharmacology.* 1999; **141**: 395–404.

20 D'Souza DC, Perry E, MacDougall L, *et al.* The psychotomimetic effects of intravenous delta-9-tetrahydrocannabinol in healthy individuals: implications for psychosis. *Neuropsychopharmacology.* 2004; **29**: 1558–72.

21 Morrison PD, Zois V, McKeown DA, *et al.* The acute effects of synthetic intravenous Delta9-tetrahydrocannabinol on psychosis, mood and cognitive functioning. *Psychological Medicine.* 2009; **1**: 1–10.

22 Barnes TR, Mutsatsa SH, Hutton SB, *et al.* Comorbid substance use and age at onset of schizophrenia. *British Journal of Psychiatry.* 2006; **188**: 237–42.

23 Caspari D. Cannabis and schizophrenia: results of a follow-up study. *European Archives of Psychiatry and Clinical Neuroscience.* 1999; **249**: 45–9.

24 Grech A, Van Os J, Jones PB, *et al.* Cannabis use and outcome of recent onset psychosis. *European Psychiatry.* 2005; **20**: 349–53.

25 Linszen DH, Dingemans PM, Lenior ME. Cannabis abuse and the course of recent-onset schizophrenic disorders. *Archives of General Psychiatry.* 1994; **51**: 273–9.

26 Fenton WS, Blyler CR, Heinssen RK. Determinants of medication compliance in schizophrenia: empirical and clinical findings. *Schizophrenia Bulletin.* 1997; **23**: 637–51.

27 Arseneault L, Cannon M, Witton J, *et al.* Causal association between cannabis and psychosis: examination of the evidence. *British Journal of Psychiatry.* 2004; **184**: 110–7.

28 Moore TH, Zammit S, Lingford-Hughes A, *et al.* Cannabis use and risk of psychotic or affective mental health outcomes: a systematic review. *Lancet.* 2007; **370**: 319–28.

29 Andreasson S, Allebeck P, Engstrom A, *et al.* Cannabis and schizophrenia: a longitudinal study of Swedish conscripts. *Lancet.* 1987; **2**: 1483–6.

30 Arendt M, Rosenberg R, Foldager L, *et al.* Cannabis-induced psychosis and subsequent schizophrenia-spectrum disorders: follow-up study of 535 incident cases. *British Journal of Psychiatry.* 2005; **187**: 510–5.

31 Hall W. Is cannabis use psychotogenic? *Lancet.* 2006; **367**: 193–5.

32 D'Souza DC, Abi-Saab WM, Madonick S, *et al.* Delta-9-tetrahydrocannabinol effects in schizophrenia: implications for cognition, psychosis, and addiction. *Biological Psychiatry.* 2005; **57**: 594–608.

33 Arseneault L, Cannon M, Poulton R, *et al.* Cannabis use in adolescence and risk for adult psychosis: longitudinal prospective study. *British Medical Journal.* Clinical Research Edition. 2002; **325**: 1212–3.

34 Hickman M, Vickerman P, Macleod J, *et al.* Cannabis and schizophrenia: model projections of the impact of the rise in cannabis use on historical and future trends in schizophrenia in England and Wales. *Addiction.* 2007; **102**: 597–606.

35 Boydell J, van Os J, Caspi A, *et al.* Trends in cannabis use prior to first presentation with schizophrenia, in South-East London between 1965 and 1999. *Psychological Medicine.* 2006; **36**: 1441–6.

36 Boydell J, Van Os J, Lambri M, *et al.* Incidence of schizophrenia in south-east London between 1965 and 1997. *British Journal of Psychiatry.* 2003; **182**: 45–9.

37 Nordstrom BR, Levin FR. Treatment of cannabis use disorders: a review of the literature. *The American Journal on Addictions/American Academy of Psychiatrists in Alcoholism and Addictions.* 2007; **16**: 331–42.

38 Stephens RS, Roffman RA, Curtin L. Comparison of extended versus brief treatments for marijuana use. *Journal of Consulting and Clinical Psychology.* 2000; **68**: 898–908.

39 Brief treatments for cannabis dependence: findings from a randomized multisite trial. *Journal of Consulting and Clinical Psychology.* 2004; **72**: 455–66.

40 Budney AJ, Higgins ST, Radonovich KJ, *et al.* Adding voucher-based incentives to coping skills and motivational enhancement improves outcomes during treatment for marijuana dependence. *Journal of Consulting and Clinical Psychology.* 2000; **68**: 1051–61.

41 Budney AJ, Moore BA, Rocha HL, *et al.* Clinical trial of abstinence-based vouchers and cognitive-behavioral therapy for cannabis dependence. *Journal of Consulting and Clinical Psychology.* 2006; **74**: 307–16.

42 Kadden RM, Litt MD, Kabela-Cormier E, *et al.* Abstinence rates following behavioral treatments for marijuana dependence. *Addictive Behaviors.* 2007; **32**: 1220–36.

43 Haney M, Hart CL, Vosburg SK, *et al.* Marijuana withdrawal in humans: effects of oral THC or divalproex. *Neuropsychopharmacology.* 2004; **29**: 158–70.

44 Haney M, Hart CL, Vosburg SK, *et al*. Effects of THC and lofexidine in a human laboratory model of marijuana withdrawal and relapse. *Psychopharmacology*. 2008; **197**: 157–68.

45 Hjorthoj C, Fohlmann A, Nordentoft M. Treatment of cannabis use disorders in people with schizophrenia spectrum disorders: a systematic review. *Addictive Behaviors*. 2009; **34**: 520–5.

46 Potvin S, Stip E, Lipp O, *et al*. Quetiapine in patients with comorbid schizophrenia-spectrum and substance use disorders: an open-label trial. *Current Medical Research and Opinion*. 2006; **22**: 1277–85.

47 Zimmet SV, Strous RD, Burgess ES, *et al*. Effects of clozapine on substance use in patients with schizophrenia and schizoaffective disorder: a retrospective survey. *Journal of Clinical Psychopharmacology*. 2000; **20**: 94–8.

TO LEARN MORE

- Castle D, Murray R. *Marijuana Madness*. Cambridge: Cambridge University Press; 2004.
- The effects of CBD and THC in healthy subjects. Available at: http://vimeo.com/13891229
- The National Cannabis Prevention and Information Website (Australia). Available at: http://ncpic.org.au/
- The Home Office guide on how to cut down and stop cannabis use. Available at: www.home office.gov.uk/materials/kc-stop.pdf
- FRANK website. Available at: www.talktofrank.com
- Support group. Available at: www.marijuana-anonymous.org
- Website for 13–19 year olds offering support. Available at: www.connexions.gov.uk

ANSWERS TO THE MULTIPLE CHOICE QUESTIONNAIRE 3.1

1   b and e are true
2   b is true, a = ~10%
3   a, b and d are true
4   a, d and e are true
5   a, b and c are true
6   e is true
7   a, c and d are true
8   c and d are true
9   b is true

CHAPTER 4

Stimulants and mental health

Richard Orr McLeod and Philip D Cooper

INTRODUCTION

Stimulants provide the professional with some of the most difficult challenges, and can have a significant impact on the individual's physical, psychological and social well-being. Anecdotally, many health professionals count stimulants as the most damaging to mental and physical well-being, as well as presenting some of the most challenging situations. In the UK, while the overall use of illicit substances has remained relatively stable, the use of certain stimulants, notably cocaine and crack cocaine, has increased in recent years.[1] The availability of stimulants, especially 3,4-Methylenedioxymethamphetamine (MDMA – ecstasy) and its derivatives, plus the marked reduction in cost, both actual and relative, of MDMA and cocaine has exacerbated the problems encountered by professionals, and the significant difficulties for the individual, family and carers.

This chapter addresses some of the challenges stimulant use presents to the individual experiencing mental health problems and considers specific issues arising from stimulant use. Two case examples are used to illustrate key points.

WHAT ARE STIMULANTS?

'Stimulants' encompass a range of different substances that includes amphetamine, methamphetamine, cocaine, crack cocaine, and MDMA, in addition to some 'legal highs' (e.g. mephedrone – Box 4.1 offers some commonly used names for stimulants). While these substances have many similarities each has differences peculiar to them. Although a brief description of these substances and their effects are given here, the reader is encouraged to refer to the 'To Learn More' section at the end of the chapter for more in-depth information.

BOX 4.1 Common stimulant street names

Cocaine hydrochloride:
- coke
- Charlie
- Columbian/Bolivian marching powder
- snow

- devils dandruff
- toot
- snort
- beak
- chisel
- Terry Farley/lemon barley (or just 'lemon')
- blow
- 'C'
- nose candy
- Nikki Lauder powder.

Crack:
- rocks
- beam me up Scotty.

Amphetamine sulphate:
- speed
- phet
- sulphate/sulf
- Billy whizz/whizz.

Methamphetamine sulphate:
- crystal meth/meth/crystal
- ice
- crank.

3,4-Methylenedioxymethamphetamine/MDMA
- ecstasy
- 'E'
- burgers
- pills
- doves
- love drug
- Jack 'n' Jills.

Stimulants activate or excite the central nervous system; in particular, they have an effect on the neurotransmitters dopamine, noradrenaline and serotonin. These neurotransmitters are thought to be involved in modulating mood, sleep, anger and aggression (serotonin) and have an important role in behaviour and cognition, motor activity, motivation and reward, sleep, mood, attention and learning (dopamine). At lower levels, stimulants produce euphoric effects, increase energy, confidence and talkativeness. At higher levels, stimulants can induce anxiety, paranoia, confusion, aggressiveness and in some cases unpleasant psychotic symptoms (delusions, hallucinations). Higher doses may also lead to serious acute physical health problems (e.g. life-threatening cardiac arrhythmia, chest pain, hypertension), particularly if the individual has an unknown underlying health problem.

As the effects of stimulants wear off ('come down') the individual is likely to experience irritability, apathy, insomnia or excessive sleep, and hunger. These effects can last for a number of days after use and can have a significant impact on an individual's level of functioning. In addition, individuals are likely to experience low mood in the days after use; weekend users may use the term 'suicide Tuesday' to describe the impact stimulants can have on their mood in the early part of the week (Box 4.2 provides a summary of the short/long-term effects).

BOX 4.2 Short-/long-term impact of stimulant use

Short-term effects of stimulant use:
- increased heart rate
- vasoconstriction/increased blood pressure
- increase in body temperature
- increase in energy levels and alertness
- euphoria
- wakefulness
- increase in confidence
- increase in talkativeness
- dilation of pupils
- decrease in appetite
- increase in sexual drive
- sweating
- flushing of skin
- rapid speech
- tightening of jaws/teeth clenching
- disinhibition
- increase in ability to concentrate
- dehydration
- nausea/vomiting
- irritability
- insomnia
- anxiety
- confusion/disorientation
- aggressiveness
- paranoid ideation
- respiratory collapse
- cardiac arrhythmias.

The long-term use of stimulants includes:
- insomnia
- irritability
- apathy
- paranoia

- panic attack
- low mood/depression
- anxiety
- weight loss/malnutrition/vitamin deficiency
- skin disorders
- immune system suppression – increased likelihood of colds, influenza, etc.
- respiratory problems ('crack lung')
- cardiovascular problems
- psychosis
- seizures
- dependence.

A major problem with stimulants, and the above risks, relates to purity of the drug. Adulteration prevents the individual from competent knowledge related to the concentration of pure ingredients, i.e. strength, which can lead to an increased risk of potential harms when purity is greater than usual. Moreover, it is unclear what other substances have been mixed with the pure substance; some of these can be, in themselves, dangerous. In addition, poly-substance use (the use of two or more substances on one occasion) can increase the risk of harm to the individual. Cocaine and alcohol are frequently used together but can produce a unique compound known as cocaethylene when they are simultaneously exposed in the liver. Cocaethylene appears to produce a heightened euphoria for the individual and prolongs the effects of the cocaine. However, it can increase an individual's heart rate and blood pressure to a greater extent than when using cocaine alone, and consequently increases the risk of cardiovascular problems.[2]

Despite the above risks and negative effects of stimulants, the short-term benefits and pleasurable effects will far outweigh the potential consequences for the individual. This is important to remember when working with individuals who use stimulants, and other substances. Often, the focus of conversation, led by the professional, can evolve around the negative impact these substances have for the individual, without acknowledging the perceived benefits. However, understanding the positive aspects of the individual's stimulant experience is essential if the professional wants to fully understand the nature of their substance use and be better placed to assist the individual in addressing any problems.

METHODS OF USE

Stimulants can be used in a variety of ways and the duration of effects can vary between substances. Table 4.1 below outlines the most common methods of use for a number of stimulants and the approximate duration of their effects. Where a number of methods of use are listed, the most common form of use is listed first and less common forms listed subsequently.

TABLE 4.1 Methods of use and duration of effects

Substance	Form	Method of use	Duration of effects
Amphetamines	Powder; tablets	Swallowed ('bombed' – powder wrapped in a cigarette paper); Inhaled ('snorted'); Injected (IV)	3–6 hours Duration less if injecting although effects more intense
Cocaine	Powder	Inhaled; Injected (IV)	20–30 minutes Duration less if injecting although effects more intense
Crack cocaine	Crystals – 'rocks'	Smoked	5–15 minutes
MDMA	Tablets; powder	Swallowed	3–6 hours

LEGAL HIGHS

Legal highs have attracted significant media interest in the past couple of years and their use is of considerable concern, mainly due to the limited understanding of the effects and potential harms of these substances. Legal highs are designed specifically to provide the individual with an experience similar to illicit substances and are freely available on the internet and in 'head shops'. The chemical structure of legal highs is often very similar to those of illicit substances, although the slight differences have enabled them to remain outside of any laws that control substances and, therefore, are considered legal. However, several countries have addressed this issue and a number of former 'legal highs' are now controlled substances. For individuals using these substances, and professionals, it is important to note that the term 'legal' is not synonymous with 'safe'.

Mephedrone is probably the most well-known 'legal high' after receiving a high level of media interest in 2009/2010. Mephedrone, often referred to as 'Meow Meow', is usually sold in powder form and swallowed either in capsules or wrapped in a cigarette paper. Mephedrone belongs to a group of substances known as cathinones. Cathinone can be extracted from the leaves of khat, although the majority of cathinones seized and tested are synthetic.[3] They are similar to amphetamine and thought to act on the neurotransmitters dopamine, serotonin and noradrenalin. Other cathinones are:

> ephedrone, which has a similar effect to methylamphetamine
> 3,4-Methylene-dioxymethcathinone (methylone), which has a similar effect to MDMA (3,4-Methylenedioxymethamphetamine)
> bupropion, which is most commonly used as a smoking cessation aid.[3]

Naphyrone (NRG-1), although not a cathinone, is structurally very similar to mephedrone and is thought to have effects similar to cocaine, although the potency is approximately 10 times greater than cocaine.[4] As with mephedrone, it usually comes in powder form and is swallowed. However, due to the potency, caution is required as only very small doses are needed to achieve the desired effects. In the UK, naphyrone and its related analogues were brought under the control of the Misuse of Drugs Act 1971 as a Class B drug in July 2010.

Legal highs are a new and rapidly changing area of substance use. As some substances are brought under control, others are developed to replace them, e.g. NRG-2/NRG-3, marketed as replacements for NRG-1 and mephedrone.

KEY POINT 4.1

It is important for professionals to stay up-to-date regarding the nature and effects of these substances.

A useful way of trying to understand the effects and potential risks associated with these substances is to utilise available anecdotal evidence. The most obvious anecdotal source is the individual. They can direct the professional in understanding the effects peculiar to them, which will subsequently assist the professional in providing a package of support specific to the individual's needs. Websites such as the Vaults of Erowid (www.erowid.org), where individuals post reports on their experience of using certain substances, can also provide a valuable source of anecdotal information on the effects of legal highs.

GENERAL POINTS ABOUT STIMULANT USE

Stimulant use has a number of specific challenges but is, on the whole, no different from other substances when it comes to mental health–substance use interventions and treatment. However, there are issues that do relate specifically to stimulant use. The differences that can occur are seen in the actual effect of the drugs, i.e. the stimulation of the nervous system and the effect that this has on therapeutic engagement and on mental health issues (e.g. psychosis and depression). It is important to recognise the effects of stimulant intoxication, especially when working in community settings. Therapeutic intervention (*see* Book 4, Chapter 2) presents difficulties when the individual is under the influence of a stimulant drug.

Attempting psychological therapies when the individual is under the influence of any drug may illicit untimely responses. For example, the individual may disclose concerns and dilemmas that at this stage they otherwise would not share due to disinhibition or abreactive responses. What can be offered at this stage is to demonstrate an unconditional regard for the individual that will hopefully maintain contact with the person so she/he can be seen again when they are not intoxicated. That is, keeping the door open until the person is ready to engage. Making a cup of tea may not be an intricate psychological intervention; however, it may be the best intervention available under the circumstances and will contribute to the therapeutic alliance.

Case study 4.1: John

John (35) was heroin dependent. He arrived in London, from his home in Bristol, during the late 1980s. John initially used heroin as a buffer after using MDMA and amphetamines but gradually moved on to heroin in combination with minor poly-drug use. After several years of stabilised drug use and methadone maintenance, John's drug use became chaotic and, consequently, he became homeless. This coincided with a sudden increase in his use of crack cocaine.

John became dependent on crack and required increasing amounts of money to support his use. As the physical and psychological impact of his crack cocaine use spiralled, John's life and ability to function became increasingly chaotic. John's substance use led to an increase in crime and he experienced several social, economic, legal, and environmental difficulties.

Analysis of John's situation showed he was dependent on crack and this required a considerably high turnover of funds to support his habit. John's increasingly chaotic lifestyle led to an increase in acquisitive crime and a flagrant disregard for self (e.g. a place to live, clothes, food). This process was exemplified by two similar events that produced very different outcomes.

While John was using only heroin he received a 'back payment' of rent to the sum of £3000. With this money, John was able to fund his drug use and lifestyle for several months and his presentation was relatively stable and orderly. Conversely, several years later, while addicted to crack cocaine, John received a similar sum from the same source. This money lasted him a weekend.

An individual using heroin might use up to £100 of the drug per day. However, usage can be limited by the nature of the drug, i.e. heroin is a central nervous system depressant and overuse of heroin will lead to unconsciousness, respiratory collapse and death. However, with cocaine and crack, there is no obvious in-built control on the amount of substance consumed. This is also true to a lesser extent for amphetamines, although the increased half-life means the need to top up is not as prevalent as with cocaine and crack.

Cocaine and crack's propensity to cause the brain to shut down dopamine receptor sites also gives rise to increasingly higher levels of drug consumption as individuals chase the 'first incredible high' they experienced from their initial use. The result of this high usage can present an increasingly complex clinical picture.

STIMULANTS AND MENTAL HEALTH

If the individual experiences stimulant–mental health problems, the complexity of problems can increase markedly. There are a number of reasons why a person experiencing mental health problems may use stimulants, as follows.

➤ The individual experiencing depression may use stimulants to combat low mood.
➤ The individual experiencing social anxiety may find stimulants provide them with confidence in social settings.
➤ The individual experiencing psychosis may use stimulants to counter the

negative symptoms of their illness (e.g. lethargy, poor self-esteem, social isolation).
➤ The individual experiencing bipolar disorder may find that stimulants curtail the rapid elevation in mood in the initial stages of mania.
➤ The individual may find a short-term reduction in the side-effects from prescribed medication.

While the use of stimulants may subjectively assist in managing these problems in the short term, they are likely, if used regularly, to worsen symptoms in the longer term and contribute to the deterioration of mental health. If the reader considers some of the long-term effects of regular and heavy stimulant use listed above, it is easy to understand the significant impact stimulants could have on the individual's mental health, level of functioning and self-care. For example, the individual using stimulants to overcome low mood, lethargy and social isolation is likely to experience a heightened level of low mood, lethargy and lack of motivation in the days following stimulant use. Subsequently, this may impact on the individual's desire to do the things that would normally be expected of him/her and less likely to interact with family and/or friends, thus increasing isolation.

It may be helpful to clarify the differences between substance-induced psychosis and serious and enduring mental illness, as both require different approaches. People using stimulants may experience drug-induced psychosis and will display the usual symptoms of a psychotic episode, but will make a good recovery following reduction of stimulants and the introduction of antipsychotic medication, usually within a few days. The antipsychotic prescription can subsequently be discontinued once symptoms have receded. However, reinstatement of stimulant use may cause a rapid relapse into substance-induced psychosis. In comparison, with serious and enduring mental illness, there is no quick resolution of psychotic symptoms following the abstinence of the substances and the prescription of antipsychotic medication. Both positive and negative symptoms of psychotic illness may also be present and the clinical picture is generally more complex.

There is increasing evidence to suggest that prolonged and heavy stimulant use can have an effect on executive functioning,[5] which has implications for those experiencing coexisting serious and enduring mental illnesses in particular. Executive function is important in planning and organisation, initiating tasks, self-monitoring, emotional control and working memory (*see* Book 3, Chapter 8). The individual experiencing lower levels of executive functioning resulting from a mental health problem may be further impaired due to ongoing stimulant use. This can impact on their ability to engage in treatment (particularly psychological approaches), increase the risk of early dropout from treatment, and impair the development of coping strategies, thus impacting on recovery. It is, therefore, important for professionals to fully assess an individual's executive functioning and adapt approaches to treatment to take into account potential deficits.

THERAPEUTIC RELATIONSHIP AND ENGAGEMENT
Engagement is an essential first step in the treatment process and its importance should not be underestimated (*see* Book 5, Chapter 7). A healthcare organisation

may have the most advanced mental health–substance use services available and its professionals may be the most skilful, knowledgeable and experienced in working with individuals experiencing these problems, but if they are unable to effectively engage individuals within services they are a redundant resource.

Engagement is about the development of trusting and mutually respecting relationships between professional and individual. Professionals should be non-confrontational and non-judgemental, and embrace recovery-focused approaches. Engagement should aim to foster partnership working between individual and professional and attempt to understand the individual's view of their problems and respond to their needs accordingly.[6] The process of engagement may often not focus on an individual's mental health and substance use problems but on address-ing issues that will have a higher level of priority for the individual, e.g. housing, finances, family relationships, social activities. Providing some stability in these areas may have a positive impact on an individual's mental health–substance use problems without directly addressing them, in addition to assisting the individual to develop trust in the professional.

Three main barriers to engagement have been identified:[7]

1 **Services**: separate systems of care (mental health and substance use); exclusion, rather than inclusion, criteria; clash of treatment philosophies; lack of resources.
2 **Professional**: lack of training; poor communication; negative attitudes; focus on 'primary' diagnosis; treatment not matched to need; policing not treating; lack of time.
3 **Individual**: services do not meet individual needs; not being listened to/heard; fear of disclosing substance use; fear of losing peers/symptom control/side-effect management.

When professionals are experiencing difficulties in engaging an individual it can often be a useful exercise to reflect on the situation from these three perspectives, either alone or with colleagues, and ask the following questions:

➤ What is it about our service that is preventing the individual from engaging?
➤ What is it about my practice, or that of my colleagues, that may be preventing the individual from engaging with me/my colleagues?
➤ How might the individual perceive the situation; what might their fears or concerns be?

This process can sometimes assist the professional in identifying barriers specific to the case and take steps to address these problems. It is important to remember that without an effective period of engagement subsequent interventions are likely to be unsuccessful.

TREATMENT

Table 4.2 outlines the psychological interventions that may be relevant to the person experiencing mental health-stimulant use problems.

TABLE 4.2 Outline of psychological interventions for differing mental health–stimulant use problems

Drug-induced psychosis	• supportive engagement • informal counselling • medication management (*see* Book 5, Chapter 13) • substance awareness • relapse prevention (*see* Chapters 15 and 16)
Serious and enduring psychotic illness	• supportive engagement • motivational interviewing (*see* Book 4, Chapters 6–8), cognitive behavioural therapy (CBT) for psychosis (*see* Book 4, Chapter 10; Book 5, Chapters 11 and 12) • psychoeducation • substance awareness training • relapse prevention – including early warning signs (EWS)
Depression (minor)	• supportive engagement • informal counselling • psychoeducation • CBT
Depression (moderate and major)	• supportive engagement • informal counselling • psychoeducation • medication management • CBT • relapse prevention – EWS
Personality disorder	• supportive engagement • CBT and/or schema-focused therapy • dialectical behaviour therapy (*see* Book 4, Chapter 11) • motivational interviewing • relapse prevention – EWS • substance awareness training

Engaging in a therapeutic relationship is helped by an accurate assessment of the person's readiness to change. Identifying the person's stage of change (*see* Book 4, Chapter 6) helps the professional to provide the right intervention at the right time. The individual in the mid-late contemplative stage may be more responsive to the introduction of ideas around reduction and cessation. However, the individual in the pre-contemplative stage may be more receptive to supportive engagement and less demanding interventions. Attempts to force the pace of change usually end up in resistance and therapeutic rupture between professional and individual. If the person is resistant to interventions, it is advisable to reassess motivation to change, re-identify the individual's priorities and base interventions on these problems instead.

Similarly, the individual's mental state will affect the type and intensity of intervention applied, especially considering the potentially rapid relapses brought about by stimulant use. Whether psychotic symptoms are substance induced or due to serious and enduring mental illness, the interventions will be mediated by the individual's mental state. The types of approaches used for psychosis are different from those used for non-psychotic situations. It is equally important to have a working knowledge of the type of psychological interventions used for mental health problems (*see* Table 4.2) as it is for substance use problems. Cognitive behavioural approaches are extremely useful in addressing mental health *and* substance use problems. There are two publications that may be useful to the reader considering this approach:

➤ *A Brief Cognitive Behavioural Intervention for Regular Amphetamine Users: a treatment guide*[8]
➤ *PsyCheck: clinical treatment guidelines.*[9]

The former adopts a cognitive behavioural approach to addressing an individual's amphetamine use, and the latter is designed to address common mental health problems in individuals who are accessing substance use services. Both are clinically focused and offer practical step-by-step guidance, in addition to a range of tools that can be used during the intervention.

Case study 4.2: Sophie

Sophie (19) was admitted to an inpatient unit due to several factors but primarily for self-harming. She had a long history of contact with services starting from the age of 11 when she was the subject of an investigation by the Children and Families Department of Social Services. The referral had been made by her school following a period of disruptive behaviour during which she disclosed to one of her teachers that she was being given amphetamines and sexually abused by a group of older boys. However, the investigation was unsuccessful as Sophie refused to name the offenders. Sophie continued her association with these boys and was subject to further abuse. Whether Sophie willingly associated with her abusers or was coerced was unclear.

Aged 16, Sophie's behaviour became extremely disruptive and she left home, partly because her parents could no longer cope with her drug taking and disruptive behaviour. Sophie briefly engaged with substance use services but soon drifted away. She was admitted to an inpatient unit aged 17 following an attempted suicide by hanging, in her flat. This attempt was uncompleted due to the unexpected arrival of a flatmate's friend. Sophie was then admitted to a specialist unit for deliberate self-harm but absconded after two weeks.

Sophie re-engaged with substance use services; however, this was for a short period only. Aged 18, Sophie was admitted to a mental health inpatient ward following a serious overdose and admission to an intensive care unit for five days.

On this occasion, Sophie engaged well with a psychology assistant and appeared to be making good progress until the assistant left. Sophie then absconded and was found in a local graveyard by a passer-by with deep lacerations to her wrists. She was returned to the ward following admission to the local general hospital and placed on a detention order under the UK Mental Health Act.[10] Sophie has been on the ward for three months but has absconded twice, returning of her own accord after three days on both occasions.

SELF-ASSESSMENT EXERCISE 4.1

Time: 10 minutes
What problems have you identified?

Presenting problems
Substance use behaviour
When not in hospital, Sophie is a regular user of amphetamines, MDMA, cocaine and cannabis. She binges on alcohol and uses 'speed' for several days before crashing. Sophie will often use benzodiazepines to help her with the 'come down'. Due to her excessive amphetamine use, Sophie is extremely malnourished.

SELF-ASSESSMENT EXERCISE 4.2

Time: 15 minutes
- What would be your plan of care?
- What issue of safety needs to be addressed?

CARE PLAN
➤ Establish a therapeutic alliance.
➤ Full assessment (*see* Book 4, Chapters 8 and 9) of current substance use – obtain a full substance use history.
➤ Undertake a thorough physical health assessment.
➤ Assess bone density – amphetamine use adversely affects calcium levels.
➤ Monitor body mass index (BMI) and encourage appropriate nutrition – refer to dietician.
➤ Complete comprehensive risk assessment.
➤ Assessment of motivation to change – for each substance.
➤ Assess locus of control (external or internal).
➤ Initiate and build a therapeutic relationship, adopting a recovery-focused approach and based on interventions using motivational interviewing techniques and cognitive restructuring.
➤ Provide brief intervention for substance use based on readiness to change.

➤ Negotiate a substance use 'contract' while an inpatient, particularly during periods of leave from ward – avoid punitive approaches to regulate substance use, i.e. withdrawal of leave following use of a substance. Controlling approaches are likely to be perceived as punishment, which will impact on the therapeutic relationship and may result in an increase of other harmful behaviours (e.g. self-harm) as a means of regaining personal control.

Deliberate self-harm

Sophie has made at least two very serious attempts at suicide and has self-harmed by cutting her arms and legs on numerous occasions. Her most recent suicide attempt was by overdose.

SELF-ASSESSMENT EXERCISE 4.3

Time: 15 minutes
With reference to Sophie's self-harm, how would your care plan evolve?

CARE PLAN
➤ Complete full assessment of self-harming behaviour and obtain full history.
➤ Complete a thorough risk assessment – collate with substance use risk assessment.
➤ Assessment of motivation to change self-harming behaviour.
➤ Ensure that Sophie is safe at all times and offer regular therapeutic contact with staff to monitor mood and develop trust.
➤ Develop a therapeutic alliance in order to improve relational security.
➤ Establish contingencies and advanced directives of care should self-harm become likely – this should include ensuring the environment is as safe as reasonably possible.
➤ Understand substance and self-harm high-risk situations.
➤ Explore triggers and situations that lead to substance use and self-harm.
➤ Identify high-risk situations (triggers) that may lead to self-harm and facilitate the development of strategies for managing stress/distress that leads to self-harming behaviour.
➤ Adopt harm reduction approaches to self-harm to ensure that if Sophie does cut herself then she does this as safely as possible to reduce the risk of long-term physical damage, e.g. tendon/nerve damage.
➤ Consider possibility of dialectical behaviour therapy (DBT) referral (*see* Chapter 13; Book 4, Chapter 11).

Note: Refer to relevant guidance for best practice on assessment and treatment of self-harm.[11–13]

Mental health

Sophie is depressed in mood and has been observed to be socially isolating herself. In addition, she experiences some auditory hallucinations of the third person command type, which tell her she is worthless and instructs self-harm. Sophie's personal hygiene is poor and she requires prompting to attend to her self-care.

SELF-ASSESSMENT EXERCISE 4.4

> **Time: 15 minutes**
> How would you develop your care plan now you have identified depression?

CARE PLAN

➤ Full assessment of existing mental health problems and symptoms – obtain full mental health history.
➤ Monitor mental state using the Brief Psychiatric Rating Scale (BPRS) weekly.[14]
➤ Complete a thorough risk assessment – collate with substance use and self-harm risk assessment.
➤ Assess motivation to change presenting mental health problem(s).
➤ Encourage Sophie to spend time in social contact and provide structure to her day – set small achievable goals/tasks.
➤ Provide psychoeducation on presenting mental health problems.
➤ Explore link between substance use and mental health.
➤ Explore psychotic phenomenon and consider cognitive behavioural therapy for psychosis.
➤ Develop strategies to manage voices, e.g. distraction and relaxation techniques – incorporate with stress management strategies adopted for self-harm behaviour.
➤ Encourage medication and monitor compliance. Initiate medication management approaches to aid compliance.

Intrusive recollections of previous traumatic events/flashbacks

Sophie describes occasions where she believes herself to be back in a room, aged 11, with her abusers. This often occurs when ward staff do their observations at night and when she is approached by men of a similar age and appearance as her abusers.

SELF-ASSESSMENT EXERCISE 4.5

> **Time: 10 minutes**
> • What would you look for?
> • How would you plan interventions to deal with Sophie's flashbacks?

CARE PLAN

➤ Assess for post-traumatic stress disorder (via trauma screening questionnaire –TSQ,[15] PTSD Checklist[16] and/or Clinician Administered Post-Traumatic Stress Disorder Scale – CAPS[17] – *see* Chapter 9).
➤ Female staff preferred.
➤ Explore and identify triggers.

➤ Reduce exposure to triggers based on risk and develop coping strategies.
➤ Liaise with psychology to identify appropriate PTSD interventions and consider referral.

Family and support networks

Sophie's family are hostile towards her and resentful of the problems that she has caused in the past. They report being happier when she had no contact with them. Sophie says she is keen to re-engage with her family and feels guilty about her past behaviour towards them.

SELF-ASSESSMENT EXERCISE 4.6

> **Time: 20 minutes**
> - What would be your aim with the family?
> - How might you achieve this?

CARE PLAN

➤ Explore possibility of family therapy.
➤ Obtain a thorough assessment of the family's needs.
➤ Support the family.
➤ Discuss level of contact Sophie would like with family.
➤ Reflect this back to Sophie.
➤ Reflect this back to the family.
➤ Collate Sophie's mental state with family involvement.
➤ Offer psychoeducation for family.

With Sophie, the initial overriding element of care is to maintain safety. This is achieved by thorough risk assessment regardless of hospital or community setting, i.e. environment does not affect risk, although the setting will provide more or fewer protective factors. In addition, it is important to set contingency plans for home treatment or hospitalisation.

When planning interventions, care should be taken not to compartmentalise the presenting problems. The plan above divides the main areas but takes into account the need to collate each area with the others – they are interrelated. Identifying problems should be undertaken using a person-centred approach.

Above all, consistency and ongoing circulatory re-evaluation of the plans based on new presentations, progress or setbacks is vital. Gauging the level of intervention will help to build a therapeutic relationship; therefore, ensuring interventions are more effective. Awareness of treatment efficacy will lead to further compliance and alliance.

CONCLUSION

The professional should maintain a therapeutic relationship to effectively provide care for the individual and family. This is especially true in the often chaotic world of the individual experiencing mental health–substance use problems. The nature of stimulants creates further difficulties due to their adverse effect on mental health and social functioning, especially with stimulants such as crack cocaine and crystal meth.

Demonstrating an expertise of mental health–stimulant use problems helps engage the individual, although engagement can be a long and difficult process with frequent therapeutic ruptures and disengagement. A consistent approach will help to overcome these problems. However, supervision and support will be essential for the professional. Group and one-to-one supervision and reflective practice allows professionals to mutually support one another, share good practice and become more emotionally and therapeutically available to the individual.

REFERENCES

1 Home Office Statistics Unit. *Drug Misuse Use Declared: findings from the 2009/2010 British Crime Survey, England and Wales.* Home Office Statistical Bulletin. Home Office; 2010. Available at: http://rds.homeoffice.gov.uk/rds/pdfs10/hosb1310.pdf (accessed 23 November 2010).

2 The Alcohol Education and Research Council (AERC). *Cocaethylene: responding to combined alcohol and cocaine use.* AERC alcohol academy briefing paper 004. London: The Alcohol Education and Research Council; 2010. Available at: www.aerc.org.uk/documents/pdfs/Cocaethylene_AERC_Academy.pdf (accessed 23 November 2010).

3 Advisory Council on the Misuse of Drugs. *Consideration of Cathinones.* London: Advisory Council on the Misuse of Drugs; 2010. Available at: www.homeoffice.gov.uk/publications/drugs/acmd1/acmd-cathinodes-report-2010?view=Binary (accessed 23 November 2010).

4 Advisory Council on the Misuse of Drugs. *Consideration of the Naphthylpyrovalerone Analogues and Related Compounds.* London: Advisory Council on the Misuse of Drugs; 2010. Available at: www.homeoffice.gov.uk/publications/drugs/acmd1/naphyrone-report?view=Binary (accessed 23 November 2010).

5 Gunn K, Rickwood DJ. The effect of amphetamine type stimulants on psychopathology, aggression and cognitive function among clients within a drug and alcohol therapeutic community. *Mental Health and Substance Use: dual diagnosis.* 2009; **2**: 120–9.

6 Rassool G. Substance use and mental health: an overview. *Nursing Standard.* 2002; **16**: 46–52.

7 Heraghty M, Anipa F, Byrant A, *et al.* The Friday Group: engaging and empowering service users with a dual diagnosis. *Health and Alcohol Misuse Project Newsletter.* Winter 2005; **9**. London: Alcohol Concern, 2005.

8 Baker A, Kay-Lambkin F, Lee NK, *et al. A Brief Cognitive Behavioural Intervention for Regular Amphetamine Users: a treatment guide.* Australian Government Department of Health and Ageing, 2003. Available at: www.health.gov.au/internet/main/publishing.nsf/Content/7BCC605BECD47DE1CA256F190003FEEE/$File/cognitive-intervention.pdf (accessed 23 November 2010).

9 Lee N, Jenner L, Kay-Lambkin F, *et al. PsyCheck: responding to mental health issues within alcohol and drug treatment. Clinical treatment guidelines.* Commonwealth of Australia; 2007. Available at: www.psycheck.org.au/download.html (accessed 23 November 2010).

10 *Code of Practice: Mental Health Act 1983.* Department of Health; 2008. Available at: www.dh.gov.uk/en/Publicationsandstatistics/Publications/PublicationsPolicyAndGuidance/DH_084597 (accessed 23 November 2010).

11 National Institute for Clinical Excellence (NICE). *Self-harm: the short-term physical and*

psychological management and secondary prevention of self-harm in primary and second-ary care. NICE, 2004. Available at: www.nice.org.uk/CG16 (accessed 23 November 2010).

12 Royal College of Psychiatrists. *Assessment Following Self-harm in Adults*; 2004. Available at: www.rcpsych.ac.uk/files/pdfversion/cr122.pdf (accessed 23 November 2010).

13 World Health Organization. *WHO Guide to Mental and Neurological Health in Primary Care.* Available at: www.mentalneurologicalprimarycare.org/content_show.asp?c=16&fid=1210&fc=011035 (accessed 23 November 2010).

14 *Brief Psychiatric Rating Scale.* Available at: www.public-health.uiowa.edu/icmha/outreach/documents/BPRS_expanded.PDF (accessed 23 November 2010).

15 Dekkers AMM, Olff M, Näring GWB. Identifying persons for PTSD after trauma with TSG in the Netherlands. *Community Mental Health Journal.* 2010; **46**: 20–5.

16 Foa EB, Cashmon L, Joycox L, *et al.* The validation of self-report measure of posttraumatic stress disorder: the posttraumatic diagnostic scale. *Psychological Assessment.* 1997; **9**: 445–51.

17 *Clinician Administered Post-Traumatic Stress Disorder Scale.* Available at: http://search-pdf-books.com/clinicianadministered-ptsd-scale-instruction-manual-pdf/ (accessed 23 November 2010).

TO LEARN MORE

• Advisory Council on the Misuse of Drugs. *Consideration of Cathinones.* Advisory Council on the Misuse of Drugs; 2010. Available at: www.homeoffice.gov.uk/publications/drugs/acmd1/acmd-cathinodes-report-2010?view=Binary

• Advisory Council on the Misuse of Drugs. *Consideration of the Naphthylpyrovalerone Analogues and Related Compounds.* Advisory Council on the Misuse of Drugs; 2010. Available at: www.homeoffice.gov.uk/publications/drugs/acmd1/naphyrone-report?view=Binary

• Baker A, Kay-Lambkin F, Lee NK, *et al. A Brief Cognitive Behavioural Intervention for Regular Amphetamine Users: a treatment guide.* Australian Government Department of Health and Ageing; 2003. Available at: www.health.gov.au/internet/main/publishing.nsf/Content/7BCC605BECD47DE1CA256F190003FEEE/$File/cognitive-intervention.pdf

• Banerjee S, Clancy C, Crome I. *Co-existing Problems of Mental Disorder and Substance Misuse (Dual Diagnosis): an information manual.* London: The Royal College of Psychiatrists Research Unit; 2002.

• Beck AT, Wright FD, Newman CF, *et al. Cognitive Therapy of Substance Abuse.* New York: Guilford Press; 1993.

• Edwards G, Dare C. *Psychotherapy, Psychological Treatments and the Addictions.* Cambridge: Cambridge University Press; 1996.

• Independent Scientific Committee on Drugs. Available at: www.drugscience.org.uk/

• Kuhn C, Swartzwelder S, Wilson W. *Buzzed: the straight facts about the most used and abused drugs from alcohol to ecstasy.* New York: WW Norton & Company; 2008.

• Lee N, Jenner L, Kay-Lambkin F, *et al. PsyCheck: responding to mental health issues within alcohol and drug treatment. Clinical treatment guidelines.* Commonwealth of Australia; 2007. Available at: www.psycheck.org.au/download.html

• Rasmussen N. *On Speed: the many lives of amphetamine.* New York: University Press; 2008.

• The Alcohol Education and Research Council (AERC). *Cocaethylene: responding to combined alcohol and cocaine use.* AERC alcohol academy briefing paper 004. London: The Alcohol Education and Research Council; 2010. Available at: www.aerc.org.uk/documents/pdfs/Cocaethylene_AERC_Academy.pdf

- Turning Point. *The Crack Report*, 2006. Available at: www.turning-point.co.uk/inthenews/Pages/TheCrackReport.aspx
- Vaults of Erowid. Available at: www.erowid.org

CHAPTER 5

Prescription drugs and mental health

Suzanne Nielsen and Nicole Lee

INTRODUCTION

There has been a substantial increase in the use of pharmaceuticals around the world, including benzodiazepines and opioid-based pain relievers. Global consumption of opioid-based pain relievers, for example, has increased by more than two and one half times over the past decade.[1]

While most pharmaceuticals are used therapeutically, some of these drugs are incorrectly used or misused, either by not being taken as directed or by being diverted to someone other than the person they were prescribed for.[1] Around 6% of the US population and 4% of the Australian population report non-medical use of a pharmaceutical in the past year.[2-4] With an increase in prescription drug misuse, there has also been an increase in reported harms.

Among those misusing prescription drugs, mental health disorders are frequently reported.[5-7] Prescription drugs are also frequently used and misused among people who are dependent on alcohol and other drugs, a population with high rates of mental health problems.[8,9]

There is a complex relationship between pharmaceutical drugs and mental health problems that present obstacles to effective treatment. For example, benzodiazepines are often prescribed for anxiety disorders, but dependence and tolerance is common and withdrawal is often characterised by symptoms of anxiety. For the individual, these withdrawal symptoms, or the lowered effectiveness of the medication because of tolerance are often interpreted as a return of the pre-existing anxiety. In this situation, it can be difficult to convince the person that it is important to withdraw from the medication and manage anxiety with non-drug measures, as a higher dose appears to resolve all symptoms.

Similarly, benzodiazepines are commonly prescribed for insomnia, but generally lose their sleep-promoting effects after two to four weeks of continuous use. However, after this time, dependence can occur and on cessation of the medication and withdrawal, insomnia may worsen, making the person less likely to continue reducing their benzodiazepine use if this worsens their sleep difficulties.

The early introduction of non-drug interventions (such as cognitive behavioural therapy for anxiety, depression or sleep problems) instead of, or as well as, pharmaceuticals may prevent or ameliorate misuse of these drugs.

TREATMENT FOR PHARMACEUTICAL DEPENDENCE

Treatment for uncomplicated benzodiazepine dependence generally consists of a period of stabilisation and then gradual reduction of benzodiazepine dose.[10,11] People are often transferred to a longer acting benzodiazepine, such as diazepam. Dose reduction can take weeks to months depending on the severity of dependence.

Although there have been few studies specifically evaluating treatments among people using prescription opioids, both methadone and buprenorphine are established as effective for treatment of opioid dependence.[12] A buprenorphinc-naloxone combination has been used for the treatment of pharmaceutical opioid dependence in the United States, with results suggesting people who use prescription opioids may have better outcomes compared to people who use illicit opioids.[13]

WORKING ALONGSIDE PEOPLE USING BENZODIAZEPINES

➤ Benzodiazepine withdrawal is a very protracted process; the individual will often need months to years of support. The end of the reduction is often the most difficult.

➤ When managing benzodiazepine dependence, before initiating prescribing it is best to develop a treatment agreement that includes only receiving benzodiazepines from one doctor and pharmacy. In some cases daily pick up of medication at a pharmacy may assist in management of medication.

➤ Strategies need to be in place to manage re-emerging mental health symptoms when medication is reduced.

➤ Benzodiazepines affect ability to learn new information. Individuals should be advised not to take benzodiazepines prior to appointments so they are able to benefit from work done, and from new skills being taught in sessions (an example is seen in Case Study 5.1).

STRATEGIES TO MANAGE MEDICATION OVERUSE

➤ If prescriptions are being collected/requested early, or reported as lost or stolen, this may indicate difficulties in managing medication. Dispensing of smaller quantities more regularly from the pharmacy may assist.

➤ The individual should be assessed to ensure reasons for aberrant drug-related behaviours are not related to under-treatment of conditions. Stockpiling medication or escalating doses can be a rational response to under-treated pain or anxiety.

SCREENING FOR PEOPLE AT RISK OF DEPENDENCE, NON-ADHERENCE OR ABERRANT DRUG-RELATED BEHAVIOURS

➤ An approach of universal precautions is recommended when drugs of dependence are prescribed. Universal precautions means applying a minimum level of precaution to all individuals when prescribing drugs of dependence, rather than relying on stereotypes to inform where extra precautions should be in place.[14]

➤ Some of the approaches that should be applied include:
  - asking about past and present use of illicit substances, alcohol and pharmaceutical drugs
  - discussing the risk of dependence and benefits of drug treatment with the person at the outset of treatment and gain informed consent
  - asking about adherence to medication
  - using objective outcome measures such as urine drug screening to monitor adherence and detect additional drug use; this may indicate treatment is not working
  - undertaking psychological assessments and regular assessment in both efficacy of treatment as well as adverse effects and aberrant drug-related behaviours.
➤ At treatment outset any medication should be considered as a trial, and if objective measures of improvement are not met, discontinuation or change in medication should be considered.

CASE STUDIES

The case studies are examples where people may present with mental health symptoms and issues relating to prescription drug use or dependence. In some cases, prescription drug use may contribute to, or disguise, the worsening of mental health symptoms (e.g. Case Study 5.1: Mary). Alternatively, medications may be taken to relieve mental health symptoms (e.g. Case Study 5. 2: Brian); though if this is inappropriate use, further problems can develop.

Case study 5.1: Mary

Background: Alprazolam, a benzodiazepine, is commonly prescribed for anxiety disorders. Best practice indicates it is for short-term use (two to four weeks) and tolerance can develop after only a few weeks of treatment.[10] It has significant impact on cognitive functioning[15] and as a result can interfere with the ability to learn new material.[16]

Introduction: Mary (30), single, is a childcare worker. Mary began having panic attacks leading up to exam time when she was studying for her certificate five years ago, which prevented her from studying. She reported failing one subject which provided impetus to seek assistance from her general practitioner (GP). Mary reported no known family history of anxiety disorders but describes herself as a nervous and shy child and adolescent.

Initial symptoms: Initially panic attacks were mild to moderate and associated with periods of increased stress. Symptoms included chest tightness and pain, hyperventilation, and fear of fainting.

Initial treatment: Mary was prescribed alprazolam by her GP, at a dose of 0.25–0.5 mg as required, which provided relief from her symptoms. Mary began to fear the onset of panic attacks and began increasing her dose of alprazolam in anticipation of anxiety symptoms and eventually increasing her dose to more than double that prescribed.

Current presentation: Mary presented with moderate benzodiazepine dependence and mild anxiety symptoms with no panic attacks. She reported that she had not had a panic attack for two months – but reported a fear of them returning. Mary's job at the childcare centre had become stressful and routine events, such as a particular child misbehaving, prompted her to increase her lunchtime dose. Mary reported difficulty sleeping and had also increased her evening dose.

Formulation: Rebound symptoms, dependence on medication, significant anxiety cognitions leading to a fear of being anxious and self-medicating in anticipation.

Treatment: Mary began an outpatient withdrawal programme with her GP and a psychologist. She was initially attending her psychology sessions after self-medicating and little progress was made, probably due to the cognitive effects of alprazolam, leading to a limitation of her ability to take on anxiety management information. Eventually, Mary agreed to cut out her daytime dose and anxiety management strategies were more successful. Withdrawal and anxiety management was undertaken over a 12-month period until Mary was no longer using alprazolam. Anxiety management continued for six months post withdrawal.

This case study highlights the risk of benzodiazepine dependence and dose escalation where anxiety disorders exist and non-drug measures are not in place to manage pre-existing anxiety symptoms. Benzodiazepines may be useful at the outset of treatment but are best used to enable the person to cope in the short term, while they are learning to manage their anxiety disorder with non-drug strategies. The risk of dependence and rebound anxiety with benzodiazepines should also be considered. In this case, when Mary returned to the GP requesting further prescriptions, questioning about medication adherence may have helped detect that things had deteriorated for her.

SELF-ASSESSMENT EXERCISE 5.1

> **Time: 5 minutes**
> What questions would you want to ask Mary?

Examples of questions that might be helpful are:
➤ What dose are you taking and how often?
➤ Have you ever needed to take a dose greater than the dose prescribed?
➤ Have you used the medication for a condition other than what it was prescribed for?
➤ Is the medication working as well as it initially did?

Objective information such as dates the medication was dispensed and whether repeat scripts were dispensed early also might indicate a problem. In some cases, it may be useful to ask the individual to keep a diary of when they use their medication and what symptoms it is being used for, particularly as benzodiazepines may impair memory and reduce the ability to recall this information accurately.

Case study 5.2: Brian

Background: Codeine, an opioid, is available in some countries (in combination with paracetamol, ibuprofen or aspirin) without a prescription for pain relief. These medications are indicated for short-term use. However, in some cases people become dependent on codeine and escalate their dose.[17] Cases of severe harms have been reported with these products.[18,19]

Introduction: Brian (37), recently divorced, is a shift worker. Brian's father was alcohol dependent, and his mother died when he was 11. Three years ago, Brian injured his back at work. Brian spent several months off work on workplace insurance. After this, Brian returned to 'light duties' at work. When Brian returned to work, he found his workplace stressful with some people he worked with accusing him of pretending to be injured. Brian begun to feel increasingly stressed about work and began spending more time at home alone.

Initial symptoms: Brian strained his back lifting some boxes. The pain worsened over several weeks. Initially, Brian was managing his pain with over-the-counter pain relievers but as the pain did not improve, he saw his GP.

Initial treatment: The GP prescribed a paracetamol-codeine prescription product for the pain initially, and diazepam as a muscle relaxant for the first week. Brian was also referred to a physiotherapist.

Current presentation: Brian continued to see his GP for several weeks. However, the GP suggested that he should stop the prescription pain relievers after 10 days. Brian found when he ceased the medication his pain worsened. He also found he was experiencing feelings of boredom and low mood and felt socially isolated. Brian started taking over-the-counter pain relievers after his GP had discontinued his prescribed pain relief. Brian found that these helped his pain, and that his mood improved. Over the next six months, Brian increased the dose he took to 24 tablets daily, and found that when he tried to cease taking the pain relievers he experienced muscle pain, agitation and diarrhoea. Brian reported he no longer enjoyed the company of the people he worked with and lost interest in participating in work social activities or his other hobbies.

Formulation: Codeine dependence and depression-like symptoms. Self-medication with codeine for dependence and mood.

Treatment: The pharmacist noticed Brian was purchasing increasing amounts of codeine and referred him back to his GP. Brian was assessed to be opioid dependent. He commenced on buprenorphine-naloxone and was referred back to the physiotherapist. Brian started attending a cognitive behavioural therapy-based recovery group where he learnt coping skills and eventually assisted in facilitating the group. Brian relapsed to codeine use after two months of treatment. He was re-established on a higher dose of buprenorphine-naloxone. After this Brian was able to abstain for codeine use and after 12 months of abstinence began to reduce his opioid maintenance treatment.

This case highlights the importance of a universal precautions approach with opioid-based pain medication. For Brian, a universal precautions approach may have resulted in the identification of some risk factors (family history of substance dependence and other psychosocial risks). This would have enabled a discussion with the prescriber about risks of prescribing opioids and safeguards could have been put in place to enable prevention or earlier detection of problematic use. If Brian was aware of the risks he may have returned to the doctor sooner rather than continuing to use non-prescription pain medication.

Case study 5.3: Joe

Background: Schizophrenia is present in just under 1% of the population.[20] Atypical antipsychotics are first line for treatment of schizophrenia. However, some case reports have been published recording misuse of atypical antipsychotic medication.[21,22]

Introduction: Joe (33) lives in a rooming house. Joe was diagnosed with paranoid schizophrenia at the age of 19. He comes from a culturally and linguistically diverse background and has few social supports (*see* Book 4, Chapters 4 and 5; Book 5, Chapter 5). Joe is currently prescribed quetiapine 400 mg daily for schizophrenia, which he collects monthly from his local pharmacy.

Initial symptoms: After a period of several years of stability, Joe was observed in the waiting room looking sedated and subsequently reported using clonazepam. He also reported that the voices in his head had recently increased. Joe's pharmacy has reported that he has been collecting his prescriptions early, and that he reported that he had lost his last supply of medication.

Initial treatment: Joe was initially prescribed quetiapine when he was transferred to a mental health service three years ago. At the time of the initial referral, the psychiatrist reviewed his medication as Joe was experiencing side-effects from chlorpromazine. At that time, the psychiatrist transferred him from an older antipsychotic to quetiapine to reduce the side-effects. Since being stabilised on quetiapine, he has had minimal psychotic symptoms and no reported extrapyramidal side-effects.

Current presentation: Joe has previously reported that he is lonely and has few friends. Recently, he has been spending time with another inpatient. Clinic staff noted another individual has been attending when Joe collected his prescriptions. When the issue of medication compliance was raised, Joe reports that he has been pressured to give his medications away.

Formulation: Re-emergence of psychotic symptoms because of non-adherence to medication; self-medication of psychotic symptoms with non-prescribed clonazepam.

Treatment: Introduction of daily dispensing of quetiapine with morning tablet supervised. Joe was linked in with a recreational day programme to increase social contact. Joe was assisted to learn refusal skills and over a six-month period takes increasing responsibility for his quetiapine and unsupervised dosing with ongoing monitoring for adherence and re-emergence of psychotic symptoms. Treatment agreement was made around seeking illicit benzodiazepines. Urine drug screening continues to be positive only for prescribed medications.

This case highlights the importance of monitoring for adherence with medications. While less commonly reported than non-medical use of drugs like opioids and benzodiazepines, misuse of antipsychotic medications has been documented. This non-medical use has been linked to the calming or anxiolytic effects of these medications.

Case study 5.4: Peter

Background: A large number of people who use illicit drugs use pharmaceuticals to either enhance the drug taking experience, or assist with withdrawal or side-effects. The practice is common among people using psychostimulants[23] but can result in dependence or an exacerbation or emergence of mental health symptoms.

Introduction: Peter (23) is a student. Peter uses ecstasy (3,4-Methylenedioxymethamphetamine – MDMA) at weekends once or twice a month (usually two pills per occasion) and 'speed' (methamphetamine) two or three times a week to stay awake to study or work (up to a gram a week). Peter has been using a friend's prescribed benzodiazepines to help him sleep.

Initial symptoms and current presentation: Peter has presented to his GP to assist with anxiety symptoms that he has developed in the last month. He reported symptoms such as sweaty palms, racing heart and 'butterflies' in his stomach which he reported were relieved by the benzodiazepines he was using but appear to be increasing. Peter did not initially report use of psychostimulants.

Initial treatment: Benzodiazepines were initially prescribed. However, after a further two weeks, it appeared that Peter's symptoms were not improving.

Current presentation: As part of ongoing benzodiazepine prescribing, Peter had agreed to routine urine drug screening. When Peter returned, a urine drug screening was positive for methamphetamine. The GP discussed this with Peter. The GP examined the onset of Peter's symptoms and the role of stimulant use in his symptoms, finding that his anxiety appeared to be linked to both his illicit substance use, and cessation of non-prescribed use of benzodiazepines. Benzodiazepines provided some initial reduction in symptoms but currently were giving decreasing relief from anxiety.

Formulation: Anxiety symptoms linked to stimulant use; tolerance to benzodiazepines resulting in reduced efficacy, and withdrawal symptoms on cessation.

Treatment: Peter was referred to a clinical psychologist that specialises in the treatment of methamphetamine users. In the first session, Peter agreed to stop using ecstasy and to reduce his stimulant use to half his regular dose with a view to reduce further. A review of lifestyle factors that led to increasing stimulant use was also addressed. Further sessions involved cognitive behavioural therapy to manage anxiety symptoms and prevent relapse to stimulant use.

This case highlights the importance of screening for current substance use and validating with objective measures such as urine drug screen. In the absence of urine drug screening it may be helpful to ask about a typical week as part of the clinical assessment to check any drug use and its potential contribution, especially when symptoms have a relatively sudden onset without a history of anxiety problems. In addition, prescribing benzodiazepines on a trial basis with regular monitoring should be considered, and where improvement is not seen or maintained, other treatment options should be undertaken. Where the individual is currently not willing to cease their substance use, harm reduction approaches should be considered, such as encouraging reductions in use or changes in patterns of use, and suggesting non-pharmacological ways to manage mental health symptoms. Care should be taken prescribing medications such as antidepressants due to the risks of interaction resulting in potentially fatal side-effects such as serotonin syndrome.[24]

CONCLUSION

Psychoactive medications have an important role to play in the treatment of many mental health conditions. While these medications are important, their use should be monitored, particularly when there are signs of overuse and where there is a known dependence liability. All prescribed drugs with a dependence liability, particularly opioids and benzodiazepines, should be provided with a universal precautions framework. Risks should be assessed prior to commencing medication. The individual and family should be made aware of the risks of these medications prior to consenting to treatment. Extra precautions may be warranted where additional risk factors are identified. Regular communication between the treatment team may assist in early detection of problematic use.

REFERENCES

1 International Narcotics Control Board (INCB). *Report of the International Narcotics Control Board for 2008*. New York: United Nations; 2008.

2 Australian Institute of Health and Welfare (AIHW). *2007 National Drug Strategy Household Survey: detailed findings*. Drug Statistics Series no. 22. Cat. no. PHE 107. Canberra: AIHW; 2008.

3 Manchikanti L. National drug control policy and prescription drug abuse: facts and fallacies. *Pain Physician*. 2007; **10**: 399–424.

4 Substance Abuse and Mental Health Services. *Results from the 2006 National Survey on Drug Use and Health: national findings*. (Office of Applied Studies, NSDUH Series H-32, DHHS Publication no. SMA 07-4293). Rockville, MD; 2007.

5 Martins SS, Storr CL, Zhu H, *et al*. Correlates of extramedical use of OxyContin® versus other analgesic opioids among the US general population. *Drug and Alcohol Dependence*. 2009; **99**: 58–67.

6 Michna E, Ross EL, Hynes WL, *et al*. Predicting aberrant drug behavior in patients treated for chronic pain: importance of abuse history. *Journal of Pain and Symptom Management*. 2004; **28**: 250–8.

7 Sullivan MD, Edlund MJ, Zhang L, *et al*. Association between mental health disorders, problem drug use, and regular prescription opioid use. *Archives of Internal Medicine*. 2006; **166**: 2087–93.

8 Marsden J, Gossop M, Stewart D, *et al*. Psychiatric symptoms among clients seeking treatment for drug dependence. Intake data from the National Treatment Outcome Research Study. *The British Journal of Psychiatry*. 2000; **176**: 285–9.

9 Ross J, Teesson M, Darke S, *et al*. The characteristics of heroin users entering treatment: findings from the Australian treatment outcome study (ATOS). *Drug and Alcohol Review*. 2005; **24**: 411–18.

10 Denis C, Auriacombe M, Fatsas M, *et al*. Pharmacological interventions for benzodiazepine mono-dependence management in outpatient settings. *Cochrane Database of Systematic Reviews*. 2006; **3**: CD005194.

11 Oude Voshaar RC, Couvee JE, Van Balkom AJLM, *et al*. Strategies for discontinuing long-term benzodiazepine use: meta-analysis. *British Journal of Psychiatry*. 2006; **189**: 213–20.

12 Mattick RP, Kimber J, Breen C, *et al*. Buprenorphine maintenance versus placebo or methadone maintenance for opioid dependence. *Cochrane Database of Systematic Reviews*. 2004; **3**: CD002207.

13 Moore BA, Fiellin DA, Barry DT, *et al*. Primary care office-based buprenorphine treatment: comparison of heroin and prescription opioid dependent patients. *Journal of General Internal Medicine*. 2007; **22**: 527–30.

14 Gourney DL, Heit HA, Almahrezi A. Universal precautions in pain medicine: a rational approach to the treatment of chronic pain. *Pain Medicine*. 2005; **6**: 107–12.

15 Barker MJ, Greenwood KM, Crowe SF. Cognitive effects of long-term benzodiazepine use: a meta-analysis. *CNS Drugs.* 2004; **18**: 37–48.

16 Curran HV. Tranquillising memories: a review of the effects of benzodiazepines on human memory. *Biological Psychology.* 1986; **23**: 179–213.

17 Sproule BAP, Busto UEP, Somer GM, *et al.* Characteristics of dependent and nondependent regular users of codeine. *Journal of Clinical Psychopharmacology.* 1999; **19**: 367–72.

18 Chetty R, Baoku Y, Mildner R, *et al.* Severe hypokalaemia and weakness due to Nurofen* misuse. *Annals of Clinical Biochemistry.* 2003; **40**: 422–3.

19 Dutch MJ. Nurofen Plus misuse: an emerging cause of perforated gastric ulcer. *Medical Journal of Australia.* 2008; **188**: 56–7.

20 McGrath J, Saha S, Chant D, *et al.* Schizophrenia: a concise overview of incidence, prevalence, and mortality. *Epidemiologic Reviews.* 2008; **30**: 67–76.

21 Christensen RC, Garces LK. The growing abuse of commonly prescribed psychiatric medications. *The American Journal of Emergency Medicine.* 2006; **24**: 137–8.

22 Pierre JM, Shnayder I, Wirshing DA, *et al.* Intranasal quetiapine abuse. *American Journal of Psychiatry.* 2004; **161**: 1718.

23 Black E, Dunn M, Degenhardt L, *et al. Australian Trends in Ecstasy and Related Drug markets.* Australian Drug Trends Series no. 10. Sydney: National Drug and Alcohol Research Centre; 2007.

24 Silins E, Copeland J, Dillon P. Qualitative review of serotonin syndrome, ecstasy (MDMA) and the use of other serotonergic substances: hierarchy of risk. *Australian and New Zealand Journal of Psychiatry.* 2007; **41**: 649–55.

TO LEARN MORE

- Gourlay DL, Heit HA, Almahrezi A. Universal precautions in pain medicine: a rational approach to the treatment of chronic pain. *Pain Medicine.* 2005; **6**: 107–12.
- Smith HS, Passik S. *Pain and Chemical Dependency.* New York: Oxford University Press; 2008.

CHAPTER 6

Tobacco and mental health

David Jones

PRE-READING EXERCISE 6.1 (ANSWERS ON P. 79)

1 Why do people who have mental health problems smoke more heavily than the rest of the population?
2 Which pharmacotherapies are available to help people quit smoking?

INTRODUCTION

Smoking is the largest cause of preventable illness and premature death in the United Kingdom. In 2002, 106 000 people died from smoking-related illnesses.[1] Twenty-two per cent of the adult population of the UK smokes, although 60% of them want to quit.[2] Encouraging as many people as possible to quit smoking has been the focus of many government initiatives in the UK since the 1998 publication of *Smoking Kills*, the government's tobacco control strategy.[3] One of those initiatives was the ban, introduced on 1 July 2007, on smoking in enclosed public places and the workplace, with a ban on smoking in adult mental health units following on 1 July 2008.[4]

People who have mental health problems tend to smoke two to three times more heavily than the general population and display a greater level of dependence,[5] although roughly half of them express a desire to quit.[6] People who have schizophrenia seem to find it more difficult to quit smoking,[7] as do people who are depressed.[8]

THE EFFECTS OF SMOKING

Mortensen and Juel[9] suggest that people who have schizophrenia have a life expectancy that is 20% lower than that of the general population, and that they experience higher rates of death from cardiovascular and respiratory disease. A study in Finland found that among people who had schizophrenia, the risk of death from respiratory disease was 10 times higher than among the general population, which the researchers attributed to smoking.[10]

Smoking also has a significant financial cost. People who have schizophrenia and smoke have been found to substantially contribute to the costs of their own care, due to them smoking more heavily, buying more cigarettes, paying more tax and being in receipt of state benefits.[11]

REASONS FOR SMOKING

BOX 6.1 Why people who have mental health problems smoke heavily

- Smoking may be a causative factor in the development of mental health problems.
- The self-medication hypothesis.
- Other factors that leave people vulnerable to both smoking and mental health problems.
- Smoking counters some of the unwanted effects of antipsychotic medication.
- The same reasons as other people – relaxation, habit, controlling nerves.
- The culture of mental health services is conducive to smoking.

There are several theories that have been put forward as to why people who have mental health problems smoke more heavily than the general population (*see* Box 6.1).

➤ Smoking may be an aetiological risk factor in the development of mental health problems.[12]

➤ Smokers may be medicating themselves – it may increase dopamine release in the pre-frontal cortex and alleviate positive and negative symptoms.[13]

➤ There may be other factors, environmental or genetic, that leave people vulnerable to both starting smoking and developing schizophrenia.[14]

➤ People who have schizophrenia may smoke more heavily to counter the sedative or dopamine-blocking actions of the antipsychotic medication that they are taking.[15]

However, qualitative research has found that people who have schizophrenia mainly cite the same reasons for smoking as the general population:

➤ relaxation
➤ habit
➤ settling nerves

. . . although smaller numbers of the people interviewed stated that their psychiatric symptoms also influenced their smoking.[16] It seems to be a common belief that smoking helps to reduce stress and anxiety,[17] although the evidence does suggest that smoking does not reduce stress[18] and that when people do quit smoking, their levels of anxiety and stress fall, not increase.[19]

Other factors that may contribute to elevated levels of smoking include boredom in psychiatric environments and the lack of other, meaningful distractions,[20] and that there is a strong culture of smoking within mental health services, with the smoking room being the hub of social activity.[21]

While it is no longer permitted to smoke within the buildings of UK mental health institutions, this culture is slow to change and, indeed, many psychiatric units appear to have ignored the ban on smoking.[22]

This can probably be explained by professional attitudes to smoking. A survey of psychiatric hospital staff[23] found that nurses were more likely to be smokers than other health professionals, and had a much more tolerant approach to smoking, regardless of whether or not they smoked themselves. They were more likely to state that smoking had a strong therapeutic value and that staff should be allowed to smoke along with the individual. These findings have significant implications for the therapeutic environment in regard to people using mental health services, and smokers are likely to find it difficult to quit in such a smoke-friendly environment. Indeed many individuals report that their smoking is not discussed with them by the health professionals, and that when they do express a desire to quit, support is not forthcoming.[24] In defence of health professionals, very few ever receive any training around smoking cessation interventions.

STOPPING SMOKING

If people try to stop smoking on their own, without any help from anyone else and without using any kind of pharmacological help, they are highly unlikely to succeed.[25] Brief interventions can be effective (especially when used in conjunction with medication), but for severely dependent people, or for people who have other complicating factors, such as mental health problems, more intensive interventions are likely to be required. The best chances of success are obtained by combining specialist, intensive support and one of the medications that are aimed at helping people quit.

WITHDRAWAL SYMPTOMS

Probably the most common reason why people fail to quit is that they struggle to deal with withdrawal symptoms (*see* Box 6.2).[26] However, most of these symptoms do not last longer than two to four weeks,[27] and can be alleviated by the use of nicotine replacement therapy (NRT).

BOX 6.2 Nicotine withdrawal syndrome

- Craving
- Headaches
- Indigestion
- Nausea
- Sore throats
- Insomnia and vivid dreams
- Constipation
- Coughing
- Irritability
- Depression
- Increased appetite and weight gain
- Tiredness and lack of concentration

THE THERAPEUTIC RELATIONSHIP

The attitude that the professional displays towards the individual is a key ingredient in any relationship (*see* Book 4, Chapter 2). An empathic, non-judgemental approach is vital. A major threat to effective working is the temptation for professionals to impose their own beliefs about the rights, wrongs, benefits and costs of smoking on the individual.[28]

ASSESSMENT

Mental health professionals should always ask whether the individual smokes, and whether they are interested in giving up. If that person states that they are interested in quitting, listed below are a number of interventions that can be offered. If the person says that they are not interested, or are not sure, a more motivational approach may be more appropriate (*see* Book 4, Chapters 6 and 7). *See* Box 6.3 for an overview of the assessment criteria.

BOX 6.3 Assessment criteria

- Number of cigarettes smoked each day
- Smoking history (age of starting smoking, age of progression to daily smoking)
- Perceived benefits from smoking (psychological, physical, social)
- Perceived barriers to change
- Readiness to quit smoking
- Reasons for wanting to quit smoking
- History of quit attempts and length of abstinence
- Related withdrawal symptoms
- Changes in psychiatric symptomatology related to previous quit attempts
- Current support

Dependence

The simplest way of assessing dependence is to ask how long it takes after waking up in a morning for the person to have their first cigarette. This question is one of six that make up the Fagerström Test for Nicotine Dependence.[29] If the individual smokes within 30 minutes of waking, they can be seen as more dependent and will probably require a higher dose of medication. The Fagerström Test for Nicotine Dependence has been validated with people who experience post-traumatic stress disorder[30] and schizophrenia.[31]

The number of cigarettes smoked each day is useful to know, but is not seen as a reliable indicator of dependence, as people may smoke a lower number of cigarettes and leave a shorter stub, thus maximising the amount of nicotine (and of harmful chemicals) that they can obtain from each cigarette.

Carbon monoxide (CO) monitoring

There are several ways of ascertaining smoking status. Asking the person if she/he is still smoking is the simplest way of getting this information, but verbal self-report is not the most foolproof of methods. Analysis of saliva cotinine is very accurate, but relatively expensive. Probably the best way is to measure the level of expired carbon monoxide by using a CO monitor. A reading of 10 parts per million or less is indicative of an individual who is not smoking. Using a CO monitor is usually very popular among people who are trying to quit as it provides instant and objective feedback that their quit attempt is on track.[32]

Decisional balance

A useful exercise to carry out with an individual expressing a desire to quit smoking is a decisional balance.[28] In this exercise, the person lists and discusses what they like and dislike about their smoking, and what will be good and not so good about stopping smoking. Getting the person to discuss the perceived benefits of their smoking will help them understand what function it plays and provide a starting point for finding alternative interventions and activities that play a similar role. This exercise can be extremely useful when trying to ascertain the person's reasons for quitting.

Previous quit attempts

It is worth exploring previous quit attempts and establishing what was helpful last time (so that it might be employed again this time), and what got in the way of change or led to relapse. If there were particular withdrawal symptoms that proved problematic, these can be identified prior to this quit attempt. It is also important to identify any changes in the person's psychiatric symptomatology during the last quit attempt, so that these can be anticipated and dealt with.

Current support

The current level of support that the person intending to quit receives is also useful to know, as this can be incorporated into any quit plan, either as a routine support or as part of an 'emergency drill' if they are tempted to smoke.

Barriers to change

It is useful to get the person to identify all the things that they think will make quitting more difficult, so that plans can be made to deal with each of those factors.

TREATMENT

Once the assessment has been conducted, and potential barriers to change have been identified, a menu of the different options for change should be presented to the person who wants to quit smoking. Treatment adherence and retention are major obstacles to overcome when working with smokers who have mental health problems,[33] so regular telephone calls to check on progress and to offer reminders about appointments should be useful.

Options for change

Medication

There are a small number of evidence-based pharmacological interventions that can help smokers in the general population quit smoking:

➤ **Champix (varenicline)** – a relatively new medication that reduces craving for and decreases the pleasurable effects of smoking. While it has been shown to be effective in helping people quit smoking, caution should be exercised for use with people who have mental health problems as it may exacerbate underlying illnesses, including depression.[34]

➤ **Zyban (bupropion)** – an atypical antidepressant that is also of use in helping people to stop smoking. Its use is contraindicated where antidepressants or antipsychotics are already being prescribed, and also in people who have a bipolar disorder.[35]

➤ **Nicotine replacement therapy** – the most widely used pharmacological aid to quitting smoking is nicotine replacement therapy. It acts as a substitute for the nicotine that is delivered by smoking tobacco, but without the harmful chemicals contained in the smoke. This is also probably the safest medication to use for people who are currently being prescribed other psychotropic drugs.

BOX 6.4 Nicotine replacement products

- **Nicotine tablet or lozenge** – put under the tongue and allowed to dissolve.
- **Nasal spray** – probably most useful for severely dependent smokers, although the effects may take some getting used to.
- **Nicotine gum** – chewed briefly and put to the side of the mouth, where the nicotine is absorbed through the buccal mucosa.
- **Nicotine inhaler** – again, the nicotine is absorbed through the buccal mucosa.
- **Nicotine patch** – the nicotine is absorbed through the skin.

For more information on the use of NRT products, *see* McEwen *et al.*[36]

Nicotine replacement therapy products are available in a variety of formats and usually double the chances of stopping smoking (*see* Box 6.4). There is little difference in the effectiveness of different types of NRT product, so the individual's preference should be the deciding consideration. They should be used for 12 weeks, possibly longer. This may be seen as a costly intervention, but the cost should be offset by the reduced cost of a lower dose of antipsychotic medication. In most areas of the UK, people who are referred to a specialist smoking cessation service can obtain NRT products from those services for a period of 12 weeks, contingent upon continued abstinence. Another option for people who have mental health problems is for their psychiatrist or GP to prescribe the NRT products, especially if the person chooses to cut down their smoking and use NRT at the same time.

Which form should treatment take?
Individual treatment
Some people who have mental health problems may find it difficult in a group situation, so individual treatment may be more appropriate for them. Individual treatment allows things to progress at the pace of the individual. It also permits greater flexibility in terms of scheduling appointments, and may make it easier for the 'support worker' to attend the session as well. Since it is not necessary to

wait for other potential quitters to be referred, treatment can commence more rapidly.

Should someone quit altogether, or should they cut down gradually?
The usual advice is that people should quit altogether and make a clean break from smoking. Switching to lower tar cigarettes, or simply smoking fewer cigarettes, usually results in compensatory smoking – people leave a shorter stub, and inhale more strongly, thus receiving a similar dose of nicotine and other chemicals. If the person thinks that they cannot stop completely, it may be worth exploring NRT products that are specifically designed to be used while still smoking.

Another useful exercise might be to encourage the person to consider which are the most, and least, important cigarettes of the day, and to encourage them to try cutting out the least important cigarettes first and substitute an appropriate NRT product.

Group treatment
Group treatment clearly requires sufficient numbers to make up a group. Waiting too long for sufficient people to be interested in joining a group may mean a loss of motivation to quit on the part of those having to wait the longest. However, if there are sufficient people who wish to quit and want to do so in a group, groups can be effective (for example in mental health day centres, group homes).

Among the general population in primary care and specialist services, group treatment has been shown to be more effective than individual treatment.[36] Whether this is true for people who have mental health problems has not been sufficiently researched. Group treatment is discussed in more detail elsewhere.[32]

Treatment content
Whether individual or group treatment is chosen, the content of treatment is very similar. The most successful treatments tend to concentrate on the management of withdrawal symptoms, and for this reason tend to be known as withdrawal-oriented therapy.[37]

After assessment, the individual is asked to set a quit date, and is offered a pre-quit session to discuss treatment options and explain what needs to happen next. They are taught how to use NRT properly and how to manage the withdrawal symptoms, and how to maximise chances of success.

The next session is scheduled for their quit date, and concentrates on reinforcing both abstinence from smoking, and use of the NRT product, along with addressing any concerns that the quitter has about the coming week.

Subsequent sessions usually happen on a weekly basis, where the previous week is reviewed, use of NRT is monitored and motivation to remain abstinent is reinforced. Smoking status is measured using the CO monitor and feedback given to the quitter. Most smoking cessation clinics tend to offer six weekly sessions, including the pre-quit session, although people with a mental health problem may require more than this in order to provide more support. The quitter's mood should be monitored closely, as there is a chance that symptoms of depression and anxiety may increase following stopping smoking. It is also important that all health professionals involved with the quitter's care remain informed about progress, so that the best possible care can be delivered.

Craving

Smokers tend to be used to dealing with craving by smoking. People who are trying to quit should be informed that craving, although unpleasant, will diminish in both frequency and intensity over time, and that each time they deal successfully with an episode of craving, it will be easier the next time it happens. Encouraging them to use NRT in response to craving is effective. Avoiding certain situations that they associate with smoking might be useful, especially shortly after the quit attempt has begun. There is no specific form of relapse prevention that has been shown to be more effective than others.[38] Thus, it is usually suggested that most of the effort and resources employed in helping someone to quit go into the initial quit attempt.

Weight gain

Weight gain is an issue for most people who quit smoking, regardless of mental health status. The average weight gain when someone stops smoking is between seven and 18 pounds (between three and eight kilos).[32] This is due to a reduction in metabolic rate.

For people who take antipsychotic medication, weight gain can be an even more significant issue, as a number of antipsychotic medications can lead to people gaining weight.[39] However, if a person who takes antipsychotic medication does quit smoking, they are likely to need to reduce the dose of their antipsychotic medication, which may offset some of normal gain in weight that people experience when they quit.

Another option might be for the individual to change the antipsychotic she/he is taking. Clozapine, olanzapine and quetiapine are associated with the greatest risk of weight gain; risperidone, zotepine and amisulpride have a lower risk, and ziprasidone does not seem to be associated with weight gain.[38] Clearly, changing medications runs the risk of leading to a period of symptom instability and it is probably a good idea to wait for the individual to be stable on their new medication before initiating an attempt to quit smoking.

Medication issues

KEY POINT 6.1

Liaison with psychiatrist and care coordinator is appropriate at any time. However, it is vital if the person is in receipt of psychotropic medication.

In case studies,[40] it was found that smokers who were prescribed clozapine and olanzapine became confused and developed significant extrapyramidal side-effects when they reduced their tobacco use, due to much higher plasma concentrations of the antipsychotic medication being present. This is because smoke constituents have an effect on the cytochrome P4501A2 system in the liver, enhancing the metabolism of antipsychotics and, therefore, requiring higher doses to have the same effect.

Other studies have found similar results.[41] Indeed, a study found that plasma concentrations of clozapine can rise up to 1.5 times in the month following cessation of smoking, and between 50% and 70% in the first four days after quitting.[42]

Once people reduce their tobacco consumption, special care and attention must be paid to dosages of antipsychotic medication in order to avoid toxicity due to elevated plasma concentrations of antipsychotics. People who are in the process of quitting smoking should be monitored closely for new and more pronounced existing side-effects, along with any signs of sedation. Thus, it may be useful to review their medication every week during the quit process using a validated side-effect rating scale such as LUNSERS.[43] For example, people who are taking clozapine and smoking between seven and 12 cigarettes per day may need to reduce their dose of clozapine by 50% when they quit.[44] Of equal importance is that if the individual relapses, their antipsychotic dose may need to be adjusted upwards. Nicotine replacement therapy is useful in that not only does it reduce cravings for tobacco but it does not affect blood plasma concentrations of antipsychotics.[45]

Care when taking prescribed medication
Care should be taken if any of the following drugs are being prescribed when the person tries to quit smoking, as their metabolism is affected by the action of tobacco smoke constituents:
➤ amitriptyline
➤ clomipramine
➤ caffeine
➤ clozapine
➤ desipramine
➤ diazepam
➤ fluvoxamine
➤ haloperidol
➤ imipramine
➤ mirtazapine
➤ olanzapine
➤ paracetamol
➤ perphenazine
➤ propranolol
➤ tamoxifen
➤ theophylline
➤ verapamil
➤ warfarin-R
➤ zotepine.

Relapse
When working alongside the person experiencing mental health–substance use problems, the long-term approach and retention of therapeutic optimism[46] is vital to helping people quit smoking. Relapse is to be expected, but this should not mean that people who have mental health problems cannot stop smoking, or that health professionals should not try to help.

CONCLUSION

While much attention is focused on co-occurring mental health and drug and alcohol use, the morbidity and mortality caused by smoking among individuals who have mental health problems is not taken seriously enough. Mental health and substance use professionals rarely receive adequate, if any, training to help people stop smoking. This issue has profound implications for the health and well-being of individuals experiencing mental health–substance use, and yet rarely receives sufficient attention from an organisational point of view. Smoking cessation treatment for people who have mental health problems is cost-effective and relatively straightforward, and deserves greater attention from both clinicians and policy-makers.

POST-READING EXERCISE 6.1 (ANSWERS ON P. 79)

---

1 What is the most common cause of relapse when a person is trying to stop smoking?
2 What is the simplest way to assess the individual's level of dependence on nicotine?
3 Which is the most effective nicotine replacement therapy product?
4 What should continue to be monitored following a successful attempt to stop smoking by a person who is being prescribed antipsychotic medication?

REFERENCES

1 Department of Health. *Smoke-free Premises and Vehicles: consultation on proposed regulations to be made under powers in the Health Bill.* London: The Stationery Office; 2006.
2 Goddard E. *Smoking and Drinking among Adults, 2006. General Household Survey 2006.* London: Office for National Statistics; 2008.
3 Department of Health. *Smoking Kills: a white paper on tobacco.* London: The Stationery Office; 1998.
4 Office of Public Sector Information. *The Smoke-free (Premises and Enforcement) Regulations.* London: The Stationery Office; 2006.
5 Kelly C, McCreadie R. Cigarette smoking and schizophrenia. *Advances in Psychiatric Treatment.* 2000; **6**: 327–31.
6 Kumari V, Postma P. Nicotine use in schizophrenia: the self medication hypothesis. *Neuroscience and Biobehavioural Reviews.* 2005; **29**: 1021–34.
7 Jochelson J, Majrowski B. *Clearing the Air: debating smoke-free policies in psychiatric units.* London: King's Fund; 2006.
8 Kinnunen T, Doherty K, Militell FS, *et al.* Depression and smoking cessation: characteristics of depressed smokers and effects of nicotine replacement. *Journal of Consulting and Clinical Psychology.* 1996; **64**: 791–8.
9 Mortensen PB, Juel K. Mortality and causes of death in first admitted schizophrenic patients. *British Journal of Psychiatry.* 1993; **163**: 183–9.
10 Joukamaa M, Heliovaara M, Knekt P, *et al.* Mental disorders and cause-specific mortality. *British Journal of Psychiatry.* 2001; **179**: 498–502.
11 Kelly C, McCreadie RG. Patients with schizophrenia who smoke: private disaster, public resource. *British Journal of Psychiatry.* 2000; **176**: 109.

12 De Leon J. Smoking and vulnerability for schizophrenia. *Schizophrenia Bulletin*. 1996; **22**: 405–9.

13 Lavin MR, Siris SG, Mason SE. What is the clinical importance of cigarette smoking in schizophrenia? *American Journal of Addictions*. 1996; **5**: 189–208.

14 Maier W, Schwab S. Molecular genetics of schizophrenia. *Current Opinion in Psychiatry*. 1998; **11**: 19–25.

15 Dawe S, Gerada C, Russell MA, *et al.* Nicotine intake in smokers increases following a single dose of haloperidol. *Psychopharmacology*. 1995; **117**: 110–5.

16 Glynn SM, Sussman S. Why patients smoke. *Hospital and Community Psychiatry*. 1990; **41**: 1027.

17 Pomerleau OF, Pomerleau CS. Behavioural studies in humans: anxiety, stress and smoking. *Ciba Foundation Symposium*. 1990; **152**: 225–35.

18 West R. Beneficial effects of nicotine: fact or fiction? *Addiction*. 1993; **88**: 589–90.

19 West R, Hajek P. What happens to anxiety levels on giving up smoking? *American Journal of Psychiatry*. 1997; **154**: 1589–92.

20 Moxham J. *Mental Health and Smoking – an opening address. Symposium report – smoking and mental health, 9 November 2001*. London: Royal Pharmaceutical Society; 2001.

21 Hackney D. *Service User Perspective. Symposium Report – smoking and mental health*. London: Royal Pharmaceutical Society; 2001.

22 Santry C. Mental health trusts ignore smoking ban. *Health Service Journal*. 22 June 2009.

23 Dickens GL, Stubbs JH, Haw CM. Smoking and mental health nurses: a survey of clinical staff in a psychiatric hospital. *Journal of Psychiatric and Mental Health Nursing*. 2004; **11**: 445–51.

24 National Health Service Smokefree. *Smoking and Mental Health*. Symposium report. 2001. Available at: www.ash.org.uk/current-policy-issues/health-inequalities/smoking-and-mental-health (accessed 3 November 2010).

25 West R, Hajek P, Foulds J, *et al.* A comparison of the abuse liability and dependence potential of nicotine patch, gum, spray and inhaler. *Psychopharmacology*. 2000; **149**: 198–292.

26 West R, Hajek P, Belcher M. Severity of withdrawal symptoms as a predictor of outcome of an attempt to quit smoking. *Psychological Medicine*. 1989; **19**: 981–5.

27 Hughes JR. Tobacco withdrawal in self-quitters. *Journal of Consulting and Clinical Psychology*. 1992; **60**: 689–97.

28 Miller WR, Rollnick S. *Motivational Interviewing: preparing people for change*. 2nd ed. New York: Guilford Press; 2002.

29 Heatherton TF, Kozlowski LT, Frecker RC, *et al.* The Fagerstrom Test for Nicotine Dependence: a revision of the Fagerstrom Tolerance Questionnaire. *British Journal of Addictions*. 1991; **86**: 1119–27.

30 Buckley TC, Mozley SL, Holohan DR, *et al.* A psychometric evaluation of the Fagerstrom Test for Nicotine Dependence in PTSD smokers. *Addictive Behaviours*. 2005; **30**: 1029–33.

31 Weinberger AH, Reutenauer EL, Allen TM, *et al.* Reliability of the Fagerstrom Test for Nicotine Dependence, Minnesota Nicotine Withdrawal Scale, and Tiffany Questionnaire for Smoking Urges in smokers with and without schizophrenia. *Drug and Alcohol Dependence*. 2007; **86**: 278–82.

32 McEwen A, Hajek P, McRobbie H, *et al. Manual of Smoking Cessation: a guide for counsellors and practitioners*. Oxford: Blackwell Publishing; 2006. p. 95.

33 Hitsman B, Moss TG, Montoya ID, *et al.* Treatment of tobacco dependence in mental health and addictive disorders. *Canadian Journal of Psychiatry*. 2009; **54**: 368–78.

34 British National Formulary. *Varenicline: 58*. London: British Medical Journal; 2008.

35 British National Formulary. *Bupropion hydrochloride: 58*. London: British Medical Journal; 2008.

36 McEwen A, West R, McRobbie H. Effectiveness of specialist group treatment for smoking cessation vs. one-to-one treatment in primary care. *Addictive Behaviours*. 2006; **31**: 1650–60.

37 Hajek P. Withdrawal oriented therapy for smokers. *British Journal of Addiction*. 1989; **84**: 591–8.

38 Hajek P, Stead LF, West R, *et al*. Relapse prevention interventions for smoking cessation. *Cochrane Database of Systematic Reviews*. 2009; **1**: CD003999.

39 Taylor DM, McAskill R. Atypical antipsychotics and weight gain: a systematic review. *Acta Psychiatrica Scandinavia*. 2000; **101**: 416–32.

40 Zullino DF, Delessert D, Eap CB, *et al*. Tobacco and cannabis smoking cessation can lead to intoxication with clozapine or olanzapine. *International Clinical Psychopharmacology*. 2002; **17**: 141–3.

41 Bozikas VP, Papakosta M, Niopas I, *et al*. Smoking impact on CYP1A2 activity in a group of patients with schizophrenia. *European Neuropsychopharmacology*. 2004; **14**: 39–44.

42 de Leon J. Atypical antipsychotic dosing: the effect of smoking and caffeine. *Psychiatric Services*. 2004; **55**: 491–3.

43 Day JC, Wood G, Dewey M, *et al*. A self-rating scale for measuring neuroleptic side-effects. Validation in a group of schizophrenic patients. *British Journal of Psychiatry*. 1995; **166**: 650–3.

44 Haslemo T, Eikeseth PH, Tanum L, *et al*. The effect of variable cigarette consumption on the interaction with clozapine and olanzapine. *European Journal of Clinical Pharmacology*. 2006; **62**: 1049–53.

45 Ashir M, Petterson L. Smoking bans and clozapine levels. *Advances in Psychiatric Treatment*. 2008; **14**: 398–400.

46 Drake RE, Mercer-McFadden C, Mueser KT, *et al*. Review of integrated mental health and substance abuse treatment for patients with dual disorders. *Schizophrenia Bulletin*. 1998; **24**: 589–608.

TO LEARN MORE

- McEwen A, Hajek P, McRobbie H, *et al*. *Manual of Smoking Cessation: a guide for counsellors and practitioners*. Oxford: Blackwell Publishing; 2006.
- Campion J, Checinski K, Nurse J. Review of smoking cessation treatments for people with mental illness. *Advances in Psychiatric Treatment*. 2008; **14**: 208–16.
- ASH – Action on Smoking and Health. ASH is a public health charity that offers a wealth of useful information around smoking and government policy, as well as cessation information. Available at: www.ash.org.uk
- NHS Centre for Smoking Cessation and Training (NCSCT) – a new web-based training resource developed to provide training around smoking cessation. Available at: www.ncsct. co.uk/index.html
- Smoking Cessation Service Research Network (SCSRN) – a very useful website that has a wide variety of clinical and research resources. Available at: www.scsrn.org
- Health Development Agency. *Standard for Training in Smoking Cessation*. London: Health Development Agency. Available at: www.nice.org.uk/niceMedia/documents/smoking_cessation_treatments.pdf

ANSWERS TO PRE-READING EXERCISE 6.1

1 It is not really known why people who have mental health problems smoke more heavily than the rest of the population, but a number of theories have been put forward:
   - that smoking somehow causes mental illness
   - that the person is self-medicating
   - that the person is countering the effects of their medication
   - that something causes both mental illness and leads the person to smoke
   - that the person smokes for the same reasons that anyone else does.
2 Bupropion (Zyban); varenicline (Champix); nicotine replacement products.

ANSWERS TO POST-READING EXERCISE 6.1

1 Failure to deal effectively with the withdrawal symptoms from nicotine is the most common cause of relapse.
2 Ask the individual how long it is after waking in a morning before he/she smokes the first cigarette.
3 There is little to choose between nicotine replacement therapy products in terms of their effectiveness, so it is best left to individual choice.
4 Following a successful quit attempt, it is vital that the side-effects caused by antipsychotic medication are monitored closely, since plasma concentrations can rise. Mood should also be monitored, since people can become depressed after stopping smoking.

CHAPTER 7

Substance use and schizophrenia

David J Kavanagh and Dawn Proctor

PRE-READING EXERCISE 7.1

Time: 10 minutes
1 How would you need to modify assessments and interventions, to deal with substance use psychosis?
2 Look at the next section for some answers.
3 Re-examine your answers at the end of this chapter.

Case study 7.1: Rebecca – part i

Rebecca (26) had her first psychiatric admission after threatening to jump off a roof, saying that a radio implant in her head had told her to do it. She told the admitting doctor that television programmes and local shopkeepers had given her coded messages. She thought she may have been chosen for a secret mission, but was unsure what it was. She had sensations of bugs crawling under her skin, and wondered if nanotechnology devices had been installed. She was oriented to time and place and did not appear either depressed or excited, but was irritated and suspicious when asked about her beliefs. Her speech was normally paced, but had pauses when she appeared distracted. She had difficulty keeping to a topic, and several questions had to be repeated before she could answer. On her first day in hospital, she stripped naked and ran through the ward, and appeared distressed and confused when staff tried to restrain her. Rebecca had been living with her boyfriend, while undertaking a visual arts degree (which she had just finished). On the second and fourth day of admission, she absconded from the ward, reportedly trying to go to her parental home ('the only safe place'). Her parents said she had been smoking cannabis daily before her admission, and drank heavily in her early 20s.

SCHIZOPHRENIA AND SUBSTANCE USE PRACTICE

KEY POINT 7.1

Screen and assess for all substances and for multiple comorbidities.

Given the high co-occurrence of schizophrenia and substance use and the significant impact on both acute risks and later outcomes,[1,2] it is imperative that mental health–substance use services routinely screen for both problems. More details about screening and assessment are provided later in the chapter.

Since the disorders are typically closely linked in a relationship of mutual influence, a single, integrated treatment by the same professional or team works best.[3]

KEY POINT 7.2

Explore the potential for mutual influence between substance use and mental health.

In practice, this means that mental health services need to address both the schizophrenia and substance use, rather than referring the substance use issues to another specialist service. This often requires a change in attitude and skill set by professionals. Furthermore, there are significant challenges for mental health–substance use practice that are posed by the presence of schizophrenia, whoever the primary caseworker may be:

➤ **Initial diagnostic uncertainty:** In first presentations of acute psychosis, it is often hard to tell if hallucinations or delusional ideas result from intoxication or withdrawal, or from schizophrenia. Depending on the substance, consumption history and amounts recently consumed, psychotic symptoms from intoxication and withdrawal usually settle over a few hours or days. The immediate focus is often on the person's physical status (e.g. assessing and managing potential overdose or withdrawal effects), prevention of harm to themselves or others, and provision of a calming and supportive environment. In the absence of other information (e.g. from collaterals or hospital files), detailed assessment and treatment planning often must wait until acute substance effects are resolved. At later stages, diagnostic uncertainty may persist for some time. Determine whether the symptoms are secondary to high levels of substance use, or if there is an underlying mental disorder that is likely to persist. As in other comorbidities, a history of symptoms in periods of abstinence can clarify the situation, but otherwise, diagnostic clarity may require weeks or months of follow-up.

> **KEY POINT 7.3**

Adapt techniques to account for any cognitive impairment.

➤ **Cognitive dysfunction:** Effects on cognition can be severe, and accentuated by neural damage from the substance use or related injury. Hallucinations compete for attention, as do noises or movements, and physical states (e.g. period pain). A quiet context and awareness of the attentional problems and of the competing stimuli is needed. Problems with attention and memory typically require that oral communication has a simple structure (e.g. avoiding double-barrelled questions and complex sentences), and that summaries, repetition, rehearsal and memory aids are used extensively. You may need to remind the individual about the topic, when their answers wander.
➤ **Difficulties communicating:** Cognitive problems may also be reflected in expressive difficulties (poverty of speech/content). Eliciting a narrative history or their perspective requires patience, and a greater reliance on closed questions and collateral reports than in most other disorders, especially in acute phases. The individual often finds it hard to politely refuse substances that are offered to them, without losing the friendship or putting themselves at risk of assault.

Several other issues also face the professional in this field:
➤ **Multiple comorbidities:** People experiencing schizophrenia and substance use problems are at heightened risk of additional co-occurring disorders (e.g. depression, social anxiety, antisocial personality disorder), which further complicate assessment. For example, there is significant overlap or similarity of symptoms between these disorders (e.g. substance use and antisocial personality can both result in antisocial activities; socially anxious cognitions and delusional beliefs may be very similar). Multiple disorders also impact on management, and substantially increase the risk of relapses, self-harm and social crises. Assertive follow-up, routine risk assessment and responsive crisis services are essential. There may also be forensic issues (e.g. a pending court hearing) that constrain choices and impede open communication.
➤ **Motivational deficits:** Multiple disorders and neuroleptic medications can detrimentally affect motivation and energy. They are associated with a sense of hopelessness about the future and likely benefits of treatment (often based on negative experiences with multiple agencies). Engagement and motivation enhancement can be challenging. Memory and motivation problems also make home practice and on-time session attendance difficult. Text messages, phone reminders, assistance from others or home visits may be needed, and some flexibility with session times may initially be necessary, while punctuality is developed.
➤ **Loss of relationships:** Previous friends and enjoyable activities are often lost over the first five years of schizophrenia, and individuals may find it hard to make new friends and establish new activities. Unemployment and financial

hardship are common. Other people who use substances may be their main social contacts outside their family, caseworkers and other people receiving treatment. Thus, substance use may be the primary source of pleasure and boredom relief. Stopping or reducing substance use may represent a major loss. We need to consider building on strengths and adding to the individual's life, rather than focusing solely on problem behaviours.

➤ **Suspicion:** Delusional ideas, as well as realistic appraisals of their situation (e.g. involuntary hospitalisation, unknown professionals) often make people experiencing mental health–substance use disorders suspicious, and patience in developing rapport and trust is even more critical in this context than in other co-occurring disorders.

➤ **Blame by others:** Families and friends are often angry when the person experiencing schizophrenia also uses substances. They may blame their disorder or relapse on the substance use, and think the person is not making sufficient effort to address their problems. A critical objective is often to further develop empathy for difficulties their friend or relative has initiating and maintaining change, and develop willingness to deliver non-intrusive support when asked. If possible, conduct a brief interview with family members before having a joint interview, to prevent it being a venue for criticising the individual.

➤ **Families need help too:** This type of mental health–substance use disorder has a particularly severe impact on the lives of families and friends. Psychotic symptoms, socially inappropriate or dangerous behaviour, the person's distress, and their increased financial, social and emotional dependence are difficult for any family to deal with. Empathy for the person's situation and shared disappointment about lost dreams for the future make others distressed. They may feel guilty or ashamed about the disorder's occurrence or about seeking involuntary treatment (if they did so). This additional stressor may exacerbate other issues in the family (e.g. marital strain). Families are often excluded from care planning and may even be discouraged from providing information and warning of impending relapses. Rarely are their own needs adequately addressed, even though their supportive role is often crucial to the success of the individual's treatment (*see* Book 3, Chapter 2; Book 5, Chapter 4).

REFLECTIVE PRACTICE EXERCISE 7.1

Time: 30 minutes
Issues for reflection
- Re-read the description of Rebecca, above.
- What primary diagnostic alternatives do you have at this point?
- What information could clarify the diagnosis?
- What do you not know about her substance use as yet?

SCREENING AND INTAKE ASSESSMENT

Intake is usually under acute time pressure, especially in busy emergency departments or other crisis services, where the priority is to triage and determine immediate treatment options. Clarification of some issues may be delayed until there are opportunities for longer interviews or observation periods. While many considerations are common to other comorbidities, several are of special importance in psychosis, as follows.

➤ **Empathise** – with the person's distress, providing reassurance in a calm, unhurried voice, avoiding sudden movements, and maintaining safe and acceptable personal distance.

➤ **Identify** – any immediate physical risk to themselves or others, and take protective action, negotiating as necessary.

➤ **Screen** – for positive, negative, disorganised and mood-related symptoms.

➤ **Ask** – about recent use of all psychoactive substances, including tobacco, prescription drugs and herbal remedies. Determine how much has been taken, and whether physical management is urgently needed.

➤ **Negotiate** – if treatment is indicated, attempt to negotiate voluntary participation (discuss available alternatives, ability of the service to provide safety and relieve distress, any concerns). If the service is at another location, check availability of transport and beds or staff. If the person is unwilling to accept treatment, determine if they fulfil criteria for involuntary treatment, and take appropriate action, minimising pharmacological or physical restriction while maintaining safety.

As soon as possible, spend time developing rapport (see subsequent section) and fleshing out aspects further, with the person and/or a close relative or friend if the opportunity arises. Confirm answers from multiple sources where possible (e.g. obtain a drug screen to check self-reports, especially where drug interaction or withdrawal pose significant risks).

> **KEY POINT 7.4**
>
> Invest time building trust and rapport in early assessment and treatment sessions.

BUILDING RAPPORT

Positive engagement involves developing trust and getting to know the whole person. In an inpatient setting, drop by regularly for brief chats. With outpatients, spend a few minutes getting to know the individual. Ask about their family, job, sport or music preferences, see if you share any interests, and briefly discuss recent relevant events (e.g. last weekend's football match). Ask about plans and hopes for the future (avoiding attempts to shape them). Apart from building rapport, these discussions have three important objectives:

1 **A basis for motivation:** Future goals are often inconsistent with continued substance use or with uncontrolled psychosis. At later stages, they can be used

to enhance motivation to address substance use and engage in treatment (*see* Book 4, Chapters 6 and 7).

2 **Incidental assessment of life issues:** The caseworker learns about issues (housing, finances and employment, interpersonal conflicts, legal problems) that may affect their mental health and substance use. Work on those issues engenders hope, strengthens the relationship and frees attention to work on mental health–substance use problems (*see* Book 4, Chapter 2; Book 5, Chapter 9).

3 **Assessment of attention span:** During these discussions and further assessment, the caseworker checks the person's ability to hold a topic of conversation for 5–10 minutes (with reminders as necessary). An attention span of at least five minutes is needed before motivation enhancement can begin effectively.

Case study 7.1: Rebecca – part ii

Rebecca huddled on a chair and avoided eye contact during initial sessions. Contacts were brief and were held at a similar time and place. The caseworker acknowledged how hard things must be at the moment, but hoped she might be able to help. She said Rebecca didn't have to talk if she did not feel like it. Over a cup of tea, they talked briefly about the ward and a TV programme that she had seen. In a later session, Rebecca mentioned she'd been to the art gallery the week before. They talked about a picture they both liked. Rebecca was worried about money, and they talked about applying for benefits. In a later meeting, they chatted about Rebecca's dream of becoming a painter, and her caseworker dropped in to an art therapy session to see her work. Rebecca was excited about a coming art exhibition where people undergoing treatment could sell their work.

ASSESSMENT

Assessment and motivation enhancement are listed separately for conceptual clarity, but they are conducted as a single process. While some questions are convergent (e.g. with yes/no answers), the interview is conducted empathically, and as a collaborative attempt to understand and address worrying issues. Provide a brief rationale for questions that may initially seem irrelevant or intrusive, summarise frequently and check the accuracy of inferences and conclusions.

Take a psychiatric and substance use history

➤ Focus on psychotic and mood-related symptoms, the nature of any suicidal thoughts or attempts, and features of dependence and abuse/harmful use.
➤ Look for periods when consumption or symptoms were better or worse.
➤ Check if increased substance use exacerbates symptoms and vice versa.
➤ Examine triggers for change, nature and outcomes of past treatments, self-control methods and their perceived utility.

Refine information about recent consumption and psychotic symptoms

➤ Ask about consumption and symptoms each day over the last week, using event-cued recall (a Timeline Followback,[4] e.g. 'Let's go through this week. You said when Joe came around yesterday afternoon, and you smoked cannabis four times. That was a bad trip – you felt really suspicious.' 'What about the day before?').

➤ Ask about other contexts when symptoms were better or worse over recent weeks, and about situations associated with less and more substance use.

➤ Confirm consumption estimates against another source, e.g. amount purchased, weekly cost, number of empty bottles, collateral reports of intoxication, urine or blood analyses.

➤ Attempt to resolve discrepancies without assuming an attempt to deceive (e.g. if her mother reported more instances of substance use, perhaps she mistook schizophrenia symptoms for intoxication. If a urine test was negative, reported consumption may have been outside detection limits of the test. If a consumption occasion was omitted, it may have been forgotten). If the person did deliberately under-report their consumption, they may fear the consequences of accurate reporting (e.g. being kept in hospital longer) – more work on rapport or other reassurance may be necessary ('Is their fear well founded?' 'How can that be addressed?').

➤ Check for regularities in symptoms and substance use ('Is that what usually happens each week?' 'Is pay week different?').

➤ Ask about the nature of current schizophrenia symptoms (e.g. who the voices are; what they say; cognitive, emotional, and behavioural responses to them).

➤ Check functional impacts of psychiatric symptoms and substance use (note the overlap with 'less good' things about substance use). Several brief instruments systematically screen across potential impacts (e.g. the DrugCheck[5]).

➤ Develop and check a functional analysis of the development and maintenance of all mental health and substance use problems, and their relationships.

Assess strengths and assets

It is easy to be lost in the complexity of problems experienced.

➤ Ask, 'What things are going well?' 'What are you good at?'

➤ Look for skills, supports and positive activities that may assist in promoting growth and recovery.

Case study 7.1: Rebecca – part iii

On treatment with 4 mg risperidone, Rebecca gradually became less distressed and was better able to respond to questions, although some thought disorder persisted. Meetings with her parents and boyfriend clarified assessments further. Rebecca's current partner introduced her to cannabis soon after they met three years ago. She had never smoked tobacco, but drank alcohol heavily (8–10 drinks, two or three times a week) from 18–21 years, apparently triggered by an untreated depressive episode. She stopped drinking following a series of alcohol-fuelled arguments with past boyfriends, and some memory blackouts after nights out with friends. She took up studying for a degree, to help her stay off alcohol. Until recently, she smoked cannabis two or three times daily with her boyfriend, and they used 1–2 g per week (with more being purchased in their pay week). She and her boyfriend said this pattern had been stable over the previous three years. Three months ago she sat the final examinations for her degree, and increased her cannabis use during this period to deal with anxiety. She began hearing occasional voices. Wondering if people were talking about her, she stopped going to her part-time job. After she increased her cannabis intake to four to six times per day, the voices and suspicion became stronger. The next week, her parents brought her to hospital. Rebecca did not have a history of suicidal thoughts, and was not currently depressed or manic. Her hallucinations included hearing a woman and man, who commented on hidden meanings in her behaviour. They said that she was a world leader in painting, but she now doubted this was true. She still puzzled about explanations of her unusual experiences.

DEVELOPMENT OF MOTIVATION

In this context, motivational interviewing retains its key characteristics of encouraging talk about change, expressing empathy and acceptance, avoiding arguing, rolling with resistance, and amplifying discrepancies between current and desired situations. A critical focus is substance use, but the approach may also be applied to treatment choices (e.g. going home prematurely vs. staying in hospital) or dysfunctional coping strategies (e.g. stripping naked when directed by the voices). Changes to the approach in schizophrenia include the following.

➤ **Divide sessions** – into several short ones or include rest breaks if the person has difficulty maintaining attention.

➤ **Summarise** – use summaries extensively and repeat steps where necessary.

➤ **Attention** – many people have difficulty holding several items in attention. Start with the implications of current behaviour, but focus written summaries on likely outcomes of change, and ask the person to highlight one or two especially important outcomes (e.g. circling them). Use visual aids to help the person see their decisional balance. Give the individual written summaries to read between sessions, and alter if they wish: this step provides additional covert rehearsal.

➤ **Dysphoria and amotivation** – undermine self-efficacy in achieving change. Several sessions may be needed to consolidate self-efficacy. Cue memories of successful self-control behaviours, and focus on hypothetical plans for the first few days of an attempt (what steps would be needed, how they would do them, who could help).

➤ **Address substances sequentially** – many people have problems with several substances. Initially, focus on one they are already concerned about (often, cigarette smoking), or with the one that they know is affecting them most (often, cannabis or amphetamines). Addressing this problem frequently alerts them to the advantages of changing other substance use, and builds their self-efficacy to do so. Accepting their choice of substance is consistent with the spirit of motivational interviewing.

KEY POINT 7.5

Revisit motivational techniques regularly to reinforce engagement in change.

Case study 7.1: Rebecca – part iv

Rebecca said cannabis had positive effects on:
- controlling thoughts and slowing them down
- anxiety
- her relationship (making it less stormy and closer, when they both smoked cannabis).

Rebecca had researched cannabis online, and had believed that it must be alright, if it was being used therapeutically. Her caseworker briefly described the usual context of therapeutic use, and (consistent with an MI approach) asked permission to give her a paper clarifying effects of cannabis. A second interview reviewed the previous discussions, and she recalled that positive effects did not always occur. The caseworker asked if any things about cannabis were not so good:
- Rebecca blamed her hospitalisation on cannabis, and was upset about the impact it made on her life.
- when Rebecca smoked a lot of cannabis, she found it hard to concentrate.
- Rebecca thought cannabis was making her current financial problems much worse, but was surprised and concerned when the annual cost was estimated.

If Rebecca stopped using, she expected a positive impact on:
- prevention of symptoms and hospitalisations
- her planned career in visual arts
- her financial situation.

Rebecca glossed over downsides of stopping cannabis use, but at the next interview, said she would miss smoking it with her boyfriend. She listed other activities they could share. Rebecca drew pictures to represent pros and cons of change, and tipped a see-saw towards stopping cannabis altogether. She wrote this in large letters across the drawing. The caseworker asked her to recall details about her previous success in stopping drinking. Rebecca said she kept busy to stay in control, and that her mother helped. Rebecca thought she could stay off cannabis without much difficulty. They talked through how she would obtain support from her mother over the first week.

ONGOING SUPPORT

Some people with psychosis are able to maintain changes in substance use after only a motivational intervention, but most need more support. As in other substance use problems, initial changes are fragile, and lapses (or full relapses) are common (*see* Chapters 15 and 16; Book 4, Chapter 13). Individuals frequently underestimate how hard it is to make major life changes, and maintain these in the face of difficult life situations and fluctuating symptoms. Dysphoria and substance refusal often represent particular challenges. Professionals should monitor and address fluctuations in motivation in all phases of treatment.

KEY POINT 7.6

Help individuals to negotiate with their family and friends to obtain effective, non-intrusive support.

While people with schizophrenia and substance use often have complex problems, their limited cognitive resources and skills make it essential that each treatment step is small and has a single focus:

➤ Look for preferred actions with potential to improve multiple targets. **Pleasurable activities** that do not involve substance use can improve mood as well as reducing consumption. Pleasurable physical activities can also improve physical health and weight control (a frequent problem with neuroleptic treatment). If the activity is with others, it may help them cope with hallucinations and improve their social skills. **Employment** limits opportunities for substance use, relieves boredom, provides a sense of achievement, gives opportunities to practise social and functional skills, and improves finances (opening new options for housing, transport, clothing purchases or recreational activity). Sometimes, **improved housing** is a key objective with multiple impacts (e.g. away from other people who use substances, reducing sleep disturbance and conflict, as well as fewer temptations to resume substance use).

➤ There may be an increased need for support from others. Help the individual to identify who will give non-intrusive and non-judgemental support when they want it. See if they would like joint sessions to explain what they are trying to do and negotiate how others can help. Work with their key supporters to develop action plans, and ensure that demands of the role do not become excessive.

KEY POINT 7.7

Assist family, friends and carers to empathise with the individual's situation, while minimising their own distress.

Consider other needs of families and friends. Help them resolve conflicts, solve problems, and deal with their own distress, loss and guilt. The family may value ideas on making an agenda for a meeting with treating staff, how to approach staff (e.g. offering information that may help), or on obtaining informed and written consent from the individual to talk about their status.

LOOKING AFTER YOURSELF

Consider your own needs (*see* Book 1, Chapter 9; Book 2, Chapters 10–12). You need to ensure you do not lose hope, even with people whose progress is slow and punctuated by severe setbacks. Make time for regular supervision and mentoring that helps you solve the difficult clinical and ethical problems posed, and addresses sources of work-related frustration and distress. Maintain a rich set of outside interests, vibrant social relationships and strong physical health, so you can continue to offer consistent support to the individual.

Case study 7.1: Rebecca – part v

Rebecca was abstinent from cannabis for two weeks, but went back to smoking it after an argument with her boyfriend. Her caseworker helped her review her reasons for change, and acknowledged how hard that situation must have been. She suggested they work out other things Rebecca could do in that situation. Rebecca thought she could listen to music. She did not want to address problems in her relationship, fearing it might precipitate a breakup, which she was not ready to deal with. During further discussion, she said her voices told her to smoke cannabis after the argument. The caseworker asked her what would happen if she did not do what they said. Rebecca said she was frightened to find out. However, she agreed to try resisting them, and planned to call the service's crisis line if she needed more help. Over the next weeks, she discovered that the voices sometimes became angry when she resisted them, but nothing bad happened.

Recalling Rebecca's response to art therapy, the caseworker searched the internet and found information on local art classes that were affordable and easily accessible by public transport. Rebecca welcomed the information, and they talked about the pros and cons of the three classes. She decided to attend a screen printing class at the local college twice per week. A month later, Rebecca had not attended any classes. She volunteered that she felt anxious about large groups. Her caseworker helped her find a smaller class, and make a plan so she woke up in time to attend. Planning weekly activities was difficult for Rebecca because of her anxiety and difficulty concentrating. She selected one 15–20 minute activity each week (e.g. walking to the park). At her request, a support worker helped her complete the weekly targets. Rebecca began feeling less anxious as she practised how to deal with social situations and test her negative cognitions about them. She gradually increased social activities and ruminated less.

With support from her caseworker and family, she dealt with a breakup with her boyfriend without returning to substance use. For a short time, Rebecca moved in with her parents, but soon after decided to live alone. Her parents were worried about that decision, and a meeting with the family developed ways they could support her. Her mother now invites her to dinner once or twice a week, and they often meet for coffee. They frequently keep in touch on the phone.

RELAPSE PREVENTION

Repetitive patterns in risk situations and prodromes may be seen in both psychosis and substance use problems. Contexts that are particularly difficult to handle (e.g. producing high craving or a need for support) or that trigger distress also offer predictive clues. While we do not want people to worry or become obsessed with tracking these indicators, it is important that the person or a family member is alert to potential risk, so that additional support and monitoring can take place:

➤ **Identify risks:** As part of the assessment, the caseworker should already have some ideas about likely warning signs and risk situations. Develop this list further throughout treatment.

➤ **Accommodate cognitive deficits:** Keep relapse prevention plans simple. Include a summary of risky situations, steps to take, and who to call. Remind the person about the plan in subsequent sessions, and rehearsing its steps. Role play variations in scenarios for substance refusal and symptom management to consolidate key skills.

➤ **Minimise negative effects of behavioural lapses and symptomatic relapse:** Respond quickly to potential lapses or relapses, to minimise their negative impacts on relationships and functional opportunities. Explain that symptomatic relapses may sometimes be hard to predict or avert, but quick action may decrease their severity or duration. For behavioural lapses, acknowledge that changing habits is hard. Minimise self-blame for behavioural lapses by saying the sessions clearly had not prepared them enough for the challenges they faced. Identify behavioural lapses and symptomatic relapses as opportunities to learn more about risky situations and gain a wider range of skills. Work collaboratively to understand factors that led to the relapse, including any relationships between their substance use and mental health.

Case study 7.1: Rebecca – part vi

Rebecca went through periods of depression, as she contrasted her previous functioning with her current abilities. Her caseworker helped her deal with the negative thoughts, and focused on her achievements. Despite continuing to take medication and remaining off cannabis, Rebecca also had problems with concentration and occasional auditory hallucinations. She had a further episode of psychosis a year later, apparently triggered by a further relationship breakup. She now continues to need a caseworker, who is working on identification of early warning signs and risk situations for relapse, and especially on dealing with relationship loss. Rebecca recently mounted an exhibition of her paintings with support from her family, and is excited about plans for a European art tour with her mother next year.

CONCLUSION

An integrated approach is required to effectively screen, assess and treat co-occurring schizophrenia and substance use, due to the close interrelationship that is typically found between these disorders. Multiple comorbidities are often seen, and a person-centred approach to the person's problems is needed. Screening and intervention are the core responsibility of mental health services, and basic comorbidity skills are essential for all mental health workers. Screening instruments and motivational procedures for substance use can be adapted from ones used in alcohol and other drug services, but need to take account of the lower levels of dependence and greater cognitive dysfunction that typify this group. Families and friends can help support change, but efforts may be needed to help them empathise with the person, and use non-intrusive strategies. Despite an often fluctuating course, many people with substance use problems and schizophrenia can successfully address the comorbidity with persistence and ongoing support, and there is every reason to maintain hope of a positive outcome.

POST-READING EXERCISE 7.1

Time: 45 minutes
Reflecting on the case of Rebecca described throughout the chapter:
- What were the strengths of the assessment and management?
- What could have been handled better?
- Consider how substance use and schizophrenia could be addressed more effectively in a clinical context you are familiar with.
- What changes to current procedures might be needed?

REFERENCES

1 Kavanagh DJ, Connolly J. Assessment of co-occurring addictive and other mental disorders. In: Miller PM, editor. *Evidence-based Addiction Treatment.* San Diego: Elsevier; 2009. pp. 89–117.
2 Kavanagh DJ, Waghorn G, Jenner L, *et al.* Demographic and clinical correlates of comorbid substance use disorders in psychosis: multivariate analyses from an epidemiological sample. *Schizophrenia Research.* 2004; **66**: 115–24.
3 Kavanagh DJ, Mueser KT. The treatment of substance misuse in people with serious mental disorders. In: Turkington D, Hagen R, Berge T, *et al.*, editors. *The CBT Treatment of Psychosis: a symptomatic approach.* London: Routledge; 2010. Chapter 12, pp. 161–74.
4 Sobell LC, Sobell MB. Timeline Followback: a technique for assessing self-reported alcohol consumption. In: Litten R, Allen J, editors. *Measuring Alcohol Consumption: psychosocial and biological methods.* Totowa, NJ: Humana Press; 1992.
5 Kavanagh DJ, Trembath M, Shockley N, *et al.* The predictive validity of the DrugCheck

Problem List as a screen for co-occurring substance use disorders in people with psychosis. In submission. Pending publication.

TO LEARN MORE

- Kavanagh DJ, Connolly J. Assessment of co-occurring addictive and other mental disorders. In: Miller PM, editor. *Evidence-based Addiction Treatment.* San Diego: Elsevier; 2009. pp. 89–117.
- Kavanagh DJ, Waghorn G, Jenner L, *et al.* Demographic and clinical correlates of comorbid substance use disorders in psychosis: multivariate analyses from an epidemiological sample. *Schizophrenia Research.* 2004; **66**: 115–24.
- Kavanagh DJ, Mueser KT. The treatment of substance misuse in people with serious mental disorders. In: Turkington D, Hagen R, Berge T, *et al.*, editors. *The CBT Treatment of Psychosis: a symptomatic approach.* London: Routledge; 2010. Chapter 12, pp. 161–74.
- Kavanagh DJ, Trembath M, Shockley N, *et al.* The predictive validity of the DrugCheck Problem List as a screen for co-occurring substance use disorders in people with psychosis. In submission. Pending publication.
- Sobell LC, Sobell MB. Timeline Followback: a technique for assessing self-reported alcohol consumption. In: Litten R, Allen J, editors. *Measuring Alcohol Consumption: psychosocial and biological methods.* Totowa, NJ: Humana Press; 1992.

CHAPTER 8

Eye movement desensitisation and reprocessing (EMDR)

Francesca Miller

PRE-READING EXERCISE 8.1

Time: 45 minutes

Before reading this chapter read 'Eye movement and desensitisation and reprocessing (EMDR): mental health–substance use', in Book 4, Chapter 12.

INTRODUCTION: FROZEN IN CHILDHOOD

Many childhood experiences are infused with a sense of powerlessness, lack of choice, lack of control and inadequacy. Even the best childhoods have moments such as when a parent goes out for the evening, in which the child feels abandoned, powerless and uncared for. The Adaptive Information Processing (AIP) model posits that even these normal experiences can be the physiologically stored causal events for many dysfunctions. Trauma from our past can be unconsciously re-enacted in the present and inhibit our future.[1]

TRAUMA

Not everyone who has a traumatic experience resorts to using substances, cutting and other forms of self-harm. What pioneers in trauma work are now helping us understand is that it is not necessarily the incident or repeated incidents of traumatic experience that causes lasting damage. It is more the significant attachments, social support and developmental age that may influence how traumatic experience affects us in later life.

Human beings are strongly dependent on social support for a sense of safety, meaning, power and control. Even our biological maturation is strongly influenced by the nature of early attachment bonds.[2]

No one could deny the obvious distress and catastrophic effects of trauma experienced by people following a disaster. The development of eye movement desensitisation and reprocessing (EMDR) within current practice has been enabled by interest in trauma and the practice of EMDR with people for whom the disaster was their childhood, and those people who may never have known anything other than the frightening physical and psychological symptoms, which can be the legacy of a disastrous childhood.

It is not the purpose here to offer a 'how to use EMDR' kit; the protocols associated with EMDR preclude this. However, web links for acquiring further information about EMDR and training courses are available at the end of this chapter (*see* To Learn More).

Case study 8.1: part i

The professional: It is 8.20 a.m. and you are sitting at the traffic lights. It is like wrestling eels into a bucket. The kids are in the car – they are falling out – but what is new! You must remember to pick up the roll of wallpaper for Saturday. How will you manage to negotiate that hour off this afternoon to pick up the birthday present you ordered for your mum? With a bit of luck you may catch the tail end of the school sports day – you felt so guilty last year when you missed it. You notice your phone is bleeping – you hope it is nothing serious. The lights change and that guy in the car behind looks none too pleased!

Eventually, you make it to work by the skin of your teeth. The receptionist is off sick, so everyone will have to cover between them – but, never mind, at least the air conditioning is on this week!

Julie: Julie is sitting in the police cells. She was picked up for criminal damage and assaulting a police officer. She jumps up with a start, covered in bruises, noticing superficial lacerations to her wrists. 'Where am I? What day is it? Oh my god, the kids!' Julie cannot remember anything. She is sweating, shaking, and feels sick. Julie has felt like this many times before. If only she had a drink, she could get her head together.

WHAT IS EMDR?

Eye movement desensitisation and reprocessing (EMDR) is a form of integrated psychotherapy created by Dr Francine Shapiro, a psychologist, and senior research fellow at the Mental Research Institute in Palo Alto, USA (*see* Book 4, Chapter 12). It is an innovative clinical treatment which has successfully treated over one million people who have experienced psychological difficulties that originate from some kind of traumatic experience, such as sexual abuse, childhood neglect, road traffic accidents and violence. EMDR is also successful in treating other complaints such as performance anxiety, self-esteem issues, phobias and other trauma-related anxiety disorders.[3]

WE HAVE ALL BEEN THERE TO A GREATER OR LESSER DEGREE

Maybe they are what EMDR therapists might refer to as a small 't' rather than large 'T' trauma, but certainly to some degree stressful pressured lifestyles and situations have a direct impact on all of us. Maybe you have experienced performance anxiety during that all-important interview. Having researched and prepared, it is almost a relief when the day of the interview arrives. There you are, knowing what you want to say, trying to calm the racing heart and shaking hands as you shuffle the papers before you go in!

In you go, the dry mouth kicks in, there is a squeak where your voice used to be and just as you are becoming aware your head has begun shaking as well . . . 'What was that question again?' 'Sorry I didn't catch that?' Your head is gone, you have forgotten everything you ever knew about anything and the papers fall to the floor . . .

It can be a fine line between the total 'buzz' of a finely tuned autonomic nervous system (ANS) delivering a 'peak performance' and the total 'unmitigated disasters' associated with speeding on nature's cocaine! Or, maybe you are one of the lucky ones, who, under pressure, somehow seems to order up just the right amount of adrenaline you need to perform well.

On a good day our neurophysiology engages smoothly via the relationship between the cortex and subcortical structures represented in Figure 8.1.

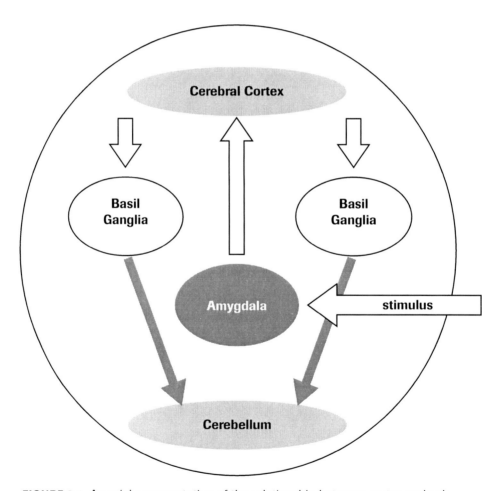

FIGURE 8.1 An axial representation of the relationship between cortex and sub-cortical structures following a stimulus

During optimum performance (Figure 8.2):

➤ The stimulus hits the amygdala (the repository of emotional experience).
➤ It is checked out in the cerebral cortex (the centre governing thought).
➤ The sympathetic mode of the autonomic nervous system kicks in via the basal ganglia ensuring optimum levels of hormones are released.
➤ Optimum performance relevant to the situation follows via the cerebellum (the centre for physical response).
➤ After the event, the parasympathetic aspect of the autonomic nervous system facilitates relaxation, we can quite literally breath again as balance is restored and we are back in 'neutral'.

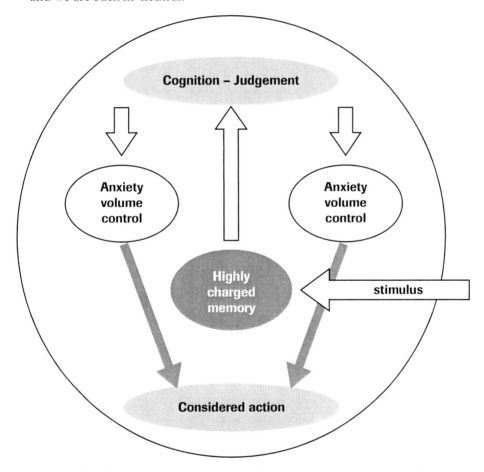

FIGURE 8.2 The interplay between cortex and sub-cortical structures in optimum conditions

Thus, for all of us, life is a series of ups and downs.

Given previous positive experiences of living and working under pressure, during periods of uncomfortable 'hyper-arousal' some of us manage to trust that the physical discomfort will pass, and our system will return to a more relaxed balanced state.

We like to think of ourselves as a pretty together intellectual society, but deep in the brain lurking just underneath our calm cool intellectualised exterior is the limbic system and the amygdala, the storehouse or hard drive that contains all our previous sensory experience. It is our survival, fight, flight and freeze centre, originally designed to save us from 'tigers' and other threatening species millennia ago. If there is perceived danger – 'bang' – on it goes. However, in an intellectualised society, there is a downside. Under pressure, it can literally cause us to act on impulse in ways that we and other people cannot always make sense of after the event.

We all have individualised 'neurological set points' that can determine our behaviour along a continuum from choice, to compulsion, to full-blown unconscious impulse.

Deprived of the opportunity and support to learn how to regulate distressing hyper-arousal, some people live on 'permanent standby': less able to relax, think in a logical way and check their experience against previous positive outcomes in highly charged situations. For some individuals, having been left unsupported in unpredictable distressing circumstances in their early years can result in a sustained, more elevated set point and lowered stress threshold.

What may be perceived by one person to be exciting can be experienced by another to be physically and psychologically overwhelming. Childhood abuse and neglect may cause a long-term vulnerability to hyper-arousal, expressed on a social level as a decreased ability to modulate strong affect states.[4]

Training in EMDR increases understanding of the unconscious neurophysiological drivers that may be driving the crisis-driven highs, lows and repetitive cycles of self-defeating behaviour that are encountered time and again by professionals working in mental health and substance use services.

Whether it is a bomb blast associated with terrorism, or the fear associated with repeated explosions in young people's lives, such as bullying or domestic violence, unpredictable threatening experiences can become encoded on the amygdala, deep within the limbic system. This associated, often unconscious, sensory information can leave individuals – as very often their parents before them – in persistent states of stress and hyper-vigilance, just as you or I may feel temporarily prior to an interview.

Case study 8.1: part ii

The professional: The phone rings again!

Emails are pouring out of the PC with those awful red tags demanding an urgent response. You can feel the irritation building amid the noise and distraction in the office. Your head is full already and it is only 11.20 (you still have not had that cup of tea), and you are struggling to think straight.

You are signing the letters amid the other rafts of paper on your desk. You answer the phone – it is a social worker from the crisis team. There is a woman in custody (Julie) who appears to have a 'primary alcohol problem'. You are alerted to a potential child protection issue amid the noise and distraction – 'Sorry can you repeat that? I wasn't quite with you'. 'What was that name again? Where?' You will be there in 20 minutes. Your plans to get through the day change in an instant.

Julie: The fearful symptoms of hyper-arousal are growing in Julie, who has just been seen by the duty social worker. 'They are going to take my children away, aren't they?' The shame, guilt and self-loathing increases. 'How could I have been so stupid? I'm pathetic!' Julie, retching, shaking and sweating, can feel 'it' building up again – getting worse. She cannot breathe, cannot think straight. Julie is terrified, needs a drink to get her head together. 'Oh my god, the children!' Julie knows they will be frightened and confused. Just one mouthful of vodka could switch this off for long enough to get through seeing the alcohol worker so she can get back to her children.

We now know that severely compromised attachment histories are associated with brain organisations that are insufficient in regulating affect states and coping with stress.[5]

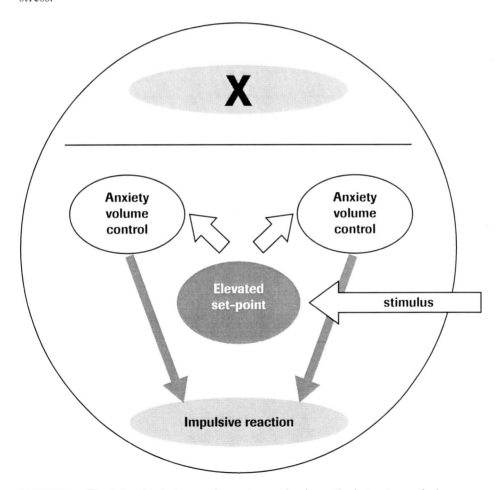

FIGURE 8.3 The interplay between the cortex and sub-cortical structures during excessive hyper-arousal

We hear the use of alcohol described:

➤ 'It helps me feel normal . . . like I can think straight . . . relax, fit in . . .'
➤ 'I don't know what came over me. It was like I couldn't breathe . . .'
➤ 'I just had to get out of there . . .'
➤ 'When I cut and hit myself, it's like I know I'm real, like I exist . . .'

For some people, given sufficiently highly charged situations, the internal dialogue necessary for effective social interaction can break down, affect people's cognition and judgement and result in compulsive and impulsive reaction.

Instead of the internal dialogue necessary to make informed choice (*see* Figure 8.3):

➤ The stimulus can hit an already elevated set point in the amygdala.
➤ The cerebral cortex is taken out of the sequence.
➤ Past distressing sensory material can be re-experienced as though in the present.
➤ Survival levels of hormones may be released resulting in 'compulsive' or in more extreme situations 'impulsive' reaction.
➤ Once the adrenaline is spent, the stimulus settles down and the already hyper-vigilant amygdala returns to 'permanent standby' until the next time.

Case study 8.1: part iii

The professional: It is 12.30, lunchtime. You gave up on the idea of the time off for sports day hours ago! You do not even notice you are hungry. There is a call from the reception desk – they are here, in reception. You head down the stairs with a million things buzzing in your head and probably quite a wad of documenta-tion that should be completed at first contact. Well, that is the theory! However, in practice . . . the waiting room is noisy and packed. Because she is dressed in inap-propriate clothing from the night before, you pick out Julie who has been brought to see you. She sits on the edge of her seat, shaking, sweating. You introduce yourself. Julie jumps. You say: '*You look terrified. Let's go somewhere a little quieter where we can talk.*'

Julie takes a massive breath in, shoulders up under her ears, hardly stopping for breath as the story pours out – her story – to yet another professional.

Julie – the past: Julie's mother had bipolar disorder; it was difficult at home. You watch the tension in her body as she describes the terror of how, at age seven, Julie often came home from school to find mother on the floor – she thought she was dead! Julie was terrified that her dad would come home and find her mother drunk. Her mother and father were always rowing. When her mother was drunk there were huge rows. Julie often stood in between her mother and father as they fought. She used to sleep with her mother to try to make sure she did not die dur-ing the night.

Such babies become children and adults with an instant exaggerated threat response, reacting to events that others would not notice as a result of the reactivation of previously sensitised neural networks. The past is not lost.[6]

> ### Case study 8.1: part iv
>
> **Julie:** Julie's parents separated when she was in her teens. She had not got on well at school. Julie always felt different from the other girls. She could not concentrate on her schoolwork, and always worried about what she would find when she got home. Julie got into trouble for being disruptive, became the class clown to try to 'fit in', and ensure she was not bullied by the others. Julie did not invite friends round to her house; she did not want people to know about her mother's drinking – it was embarrassing.

The traumatised child lives in an aroused state, ill prepared to learn from social, emotional and other life experiences.[7]

> ### Case study 8.1: part v
>
> **Julie:** By 13 years of age, Julie had been referred to an educational psychologist and her mental health file was commenced. Over the years the file had grown, she became well known to services having presented not infrequently to the Accident and Emergency department following an overdose. Julie had numerous admissions to psychiatric wards. She has numerous superficial scars from cutting and cigarette burns on her forearms.

Repeated experiences of terror and fear can be ingrained within the circuits of the brain as states of mind. With chronic occurrence, these states can become more readily activated (retrieved) in the future, such that they become characteristic traits of the individual.[6]

> ### Case study 8.1: part vi
>
> **Julie:** When Julie first drank alcohol she felt 'normal', more confident, and able to speak with people and fit in. She began hanging around with a bad crowd. Consequently, Julie tried most things, but alcohol was her main stay. 'Sometimes' it got out of hand and she would get into trouble with the police. On one occasion, Julie was charged with an offence of drunk and disorderly – but nothing too serious. All that changed when she got pregnant.
>
> As Julie speaks, she is distracted, feeling the build-up of the physical symptoms associated with her fear and alcohol withdrawal. Her mouth is dry and she is shaking.
>
> Julie is now a mother with two young children. She has made massive changes over the years and is determined to be a good mum. Julie is determined not to

put her children through what she went through as a child. Two years ago Julie undertook a detoxification on a mental health ward. Since then, Julie has detoxified herself many times – without help – because she feels so guilty.

Julie – the present: A couple of days ago Julie had to see her GP and was given a chlordiazepoxide prescription to help with alcohol withdrawal because she was finding it harder to stop this time. Julie has not taken the tablets as the GP suggested – she keeps some spare for emergencies. She had some yesterday morning so she could get the kids to school without having to have a drink, and had a few more at teatime. Julie had been doing well, and then her partner came home furious about the credit card statement that showed she had been buying alcohol. There had been a massive row, the kids were crying; she could feel 'it' building up, felt like she could not breathe, could not think straight, all she knew was that she had to get out of there. Julie ran from the house, and before she knew it she had bought a half bottle of vodka – and drank it fast behind the off licence because 'it always works'. That was the last thing Julie can remember.

> *I don't know what came over me. I feel so guilty I can see what I'm doing. They're going to take my children away, aren't they? I'm pathetic. It's all my fault.*

As Julie speaks you can tell from her posture, her distracted hurried speech, and the fearful expression on her face, the fear is commencing again, worsened by the alcohol withdrawal. Despite what Julie is saying and wanting to do, in this moment she feels sick and cannot think straight.

Julie – the future? Julie knows if she can just have a small amount of vodka, it will switch it off so she can think straight and get back home to the children. 'They must be terrified and wondering where I am.'

In the absence of a caregiver, children experience extremes of under- and over-arousal that are physiologically averse and disorganising.[8]

WHERE DO WE GO FROM HERE?
Management

Case study 8.1: part vii

The professional: You listen. Listen and notice. Once you have developed an understanding of trauma, you hear and see in a different way. Listening is reflective of the first parts of the eight phase EMDR protocol and of positive psychology (*see* Book 4, Chapter 12). You offered Julie a safe place to talk. You listen intently to her traumatic story, watching her body language, noting hot spots of hyper-arousal and discomfort as she describes terrifying images. You note the triggers for the fear and other hyper-aroused affect states Julie experiences in her body. You listen closely for self-deprecating references (negative cognitions) associated with Julie not feeling able to cope. You hear how all that Julie described happened in the absence of a caregiver who could help her learn to modulate her hyper-arousal as a child.

You consciously avoid responses that might further reinforce Julie's fear and heighten her physically experienced hyper-arousal, and need for a drink to switch it off. You hear how the legacy of her past is impacting on her experience of herself in the present, and how what used to help her feel safe (alcohol) was now keeping her stuck in self-defeating cycles of behaviour that impeded her future.

The responses interweave Julie's past with her present. You remind Julie of her resilience over the years. You point to the evidence of past success and achievement that Julie has lost sight of in her latest episode of disintegrating fear. You work alongside Julie to help her to get back in touch with her capable adult in the present, and not the powerless child she had been years ago. You help Julie experience containing her fear.

As the professional you were able to be with Julie confidently, because rather than hearing a problem, you could hear an opportunity. Alongside Julie you built on your first contact. Using EMDR in a focused therapeutic way in future sessions you could increase Julie's resilience – build on her existing resources, and move towards treating her traumatic condition, rather than just attempting to manage the cycles of behaviour that arise from it.

ENCOUNTERS

The above example is based on numerous encounters with individuals under such circumstances over the years. Hyper- and hypo-arousal can take many forms. Some people cry uncontrollably, struggle to express themselves coherently or perhaps occasionally (but rarely) shout angrily – blaming and hostile. Others present in childlike states, sitting shamefully without speaking. However, behind whatever form of behaviour the original traumatic story, the fear, the attempts to self-regulate and the distressing hyper- and hypo-arousal keep the person trapped in cycles of self-defeating behaviour.

WHAT EMDR OFFERS THE INDIVIDUAL

Prior to unearthing the traumatic roots of the current behaviour, people need to gain reasonable control over the long-standing secondary defences that were originally elaborated to defend against being overwhelmed by traumatic material. This includes substance use problems and violence against self or others. The trauma can only be worked through after a secure bond is established with another person.[2]

During thorough comprehensive trauma history, treatment planning and preparation stages of the EMDR protocol, individuals are reassured by receiving information that permits them to comprehensively understand their own actions and reactions. Many people report a great sense of relief in feeling heard and understood.

As in the above case studies, the professional cared to know Julie was frightened. Julie knew the professional cared and understood her distress. As the hyper-arousal reduced, Julie returned to a balanced physical state. As the physical manifestations of her fear lessened, Julie began to think more clearly. Having a balanced perspective enabled Julie to process information adaptively in her present situation.

Julie was less frightened of herself, and assured that this time she was not alone in her fear. There were still some pressing practicalities to deal with, but Julie no longer felt the urgent need to have a drink to manage her fear. Julie and her children had greater hope of breaking the cycle.

In the later phases of the EMDR protocol, Julie and the professional establish target memories, assess levels of subjective distress to be processed, and moved to the desensitisation phase. This was facilitated with further use of patterned eye movements and other forms of bilateral stimulation, targeting images from the past. There is mounting evidence to support findings that this facilitates the individual in desensitising unprocessed memories, blocked emotions, thoughts and physical sensations that may have been imprinted on their physiology years ago.

Throughout, the professional continually checks with the individual, interweaving through the blocked processing with the use of talking therapies, re-evaluating and checking for bodily held sensations associated with other unconscious target material.

Julie and the professional worked together to:
➤ develop containment and effective self-management of hyper- and hypo-arousal
➤ develop confidence associated with being able to integrate or more effectively manage previously overwhelming experiences
➤ challenge the validity of negative cognitions such as 'I'm pathetic' and the distorted beliefs 'it's all my fault'
➤ develop personal resources that increase resilience, dependable self-referencing and internal locus of evaluation
➤ develop reinforcement of a more balanced worldview and self-concept, by enabling Julie to begin to weave her past and present experiences together
➤ develop adaptive responses in the present to previously disorganising stimulus.

For some individuals whose lives are disrupted by unpredictability, treatment enables them to have contact with a stable caregiver who can help them begin to learn to manage what were previously overwhelming emotional experiences. The individual receives and learns from this, thereby increasing their parenting skills and the likelihood that they can offer the same to their own children.

WHAT EMDR PROVIDES FOR THE PROFESSIONAL

It seems like a travesty to have to say this, but despite 15 years of acute mental health work, and 17 years of substance use work, it is only since training in EMDR that this author identified answers to long-held questions. EMDR training increased the author's depth of understanding of, and the therapeutic framework needed to respond effectively to, the distress she encountered in her work. Such training enables the professional to empathise with the self-loathing and frustration of a significant number of chronically lapsing individuals who may well be unrecognised, untreated, adult children of trauma attempting to self-regulate debilitating hyper- and hypo-arousal, with the use of substances, and self-harming behaviours.

Although we may become desensitised to the horrific stories we hear over time, the limbic system will not. Whether inherited, acquired because of life experience, or invited by regular excessive use of substances and processes, autonomic nervous system imbalances undermine cognitive ability, learning, motivation and behaviour. Thus, it leaves some people condemned to a life determined by avoidance of potentially overwhelming situations rather than choice.[9]

Eye movement desensitisation and reprocessing training provides an understanding that some people may never have experienced the luxury of a sense of peace, belonging and safety that others may take for granted. EMDR training allows the professional to:

➤ appreciate the importance of safe, secure attachment in childhood, and the devastating legacy of uncertainty and abandonment
➤ understand the physiology behind the bodily held tension, and breathing patterns
➤ work therapeutically with the lowered emotional tolerance and outbursts, and appreciate the power of the overwhelming triggers
➤ make sense of, and explore with the individual in a therapeutic way, seemingly incongruous statements like, 'If I could just have a drink I know I could get my head together to look after the children'.

The hyper-arousal interferes with the ability to make calm and rational assessments and prevents resolution and integration of the trauma.[2]

FUTURE SERVICES

How effective have we been over recent years in responding to the increasing levels of distress, alcohol and substance use and self-harming we encounter? Are we enslaved by our past, or can we embrace what we have available to us in the present and move towards fully integrated treatment services for the future?

With EMDR we have in our grasp what we have needed for many years: an opportunity to help individuals cross that paradoxical chasm of 'they need to be stable before we can effectively assess and treat them'. Embracing the evidence from trauma and EMDR research and with just a slight change in theoretical perspective could lead to a change in the way we develop and offer first point of contact services to distressed individuals. The challenge to change is ours! There is more to integrated services than putting multidisciplinary teams in a new building together! If we can embrace the wealth of research emerging from the neuropsychiatry and neuropsychology movement, we will find that we are on the threshold of a new understanding that could transform health and social policy for the future. We could actively ensure every child really does matter.

We have a responsibility to increase our understanding, develop our skills and begin to actively treat, rather than attempt to manage, the increasing numbers of 'high risk' distressed individuals we encounter in front-line practice.

We know that alcohol works, as do other powerfully depressant and stimulant drugs and processes that 'switch off' the hyper-arousal or 'switch us back on' during periods of hypo-arousal. We also need to be aware that when suggesting to the individual that she/he stops drinking or engaging in other potentially injurious behaviours, we may in fact be asking some of them to let go of their coping strategies.

Rather than the problem we perceive it to be, for some individuals excessive use of substances and self-harming may well be an attempt at a solution. Or, as one person put it: 'I don't have a problem with alcohol; alcohol is the solution to my problem. It lets me function; it does what it says on the box.' Little wonder some people attach to these powerful substances and processes in the absence of other reliable attachments that can enable them to modulate their distress.

Advanced imaging and technology now enables us to measure the real hidden harm and long-term damage associated with neurological imbalance. EMDR, and other more integrated therapeutic approaches such as Heart Math[10] and Bowen therapy,[11] respond therapeutically to the cognitive, affective, somatic and behavioural whole person experiences. They influence autonomic nervous system imbalances, and dovetail easily and effectively with the evidence-based cognitive mapping approaches increasing in popularity in recovery work.

It is paramount that we provide environments that are relationally enriched, safe, predictable and nurturing. Failing this, our conventional therapies are doomed to be ineffective.[7]

Indeed, to minimise or disregard another human being in the height of their subjective distress can be re-traumatising, and a further re-enactment of the original wounding experienced by people who may have been denied stability and secure loving attachments in childhood.

LOOKING AFTER THE PROFESSIONAL

What may be perceived as exciting by some could prove to be physically and psychologically overwhelming for others. Traumatisation occurs when both internal and external recourses are inadequate to cope with external threat.[2]

Many frontline professionals are working in persistent states of hyper-arousal, required to be hyper-vigilant in the management of high-risk, emotively distressing cases amid pressured work environments.

We too have our stories. Indeed many of us may be deemed to be successful in the workplace because of them. Some of us can be found at the coalface, in crowded noisy hyper-arousing work environments, wrestling the modern day 'tigers' of incessant emails, deadlines and risk management. Others are in the boardrooms, wrestling with tender submissions, contracts and service level agreements. At home, or at work, for all human beings, whatever the situation in pressured work environments, the limbic system makes little distinction. Bombarded with sufficient or sustained levels of hyper-arousal, our autonomic nervous system can impact directly on our physical and psychological well-being and functioning.

The traumatic response is plainly evident in the workplace. The same hyper-arousal and neurological responses can be witnessed in professionals as those they encounter in the individual:

➤ feeling physically sick looking at computer screens
➤ irritability
➤ poor concentration
➤ ruminating thought
➤ disorientation
➤ losing whole chunks of time
➤ panic/fear
➤ increased startle response
➤ sleep disturbance.

All of the above are classic indicators of autonomic nervous system imbalance associated with stress in the workplace (*see* Book 2, Chapters 10–12). As professionals our past can be triggered by our work in the present, and can serve to undermine the future for ourselves and our families.

We hear: 'I can't wait to get home; I'm going to call and pick up a nice bottle of wine, put my feet up and relax.' We increasingly hear of dedicated professionals who are turning to the use of substances, including prescribed medication, in attempts to regulate work-related stress and unwind at the end of a hectic day.

Some professionals – innovative and dedicated – who have given their lives to their work, run the risk of ending their careers burned out, or entrenched in the indignity of substance use dependence themselves.

It is essential that we offer professionals the conditions we require of them to offer each individual. We need to ensure that the professionals' resilience is monitored and supported through effective supervision, careful monitoring of workload, and options for time out.

Take time for you to explore the concept of vicarious traumatisation in the workplace.[12]

POST-READING EXERCISE 8.1

Time: 45 minutes
- What brings you to this book – to this page?
- Notice what happens inside of you next time you are confronted with a person in hyper-arousal:
  - What thoughts and feelings are in you as you listen?
  - On a scale of 0 to 10 – where 0 is no disturbance at all and 10 is the most disturbing – how would you rate your own level of disturbance as you listen?
  - Notice as you move out of a highly charged space like that – how do you let go of encounters with that traumatic energy?
  - How do you return your own system to a balanced set point?
  - Make a list of the relationships and support networks where you can receive support.

REFERENCES

1 Shapiro F. Frozen in childhood. In: *Eye Movement Desensitization and Reprocessing: basic principles, protocols, and procedures*. New York: Guilford Press; 2001. p. 47.
2 Bessel A, van der Kolk MD. Social attachments and the traumatic response. *Psychiatric Clinics of North America*. 1989; **12**: 389–411.
3 Eye movement desensitisation and reprocessing. Europe Website: Available at: www.emdr. org (accessed 9 November 2010).
4 Bessel A, van der Kolk MD, Perry JC, *et al*. Childhood origins of self-destructive behaviour. *American Journal of Psychiatry*. 1991; **148**: 1665–71.
5 Schore AN. The effects of early relational trauma on right brain development, affect regulation and infant mental health. *Infant Journal of Mental Health*. 2001; **22**: 201–69.
6 Balbernie R. Circuits and circumstances. *Journal of Child Psychotherapy*. 2001; **27**: 237–55.
7 Larrieu JA, Zeenah CH. Treating infant parent relationships in the context of maltreatment: an integrated systems approach. In: Saner A, McDonagh S, Rosenblum K, editors. *Treating Parent-Infant Relationship Problems*. New York Guilford Press; 1998. pp. 243–64.
8 Finkehorn D, Brown A. The traumatic nature of child sexual abuse. *American Journal of Orthopsychiatry*. 1985; **66**: 390–400.
9 Miller F. The Big Bang. *Drink and Drug News*. 2009; 12 Jan. p. 14.
10 Lloyd A, Brett D, Wesnes K. Coherence training in children with Attention Deficit Hyperactivity Disorder. *Alternative Therapies*. 2010; **16**: 34–42.
11 Mallieu C. Body talk. *Drink and Drug News*. 2009; March. p. 12.
12 Rothschild B. *Help for the Helpers: the psychophysiology of compassion fatigue and vicarious traumatization*. New York: WW Norton; 2006.

TO LEARN MORE

- Substance misuse, online and hard copy magazine. Available at: www.drinkanddrugnews.com
- American website for papers and research info. Available at: www.emdria.org
- UK and Ireland training programmes lists of UK practitioners. Available at: www.emdr-europe.org
- Humanitarian Assistance programme. Available at: www.emdrhap.org
- Self-care books visualisation and holidays. Available at: www.joyofburnout.com
- Child development information and research. Available at: www.zerotothree.org
- Contact the author. Available at: www.nrgbalance.co.uk
- Information about Bowen Therapy and UK practitioners. Available at: www.thebowen technique.com
- Information about Heart Math and UK practitioners. Available at: www.heartmathsolutions. com

CHAPTER 9

Post-traumatic stress disorder and substance use

Walter Busuttil

INTRODUCTION

Some people exposed to an overwhelming traumatic experience involving intense fear, horror and helplessness may go on to develop post-traumatic stress disorder (PTSD). PTSD is characterised by three stereotypical symptom clusters comprising:

➤ Re-experiencing
➤ Hyper-arousal
➤ Avoidance phenomena.[1]

Alcohol and illicit drug misuse and dependence are common comorbid presentations in many people experiencing PTSD. If there has been exposure to multiple traumatic experiences, and the more chronic the PTSD is, the more likely it is that individuals will present with comorbid histories of substance use problems. The environment and culture of the individual are also important determining factors relating to PTSD–substance use problems after traumatisation. Pre-trauma characteristics including pre-exposure substance misuse also predicts that an individual will be more likely to be exposed to traumatic experiences and may go on to develop PTSD.

Comorbid substance use problems and dependence have implications in the treatment and clinical management of PTSD.

PTSD GENERAL
Aetiology of PTSD

Information processing models incorporate the notion that it is the inability to work through the psychological traumatic experience at the time of or in the immediate aftermath of exposure that causes PTSD.[2-4] Behavioural models stipulate that sensory perceptions experienced during traumatisation can later, by the process of stimulus generalisation, act as triggers for re-experiencing symptoms.[5] Good social support before, during and after traumatisation has been shown to be protective or to diminish the psychological impact of the trauma and its symptomatology.[6-9] Cognitive models dictate that the traumatic information must be worked through, and cognitive distortions challenged, before being accommodated within cognitive schema.[10-12] Biological theories mirror cognitive theories with malfunction of the limbic system including the amygdala and hippocampus, thought to feature prominently.[13-15] Biological-cognitive models including the dual representational theory view PTSD as a memory disorder characterised by an inability to lay down traumatic memories and express the traumatic material as a cohesive verbal narrative.[13,16-18]

Risk factors

Research consistently demonstrates that the primary predictive factor relating to the development of PTSD is a dose-response effect related to traumatic exposure.[19-21] The nature of the trauma is also of primary importance.

> **KEY POINT 9.1**
>
> The more personal and 'man-made' the trauma is (such as an assault) the more likely PTSD will develop.[22]

This is in contrast to 'Acts of God', such as in a disaster situation where the trauma is not directed personally at the victim, where PTSD is less likely to result. Secondary factors leading to the development of PTSD include the level of preparedness – perceived ability to counter threat;[23] support networks during and after exposure;[6,24,25] and peri-traumatic dissociation.[26] Personality variables including high levels of neuroticism and introversion are also related to the development of PTSD after the traumatic exposure.[27-30] Conflicting outcomes are evident for other factors including a past psychiatric history, personality deficits;[31] gender[32-34] – it is thought that women are more vulnerable by an increased factor of 20% as compared to men. A high status of educational standard has been found to be protective.[35] There is evidence that previous exposure to trauma may actually be protective in younger (military) populations[36] but is not so in the elderly.[37] Traumatic exposure in old age is thought to be a vulnerability.[38] Studies that evaluate the interaction between gender and personality traits, subsequent traumatic exposure, and the development of PTS symptoms, suggest that there may be a reciprocal relationship between personality traits of antisocial behaviour in men and borderline personality traits in women. Experiencing a traumatic event may produce elevated levels of these traits, which may in turn increase the probability of exposure to subsequent (multiple) trauma.[39,40]

Classification: single versus multiple traumatic exposure – simple and complex PTSD

The Diagnostic and Statistical Manual (DSM-IV)[1] defines PTS syndromes more rigidly than the International Classification of Diseases (ICD-10).[41] Both classifications include an immediate onset acute stress disorder or reaction characterised by extreme anxiety features and dissociative symptoms together with features of the three PTS core symptom clusters. DSM-IV defines acute PTSD as being present if the duration of symptoms is less than three months immediately following trauma- tisation. Chronic PTSD is said to be present if symptoms last for over three months. Delayed PTSD is said to be present if symptoms present after six months following traumatisation. Both DSM-IV and ICD-10 do not clearly distinguish between the effects of exposure to single (e.g. one road traffic accident), versus multiple trauma (e.g. being exposed to a war zone, being kidnapped and subjected to prolonged torture), although ICD-10 alludes to this in the definition of the category 'Enduring personality change following subjection to catastrophic stress' (ICD Code F62.0[41]). This is said to be more likely to present in those subjected to multiple trauma in adulthood who develop chronic PTSD. These trauma victims then go on to develop enduring personality changes characterised by:

➤ a hostile or mistrustful attitude towards the world
➤ social withdrawal
➤ feelings of emptiness or hopelessness
➤ a chronic feeling of being on edge as if constantly threatened
➤ estrangement.

In 1994, the DSM-IV working party investigated the concept of Complex PTSD (CPTSD).[42,43] Complex PTSD is postulated to be generated by exposure to repeated multiple traumatic exposure in early development, and most likely to develop in those exposed to multiple trauma below the age of 26 years.[44-46] Typically, many CPTSD sufferers are adult survivors of sexual abuse. Complex PTSD is character- ised by three areas of disturbance:[49]

1 **Symptoms:** of PTSD, Affective, Dissociative and Somatic.
2 **Characterological changes:** relating to control, relationships, and self-perception.
3 **Repeated harm:** a propensity to repeat harm: to the self; by others and of others.

At face value, similarities exist between CPTSD and borderline personality disor- der; however, clear, distinctive phenomena have been deduced.[50,51] Complex PTSD may be included in some form in the forthcoming DSM-V. It should be noted that studies have demonstrated that victims of childhood sexual abuse are more likely to misuse drugs and alcohol in adult life, as well as suffer from Complex PTSD.

Comorbidity

Comorbid disorders are usually commonly present alongside PTSD. General population and specific disaster and combat veteran sample studies demonstrate consistent comorbid patterns with variable ranges, including:

➤ depressive illness 50–75%
➤ anxiety disorder 20–40%
➤ phobias 5–37%
➤ alcohol abuse/dependence 6–55%
➤ illicit drug abuse/dependence 25%.

Divorce, unemployment, accident rates and suicide rates are all increased in PTSD sufferers.[30,50-55]

The interrelationship between traumatic exposure (TE), PTSD and substance use: vulnerable groups

In British combat veteran populations the commonest comorbid patterns are PTSD present with depression and alcohol abuse or dependence.[56-58] To date there is a paucity of British studies looking at the extent of traumatic life events and PTSD among substance misusers.[59] Most studies have been conducted in non-British populations. Nearly 40% of US Vietnam veterans had a lifetime prevalence of alcohol abuse or dependence.[30] Comorbid psychotic depression or psychoses generated from substance misuse are common in those who have been exposed to psychological trauma.[60]

The US national comorbidity study demonstrated that females with PTSD were 2.48 times more likely to have a diagnosis of alcohol abuse or dependence and 4.46 times more likely to have a diagnosis of drug abuse or dependence as compared to females without a diagnosis of PTSD.[61]

Adult survivors of sexual abuse have higher lifetime prevalence rates for alcohol dependence.[62-64] A history of childhood physical abuse is associated with past year alcohol abuse or dependence[65] and drug-related problems.[66] Studies of female populations both in mental health treatment and outside mental health treatment who have alcohol-related problems demonstrate higher rates of past histories of childhood sexual abuse.[67,68] Female patients who were subjected to interpersonal violence (IPV) have higher rates of PTSD by 2.9–5.9 times and substance abuse by 5.6 times compared to females who have no history of IPV.[69] Females using drugs with a history of IPV were found to have higher PTSD severity scores compared to females who had no drug use or alcohol use only.[70] Offspring of alcohol dependent individuals have a high risk of a variety of psychosocial problems including increase in the use of illicit drugs and alcohol, and behavioural and emotional problems including running away from home. Exposure to alcoholism and family violence is also associated with psychosocial functioning of children during adolescence including increasing lifetime levels of substance use, conduct disorders and low self-esteem.[71]

CLINICAL PRESENTATION OF PTSD WITH COMORBID ALCOHOL AND/OR ILLICIT DRUG USE

KEY POINT 9.2

The effect of substances on PTSD is not straightforward.

As a rule, stimulant drugs will tend to increase the hyper-arousal symptom cluster of PTSD; with anger impulsivity anxiety, hyper-arousal and hyper-vigilance all increasing. Depressant substance will in theory reduce hyper-arousal symptoms at first, at least giving relief from anxiety and promoting sleep for example; however, then as the substance is metabolised and blood levels fall, hyper-arousal symptoms may be increased through the development of withdrawal symptoms.

Cultural and behavioural factors are important considerations. Individuals experiencing alcohol use disorders prior to traumatic exposure may be more vulnerable to the development of PTSD symptoms following exposure to traumatic events. The culture within which the individual operates is an important consideration. For example, levels of alcohol intake are higher than the general population in the military and emergency services as part of a macho image.[58]

KEY POINT 9.3

The level of alcohol use prior to, and at the time, immediately following traumatic exposure is an important consideration. It is postulated that information processing of the traumatic event is impeded by excessive alcohol use in the aftermath of the trauma.

One study demonstrated that in the acute phase following exposure to psychological trauma, females who had pre-existing alcohol use disorders had higher levels of PTSD symptoms and remained more symptomatic at three months post exposure than those who did not use alcohol.[72]

People experiencing PTSD may use drugs including cannabis and alcohol to specifically target PTSD symptoms, e.g. in order to avoid trauma reminders or distressing re-experiencing symptoms including intrusive memories, nightmares and flashbacks. Sedation is desired in the hope that nightmares might also be avoided. Individuals may also use substances in the hope of reducing hyper-arousal symptoms. Many do not realise that substance use, and in particular alcohol and cocaine, can amplify symptoms of hyper-arousal including irritability, anger and violence including marital violence.[73,74] In the case of alcohol, hyper-arousal symptoms are amplified especially through withdrawal due to reducing blood alcohol levels.[75] This heightened arousal in turn may amplify the frequency and intensity of re-experiencing symptoms including nightmares and flashbacks as well as dissociative symptoms. Alcohol changes sleep stage patterns and is thought to lead to an increase in nightmares by this mechanism as well.[76]

Some people manage to mask their PTSD symptoms for many years especially through heavy drinking of alcohol. Their PTSD symptoms re-emerge once they have been through detoxification. In a cohort of female adult survivors of sexual abuse, two coping models were described.[77]

1 **The Distress Coping Model:** described those who drank alcohol to cope with negative emotions.
2 **The Emotion Regulation Model:** described those who drank to cope with negative emotions as well as drinking to enhance positive emotions.

In another study, lower educational levels and a history of childhood trauma was associated with an increase in substance abuse and higher levels of distress and avoidant coping in adult females.[78] PTSD is a syndrome that incorporates avoidance as the main coping mechanism, as well as hyper-arousal symptoms including impulsivity. Sensation-seeking and risk-taking behaviours are also commonly seen in the context of an unstable mood. Alcohol and drug use problems may be seen as a manifestation of these symptoms and coping behaviours which are part and parcel of PTSD.

TREATMENT STRATEGIES FOR PTSD GENERAL PRINCIPLES

The treatment of PTSD will ultimately require the individual to process the traumatic experiences by undertaking trauma-focused therapy. For this to be facilitated, the individuals must be safe and stable enough to cope with confronting the trauma. The most efficacious trauma-focused therapies are trauma-focused cognitive behavioural therapy (TF-CBT) and eye movement desensitisation and reprocessing.[79] NICE Guidelines were primarily written with Simple PTSD in mind, although some randomised controlled studies of people experiencing Complex PTSD were also referred to.[80]

For the treatment of Simple PTSD, psychotherapy is recommended first followed by adjunctive antidepressant therapy if therapy alone fails.[79] Simple PTSD without comorbid psychiatric disorders or substance misuse can be relatively straightforward to treat. However, away from research studies, commonly PTSD sufferers present with comorbid psychiatric illness including concomitant substance use, as well as the social ramifications of these mental health illnesses and substance use. Commonly, there can also be a history of chronicity and exposure to multiple traumas. Treatment is more complicated and difficult in cases of Complex PTSD.[80,81] These individuals will also require much more intensive and multiagency input.[82]

Alcohol or illicit drugs interfere with information processing. They will consequently impede trauma-focused therapies which are aimed at enhancing information processing of the traumatic material. Trauma-focused therapy is therefore of little value and individuals will require to reduce and abstain from using the illicit substance or alcohol before treatment can be effective for PTSD.

Some professionals have debated the concurrent treatment of substance use and that of comorbid PTSD.

KEY POINT 9.4

Questions must be asked at the initial assessment in order to determine the extent of the substance use problems.[83]

In all these cases, clinical judgement must be exercised. More recent evidence demonstrates that abstinence should be achieved before trauma-focused therapy is delivered. This strategy predicts better outcome for both PTSD and the comorbid substance abuse and dependence. Abstinence from these substances should ideally be a prerequisite to trauma treatment. At present it is recommended that abstinence from substances should be achieved before trauma-focused treatment begins.[75]

Psychoeducation for PTSD and for substance use problems should be dovetailed, and issues concerning addiction and misuse, as well as relapse prevention (*see* Chapters 15 and 16; Book 4, Chapter 13), should be integrated within the intervention for PTSD. Detoxification from substances should lead directly to psychoeducation followed by trauma-focused work in an uninterrupted sequence. The Australian combat veterans' services use the following model for veterans suffering from alcohol dependence and PTSD.

1 The individual is detoxified over a period of 10 days.
2 Followed immediately by an intensive alcohol education programme.
3 Followed by a residential group programme incorporating psychoeducation for PTSD and trauma-focused CBT lasting for about five weeks.
4 Followed by outpatient group and individual therapy including relapse prevention spread over a period of a year.[84]

Individuals with a history of substance dependence may require long-term support and treatment and should be encouraged to attend self-help treatment groups such as the AA in the long term (*see* Book 4, Chapters 14 and 15).[83]

While cases of Simple PTSD respond well to outpatient sessions of trauma-focused therapy with little stabilisation required, those suffering from Complex PTSD or severe chronic PTSD will require much preparation and stabilisation before they are able to engage in treatment. Some will require inpatient treatment programmes. These are most commonly utilised by adult survivors of sexual abuse and combat veterans. The prognosis of untreated CPTSD is poor. The additional comorbid substance use problems further complicate clinical management. Box 9.1 summarises interventions for complicated cases of PTSD, which also present with substance use problems.

BOX 9.1 General treatment strategies for those suffering from complex or chronic PTSD with substance use problems

Four main stages of treatment are used:
1 Preparation
2 Stabilisation and safety
3 Disclosure and working through traumatic experiences
4 Rehabilitation

1 Preparation
- Multimodal assessment: clinical history and mental state examination; psychometric tests for PTSD and comorbidity: subjective and objective. Assessment of substance use.
- If required detoxification from alcohol and drugs followed immediately by alcohol and drug psychoeducation tailor made for those also suffering from PTSD. Start relapse prevention.
- Prescription of appropriate medications to ensure abstinence from alcohol: disulfiram, acamprosate. Ensure safety: supports, basic welfare needs – homelessness, isolation, etc.

2 Stabilisation and safety
- Prepare for trauma-focused therapy: ensure motivation, support and safety.
- Prescribe appropriate medications for the treatment of PTSD and comorbid illness including depression: selective serotonin re-uptake inhibitors (SSRI) and related antidepressants aimed at reducing re-experiencing and hyper-arousal symptoms of PTSD as well as treating depression; mood stabilisers which are useful in reducing re-experiencing and dissociative symptoms and stabilising mood and reducing impulsivity; anti-impulse medications including clonidine; major tranquillisers for pseudo psychotic symptoms including psychotic symptoms generated by illicit drugs.
- Appropriate treatment for any other comorbid disorders
- Stabilisation through bespoke psychoeducation sessions usually delivered in a group; followed by individual or group trauma-focused psychotherapy including TF-CBT; Exposure; EMDR followed by rehabilitation.

3 Disclosure and working through traumatic experiences
- Therapy: outpatient trauma-focused cognitive behavioural therapy; eye movement desensitisation and reprocessing (TF-CBT; EMDR) – single trauma (Simple PTSD) much easier!
- Residential specialist services: group programmes that include initial phasic psychoeducation, individual trauma-focused therapy which is carried on longer term after programme has ended, and rehabilitation are commonly used in specialist centres for combat veterans and adult survivors of sexual abuse.

4 Rehabilitation
- Work retraining, maintenance.
- Family and spouse interventions – carer's groups, family and couple therapy.
- Alcohol and drugs relapse prevention and follow-up.
- Specialist alcohol and drug services and AA long term.

CLINICAL SERVICES AND TREATMENT LIMITATIONS
The ideal clinical care plans stipulate that drug and alcohol services must work in tandem with psychological trauma services. Moreover, they also stipulate that the following must be available at all times to provide uninterrupted clinical pathways to the patient's recovery:
➤ psychiatrists who prescribe appropriate medications
➤ inpatient beds for detoxification or home community detoxification services
➤ traumatic stress specialist psychiatrists, therapists and/or psychologists
➤ in some cases, inpatient specialist programmes.

Translation of theoretical clinical management into actual practice can be very difficult because of a lack of specialist psychological trauma and drugs and alcohol services. This is highlighted by the clinical case studies 9.1 and 9.2.

Case study 9.1: Nazim

Nazim (45) was forced to see his GP by his wife who threatened to leave him. He was assessed as suffering from acute alcohol withdrawal symptoms. He gave a history of drinking a whisky on a daily basis for the previous three years with bouts of heavy drinking spanning 25 years in all.

Nazim had served in the military and gave a history of being a Falkland Islands war veteran. Prior to the war in 1982, he had served in the army for four years including a six-month tour in Northern Ireland where he had used alcohol to cope with the stress of patrolling the streets. Nothing untoward had happened during his six-month tour there, although he felt constantly under threat. During the Falklands War, Nazim had been involved in many hours of close combat. His friend had been killed next to him.

On his return to the UK, Nazim was supported by his wife. Soon after the war, his alcohol intake increased from previous levels of perhaps five pints of beer on Friday and Saturday nights to five pints of beer most nights. He did this to reduce the nightmares and panic attacks. Nazim managed to hide his alcohol problems from his family and his superiors in the army until one day he was arrested for fighting. He was admitted to a military psychiatric hospital for alcohol detoxification on two occasions after this but he could not stop drinking. In the end, he was discharged from the army administratively. His nightmares and panic attacks were not picked up as they were masked by his alcohol consumption and the army took the view that alcohol dependence should lead to an administrative rather than a medical discharge.

After his discharge, Nazim worked briefly in a warehouse but it was soon felt that he was too disruptive at work. He was irritable and difficult to work with. He became more and more aggressive at home and his wife decided to leave him after he became aggressive towards her. Nazim lost his house and lived on the streets for a few months but then he found accommodation in a hostel for many months. Eventually, he was able to find accommodation in a bedsit thanks to an ex-service charity. He continued to live alone and drink heavily for many years until he met his second wife 10 years later. She too was recovering from alcohol dependence. Nazim continued to drink heavily, but was emotionally supported by his wife.

After assessment by his GP, Nazim was admitted to his local NHS medical ward where he received medical care and where he underwent a detoxification from his alcohol. He had vitamin deficiencies that were corrected using vitamin B supplements. He remained in hospital for six weeks.

After his detoxification, Nazim complained of progressively severe nightmares, flashbacks and intrusive memories pertaining to his military service in the Falklands. He became increasingly hyper-vigilant and irritable, avoided company, and became more isolated. Unfortunately, no NHS psychological trauma services were available and Nazim was referred locally to psychology services – but this had a waiting list of around 18 months. Fortunately, he was also known to the national charity Combat Stress that offers specialist services for ex-servicemen and combat veterans.

Nazim was able to attend for an initial five-day assessment admission to a treatment centre where multidisciplinary assessment confirmed his diagnosis of PTSD comorbidly present with depression in the context of long-standing alcohol dependence. Following this, he was seen in outpatients by a Combat Stress consultant psychiatrist who encouraged absolute abstinence from alcohol and who started Nazim on acamprosate to reduce alcohol cravings, as well as vitamin B supplements and mirtazapine in order to reduce PTSD symptoms and help to contain his depression. This was followed quickly by a 10-day admission where he received specialist alcohol and PTSD psychoeducation sessions as well as sessions of anger management, anxiety management, coping skills groups and preparation for trauma-focused psychotherapies. Nazim is now fully engaged in outpatient trauma-focused CBT. He has continued working as an administrator. Nazim's driving licence was taken away for a year – but then reinstated. His family, including his wife, have stood by him. Nazim understands he must remain abstinent from alcohol. His symptoms of PTSD, including nightmares and flashbacks, are being worked with in therapy and are improving.

Case study 9.2: Jane

When Jane was aged between five and 14 years, a neighbour repeatedly sexually abused her. She gave a history of 'sending' her mind to a safe place while she was being abused. As an adult, Jane presented to general mental health services with a history of deliberate self-harm by cutting, which was occurring twice a week. Jane also said she had periods where her mind would go blank. She had 'visions' of the abuse when she could also feel something painful inside her vagina, nightmares of the abuse, which occurred every night, and she could hear derogatory voices outside her head that turned out to be the voice of her perpetrator telling her she was worthless and that she should die. Jane had poor self-esteem, and suicidal ideas with plans to jump from a bridge. She also gave a two-year history of drinking between three and five (UK) units of alcohol every night in order to help herself sleep, as well as using amphetamines intermittently as this made her feel alive. She complained she felt emotionally numb otherwise.

Jane was initially assessed by the crisis team and a working diagnosis of schizoaffective disorder with borderline personality disorder and alcohol and drug abuse was made. She was admitted to a general adult ward because of her suicidal risk. She stopped using amphetamines. This together with the prescription of antipsychotic medication reduced the derogatory voices but did not stop her visions (flashbacks) and vaginal (somatic pain and tactile flashbacks) sensations and pain. This reduced over a period of weeks following the prescription of an antidepressant.

A second opinion was sought, and a diagnosis of PTSD (complex type) with comorbid depression and alcohol and amphetamine abuse was made. Following discharge from hospital, community psychiatric nurse (CPN) support did not stop her self-harming, nor did she stop her drug and alcohol misuse. Jane was admitted to a tertiary private sector specialist unit where she initially received individual and group sessions of mindfulness and other techniques used in dialectic behaviour therapy (DBT[85]– *see* Chapter 13; Book 4, Chapter 11) but not amounting to a full course of DBT. This was because her self-harming behaviours reduced and stopped quickly. With this support, Jane was also able to reduce and stop her alcohol and drug misuse. At the same tertiary private sector specialist unit, Jane then attended a highly structured 90-day programme comprising one month of psychoeducation about PTSD, including individual sessions of psychoeducation aimed at helping her to cope without self-harming, drinking and using illicit drugs. This was followed by a second month of trauma-focused CBT and then a final month of cognitive restructuring delivered through individual and group work and rehabilitation.[86] Jane was transferred back to her National Health Service (NHS) community mental health team (CMHT) and reviewed by the specialist PTSD service at six weeks, six months and over year follow-up points. By this time, Jane's PTSD, dissociative, affective and somatic symptoms had reduced and this was maintained over the follow-up period. There had been no further deliberate self-harm, and she had stopped abusing alcohol and illicit drugs. Jane continued to have support from her CMHT.

CONCLUSIONS

KEY POINT 9.5

PTSD commonly presents with comorbid substance use problems, especially with alcohol.

Treatment of PTSD can be difficult, especially if the individual has been exposed to multiple trauma. These presentations are more likely to also involve comorbid alcohol and substance use problems, including dependence, which can further complicate treatment and worsen the prognosis. Trauma-focused psychotherapies are essentially the treatment that reduces PTSD symptoms. Trauma-focused therapies will not work if information processing is impeded by illicit drug and alcohol use problems. Treatment of substance use problems must be undertaken before trauma-focused work can be performed.

KEY POINT 9.6

Specialist services for the treatment of these PTSD and substance use disorders must work together in order to facilitate clear smooth clinical pathways in order to ensure thorough intervention and treatment.

REFERENCES

1 American Psychiatric Association. *Diagnostic and Statistical Manual of Mental Disorders.* 4th ed. Washington, DC: American Psychiatric Association; 1994.

2 Rachmann S. Emotional processing. *Behaviour Research and Therapy.* 1980; **18**: 51–60.

3 Horowitz MJ. *Stress Response Syndromes.* 2nd ed. New York: Jason Aronson; 1986.

4 Horowitz MJ. Stress response syndromes. A review of posttraumatic stress and adjustment disorders. In: Wilson JP, Raphael B, editors. *International Handbook of Traumatic Stress Syndromes.* New York: Plenum Press; 1993. pp. 145–55.

5 Keane TM, Fairbank JA, Caddell RT, *et al.* A behavioural approach to assessing and treating PTSD in Vietnam veterans. In: Figley CR, editor. *Trauma and its Wake: the study and treatment of post traumatic stress disorder.* Vol. 1. New York: Brunner Mazel; 1985. pp. 257–94.

6 Green BL, Wilson JP, Lindy JD. Conceptualizing post-traumatic stress disorder: a psychosocial framework. In: Figley CR, editor. *Trauma and its Wake: the study and treatment of post traumatic stress disorder.* Vol. 1. New York: Brunner Mazel; 1985. pp. 53–69.

7 Green MA, Berlin MA. Five psychosocial variables related to the existence of post-traumatic stress disorder symptoms. *Journal of Clinical Psychology.* 1987; **43**: 643–9.

8 Green BL. Identifying survivors at risk. In: Wilson JP, Raphael B, editors. *International Handbook of Traumatic Stress Syndromes.* New York: Plenum Press; 1993. pp. 135–44.

9 Green BL, Lindy JD, Grace MC, *et al.* Multiple diagnosis in posttraumatic stress disorder. The role of war stressors. *Journal of Nervous and Mental Disorders.* 1989; **177**: 329–35.

10 Follette MV, Ruzek IJ, Aburg RF. *Cognitive Behaviour for Trauma.* New York: Guilford Press; 1998.

11 Foa EB, Rothbaum BO. *Treating the Trauma of Rape: cognitive-behavioural therapy for PTSD.* New York: Guilford Press; 1998.

12 Elhers A, Clark D. A cognitive model of post traumatic stress disorder. *Behaviour Research and Therapy.* 2000; **38**: 319–45.

13 van der Kolk BA, McFarlane AC, Weisaeth L. *Traumatic Stress: the effects of overwhelming experience in the mind, body and society.* New York: Guilford Press; 1996.

14 Pitman R. Neuroimaging findings in PTSD. Conference presentation: trapped by trauma; dissociation and other responses. Defence Medical Services Psychological Injuries Unit. International Conference. York, 26–27 October 2000.

15 Shalev A. Keynote address. *ESTSS Seventh European Conference on Traumatic Stress Studies.* Edinburgh, 26–29 May 2001.

16 Brewin CR. A cognitive neuroscience account of post traumatic stress disorder and its treatment. *Behaviour Research and Therapy.* 2001; **39**: 373–93.

17 Brewin CR, Holmes EA. Psychological theories of post traumatic stress disorder. *Clinical Psychology Review.* 2003; **23**: 339–76.

18 Brewin CR, Dalgliesh T, Joseph S. A dual representation theory of post traumatic stress disorder. *Psychological Review.* 1996; **103**: 670–86.

19 Goldberg J, True WR, Eisen SA, *et al.* A twin study of the effects of the Vietnam War on post-traumatic stress disorder. *Journal of the American Medical Association.* 1990; **263**: 1227–32.

20 Kulka R, Schlenger WE. Survey research and field designs for the study of posttraumatic stress disorder. In: Wilson JP, Raphael B, editors. *International Handbook of Traumatic Stress Syndromes.* New York: Plenum Press; 1993. pp. 145–55.

21 True WR, Rice J, Eisen SA, *et al.* A twin study of genetic and environmental contributions to liability for post traumatic symptoms. *Archives of General Psychiatry.* 1993; **50**: 257–64.

22 Janoff-Bulman R. The aftermath of victimisation: rebuilding shattered assumptions. In:

Figley CR, editor. *Trauma and its Wake: the study and treatment of post traumatic stress disorder.* Vol. 1. New York: Brunner Mazel; 1985. pp. 15–35.

23 Creamer M, Morris P, Biddle D, *et al.* Treatment outcome in Australian veterans with combat related posttraumatic stress disorder: a cause for cautious optimism? *Journal of Traumatic Stress.* 1999; **12**: 625–41.

24 Parkes CM. Psycho-social transitions: a field for study. *Social Science and Medicine.* 1971; **5**: 101–15.

25 Flannery RB. Social support and psychological trauma: a methodological review. *Journal of Traumatic Stress.* 1990; **3**: 593–611.

26 Marmar CR, Weiss DS, Metzler T. Peritraumatic dissociation and post traumatic stress disorder. In: Bremner JD, Marmar CR, editors. *Trauma Memory and Dissociation.* Washington, DC: American Psychiatric Press; 1998. pp. 229–52.

27 Davidson JRT, Kudler H, Smith R. Personality in chronic post-traumatic stress disorder: a study of the Eynseck inventory. *Journal of Anxiety Disorders.* 1987; **1**: 295–300.

28 McFarlane AC. The longitudinal course of post traumatic stress morbidity: the range of outcomes and their predictors. *Journal of Nervous and Mental Disorders.* 1988; **176**: 30–9.

29 McFarlane AC. The aetiology of post traumatic stress disorders following a natural disaster. *British Journal Psychiatry.* 1988; **152**: 116–21.

30 Kulka R, Schlenger WE, Firbank JA, *et al. Trauma and the Vietnam War Generation: report of findings from the National Vietnam Veterans Readjustment Study.* New York: Brunner Mazel; 1990.

31 Schnurr PP, Friedman MJ, Rosenberg SD. Premilitary MMPI scores as predictors of combat-related PTSD symptoms. *American Journal of Psychiatry.* 1993; **150**: 479–83.

32 Smith EM, North CS. *Aftermath of a Disaster: psychological response to the Indianapolis Ramda jet crash. Quick Response Research Report 23.* Boulder, CO: Natural Hazards Research and Applications Information Center; 1988.

33 Steinglass P, Gerrity E. Natural disasters and post-traumatic stress disorder: short-term versus long-term recovery in two disaster-affected communities. *Journal of Applied Social Psychology.* 1990; **20**: 1746–56.

34 Green BL, Lindy JD, Grace MC. Buffalo Creek survivors in the second decade: stability of stress symptoms. *American Journal of Orthopsychiatry.* 1990; **60**: 43–54.

35 Chemtob CM, Baner GB, Neller G. Post-traumatic stress disorder among special forces Vietnam veterans. *Military Medicine.* 1990; **155**: 16–20.

36 Noy S. Stress and personality as factors in the causation and prognosis of combat reactions during the 1973 Arab-Israeli war. In: Belenky GL, editor. *Contemporary Studies in Combat Psychiatry.* Westport, CT: Greenwood Press; 1987. pp. 21–9.

37 Solomon Z, Prager E. Elderly Israeli Holocaust survivors during the Persian Gulf War: a study of psychological distress. *American Journal of Psychiatry.* 1992; **149**: 1707–10.

38 Bell P, Kee M, Loughrey G. Post-traumatic stress disorder in Northern Ireland. *Acta Psychiatrica Scandinavica.* 1988; **77**: 166–9.

39 Chu JA. The victimisation of adult women with histories of childhood abuse. *Journal of Psychotherapy, Practice and Research.* 1992; **1**: 259–69.

40 Lauterbach D, Varna S. The relationship among personality variables, exposure to traumatic events and severity of post traumatic stress symptoms. *Journal of Traumatic Stress.* 2001; **14**: 29–45.

41 International Classification of Diseases. *Classification of Mental and Behavioural Disorders: Clinical Descriptions and Diagnostic Guidelines.* 10th ed. Geneva: World Health Organization; 1992.

42 Herman JL. Complex PTSD: a syndrome in survivors of prolonged and repeated trauma. *Journal of Traumatic Stress*. 1992; **1**: 377–91.

43 Herman JL. Sequelae of prolonged and repeated trauma: evidence for a complex post traumatic syndrome (DESNOS). In: Davidson JRT, Foa ED, editors. *Posttraumatic Stress Disorder. DSM-IV and Beyond*. Washington, DC: American Psychiatric Press; 1993. pp. 213–28.

44 van der Kolk BA, Roth S, Pelcovitz D, *et al. Complex Post Traumatic Stress Disorder. Results from the DSM-IV Field trial for PTSD*. New York: American Psychiatric Association; 1994.

45 van der Kolk BA, Roth S, Pelcovitz D, *et al.* Disorders of extreme stress: the empirical foundation of a complex adaptation to trauma. *Journal of Traumatic Stress*. 2005; **18**: 389–99.

46 Roth S, Newman E, Pelcovitz D, *et al.* Complex PTSD in victims exposed to sexual and physical abuse: results from the DSM-IV field trial for posttraumatic stress disorder. *Journal of Traumatic Stress*. 1997; **10**: 539–56.

47 Bloom S. *Creating Sanctuary: toward the evolution of sane societies*. London: Routledge; 1997.

48 Gunderson J. The borderline patient's intolerance of aloneness: insecure attachments and therapist availability. *American Journal of Psychiatry*. 1996; **153**: 752–8.

49 Gunderson J, Sabo AN. The phenomenological and conceptual interface between Borderline Personality Disorder and PTSD. *American Journal of Psychiatry*. 1996; **150**: 19–27.

50 Helzer JE, Robins LN, McEvoy L. Post-traumatic stress disorder in the general population. Findings of the epidemiological catchment area survey. *New England Journal of Medicine*. 1987; **317**: 1630–4.

51 Hryvniak MR. Concurrent psychiatric illness in inpatients with post-traumatic stress disorder. *Military Medicine*. 1989; **154**: 399–401.

52 Shore JH, Vollmer WM, Tatum E. Community patterns of post traumatic stress disorders. *Journal of Nervous and Mental Disorders*. 1989; **177**: 681–5.

53 Davidson JRT, Hughes D, Blazer D, *et al.* Post-traumatic stress disorder in the community: an epidemiological study. *Psychological Medicine*. 1991; **21**: 713–21.

54 McFarlane AC, Papay P. Multiple diagnoses in posttraumatic stress disorder in the victims of a natural disaster. *Journal of Nervous and Mental Disorders*. 1992; **180**: 498–504.

55 Davidson JRT, Fairbank JA. The epidemiology of post traumatic stress disorder. In: Davidson JRT, Foa EB, editors. *Posttraumatic Stress Disorder. DSM-IV and Beyond*. Washington, DC: American Psychiatric Press; 1993. pp. 147–69.

56 Busuttil W. *Psychometric Data Analyses and Clinical Audit Data for Combat Stress 2005–2009*. Internal publication. Leatherhead, England: Combat Stress; 2009.

57 Fletcher KD. Combat Stress (the Ex-Servicemen's Mental Welfare Society) and War Veterans. In: Lee H, Jones E, editors. *Lessons from the Gulf War*. London: Wiley; 2007.

58 Iversen AC, Greenberg N. Mental health of regular and reserve military veterans. *Advances in Psychiatry*. 2009; **15**: 100–6.

59 Reynolds M, Mezey G, Chapman M, *et al.* Co-morbid post-traumatic stress disorder in a substance misusing clinical population. *Drug and Alcohol Dependence*. 2005; **77**(3): 251–8.

60 Sareen J, Cox BJ, Goodwin RD, *et al.* Co-occurrence of posttraumatic stress disorder with positive psychotic symptoms in a nationally representative sample. *Journal of Traumatic Stress*. 2005; **18**: 313–22.

61 Kessler RC, Sonnega A, Bromet E, *et al.* Posttraumatic stress disorder in the National Comorbidity Survey. *Archives of General Psychiatry*. 1995; **52**: 1048–60.

62 Kendler KS, Bulik CM, Silberg J, *et al.* Childhood sexual abuse and adult psychiatric and

substance misuse disorders in women: an epidemiological and co-twin analysis. *Archives of General Psychiatry*. 2000; **57**: 953–9.

63 Monlar BE, Buka SL, Kessler RC. Child sexual abuse and subsequent pathology: results from the national comorbidity survey. *American Journal of Public Health*. 2001; **91**: 753–60.

64 Langeland W, Drajjer N, van den Brink W. Assessment of lifetime physical and sexual abuse in treated alcoholics. Validity of the Addiction Severity Index. *Addictive Behaviors*. 2002; **28**: 871–8.

65 Kilpatrick DG, Acierno R, Saunders B, *et al*. Risk factors for adolescent substance abuse and dependence: data from a national sample. *Journal of Consulting and Clinical Psychology*. 2000: **68**: 19–30.

66 Duncan RD, Saunders BE, Kilpatrick DG, *et al*. Childhood physical assault as a risk factor for PTSD, depression, and substance misuse: findings from a national survey. *American Journal of Orthopsychiatry*. 1996; **66**: 437–48.

67 Miller BA, Downs WR, Gondoli DM, *et al*. The role of childhood sexual abuse in the development of alcoholism in women. *Violence and Victims*. 1987; **2**: 157–72.

68 Miller BA, Downs WR, Testa M. Interrelationships between victimisation experiences and women's alcohol use. *Journal of Studies on Alcohol*. 1993; **11**: 109–17.

69 Golding JM. Intimate partner violence as a risk factor for mental disorders: a meta-analysis. *Journal of Family Violence*. 1999; **14**: 99–132.

70 Sullivan TP, Holt L. PTSD symptom clusters are differentially related to substance misuse among community women exposed to intimate partner violence. *Journal of Traumatic Stress*. 2008; **21**: 173–80.

71 Ritter J, Stewart M, Bernet C, *et al*. Effects of childhood exposure to familial alcoholism and family violence on adolescent substance use, conduct problems, and self-esteem. *Journal of Traumatic Stress*. 2002; **15**: 113–22.

72 Kaysen D, Simpson T, Dillworth T, *et al*. Alcohol problems and posttraumatic stress disorder in female crime victims. *Journal of Traumatic Stress*. 2006; **19**: 399–403.

73 Parrott DJ, Dorbes J, Saladin ME, *et al*. Perpetration of partner violence: effects of cocaine and alcohol dependence and posttraumatic stress disorder. *Addictive Behaviors*. 2003; **9**: 1587–602.

74 Savarese VW, Suvak MK, King LA, *et al*. Relationships among alcohol use, hyperarousal and marital abuse and violence in Vietnam veterans. *Journal of Traumatic Stress*. 2001; **14**: 717–32.

75 Stewart SH. Alcohol abuse in individuals exposed to trauma: a critical review. *Psychological Bulletin*. 1996; **120**: 83–112.

76 Abueg FR, Fairbank JA. Behavioural treatment of post traumatic stress disorder and co-occurring substance abuse. In: Saigh PA, editor. *Post Traumatic Stress Disorder: a behavioural approach to assessment and treatment*. Boston: Allyn & Bacon; 1992. pp. 111–46.

77 Grayson CE, Nolen-Hoeksema S. Motives to drink as mediators between childhood sexual assault and alcohol problems in adult women. *Journal of Traumatic Stress*. 2005; **18**: 137–45.

78 Min M, Farkas K, Minnes S, *et al*. Impact of childhood abuse and neglect on substance abuse and psychological distress in adulthood. *Journal of Traumatic Stress*. 2007; **20**: 833–44.

79 National Institute of Health and Clinical Excellence (NICE). *Guideline No 26: post traumatic stress disorder in adults and children in primary, secondary care*. London and Leicester: Gaskill and British Psychological Society; 2005. Available at: www.nice.org.uk/nicemedia/pdf/CG026fullguideline.pdf (accessed 7 March 2011).

80 Busuttil W. Complex post-traumatic stress disorder: a useful diagnostic framework? *Psychiatry*. **8**(8): 310–14.

81 United Kingdom Trauma Group (UKTG). *Statement on Complex PTSD*. London: United Kingdom Trauma Group; 2009.

82 Hill DM, Busuttil W. Dual diagnosis in service veterans with post traumatic stress disorder and co-existing substance abuse. *Advances in Dual Diagnosis*. 2008; **8**: 33–6.

83 Jelinek JM, Williams T. Post-traumatic stress disorder and substance abuse: treatment problems, strategies and recommendations. In: Williams T, editor. *Post Traumatic Stress Disorders: a handbook for clinicians.* Ohio: Disabled American Veterans; 1987. pp. 103–15.

84 Steindl SR, Young RM, Creamer M, *et al.* Hazardous alcohol use and treatment outcome in male combat veterans with post traumatic stress disorder. *Journal of Traumatic Stress.* 2003; **16**: 27–34.

85 Linehan MM. *Cognitive Behavioural Treatment of Borderline Personality Disorder*. New York: Guilford Press; 1993.

86 Busuttil W. The development of a 90 day residential program for the treatment of Complex Post Traumatic Stress Disorder. *Journal of Aggression, Maltreatment and Trauma.* 2006; **12**: 29–55.

TO LEARN MORE

- Combat Stress. Available at: http://combatstress.org.uk/
- International Society for Traumatic Stress Studies. Available at: http://istss.org/
- European Society for Traumatic Stress Studies. Available at: http://estss.org/
- UK Trauma Group. Available at www.uk.trauma group.org/
- UK Psychological Trauma Society. Available at: www.ukpts.co.uk/
- Bloom S, editor. *Creating Sanctuary: toward the evolution of sane societies*. London: Routledge; 1997.
- Foa EB, Keane TM, Friedman MJ, *et al.*, editors. *Effective Treatments for PTSD: practice guidelines from the International Society for Traumatic Stress Studies*. New York: Guilford Press; 2009.
- Nasser M, Baistow K, Treasure J, editors. *When the Body Speaks its Mind: the interface between the female body and mental health*. London: Routledge; 2007.
- Teherani N, editor. *Managing Trauma in the Work Place: supporting workers and organisations*. Oxford: Routledge; 2010.
- van der Kolk BA, McFarlane AC, Weisaeth L, editors. *Traumatic Stress: the effects of overwhelming experience in the mind, body and society*. New York: Guilford Press; 1996.
- Williams MB, Garrick J, editors. *Trauma Treatment Techniques: innovative trends*. New York: Haworth Press; 2006.

CHAPTER 10

Attention deficit hyperactivity disorder and substance use

Arthur G O'Malley

INTRODUCTION

This chapter examines the role in which substance use may play prenatally in the aetiology of attention deficit hyperactivity disorder (ADHD), and how this can lead to problems with both attention and impulsivity. In addition, it outlines the pre- and peri-natal environmental risks for ADHD, and the potential role of genetic processes in mediating susceptibility. The evidence linking substance use to early behavioural problems, and how this links with both emotional regulation and dys-regulation, is reviewed. The latter is now assumed to be a precursor to ADHD. The chapter concludes with a therapeutic approach developed by the author which can help alleviate many of the symptoms of emotional dysregulation, which underlie the later development of ADHD.

EMOTIONAL DYSREGULATION BRAINSTEM FUNCTIONING AND ADHD

Geva and Feldman[1] have proposed a neurobiological model for the effects of early brainstem functioning on the development of behaviour and emotional regulation in infants. The model proposes links between functions that are mediated by the brainstem, such as cardiac regulatory tone with higher order cognitive and social self-regulatory outcomes, which may be directly mediated by attention modula-tion and stress management. It is crucial to do further research in the area between brainstem dysfunction and higher order prefrontal mediated functions linking the limbic system and the cortical system. The links between brainstem disorders and deficits in higher cortical skills underlies evidence for the development of attention deficit hyperactivity disorder and potentially conduct disorder.

WHAT EVIDENCE EXISTS FOR SUBSTANCE USE DISORDERS CAUSING ADHD?

Evidence for early damage to the foetal brain comes from several studies. One study[2] examined possible neurotoxic effects of prenatal methamphetamine (meth) on the developing brain and on cognition. Ten meth-exposed and nine unexposed chil-dren had magnetic resonance imaging (MRI) scans and completed neurocognitive assessments. Meth-exposed children scored lower on measures of visual motor integration, attention, verbal memory and long-term facial memory. Despite having similar whole brain volumes in each group, the meth-exposed children had smaller volumes in the following areas:

➤ putamen
➤ globus pallidus
➤ hippocampus
➤ caudate.

These structures, if small, will have less integration with brainstem structures and these abnormalities correlate with poorer performance on sustained attention and delayed verbal memory. Thus, compared to the controlled group, this small number of children exposed to meth prenatally exhibited smaller sub-cortical volumes and had some associated neurocognitive deficits in attention and impulsivity. These preliminary findings suggest prenatal meth exposure may be neurotoxic to the developing brain and lead to the development of either ADHD or conduct disorder.

Another study[3] assessed a component of attention known as **selective attention** in a large poly substance cocaine-exposed cohort of four-year-olds. Studies of maternal pregnancy with use of cocaine and cigarettes showed both were associated with increased number of commission errors indicating inferior selective attention. Severity of maternal use of marijuana during pregnancy was positively correlated with omission errors suggesting impaired sustained attention. Substance exposure effects in pregnancy were independent of:

➤ maternal post-partum state
➤ psychological distress
➤ birth mother cognitive functioning
➤ caregiver functioning
➤ other substance exposure
➤ the child's verbal IQ.

This research suggests that exposure to substances such as cocaine and marijuana interferes with children's attentional abilities at four years of age, and that this could easily lead to the development of symptoms of ADHD or conduct disorder.

RISK FACTORS ASSOCIATED WITH ADHD-LIKE DEFICITS

Examples of specific *in utero* risk factors associated with ADHD-like deficits include prenatal exposure to:

➤ nicotine[4]
➤ alcohol[5]
➤ recreational drugs[6]
➤ polychlorinated biphenyls (PCBs)[7]
➤ hexachlorobenzene[8]
➤ glucocortocoids[9]
➤ maternal stress during pregnancy[10]
➤ poor maternal diet[11]

In addition, prematurity resulting in small size at birth is a very strong environmental predictor of ADHD symptoms in childhood.[12]

Many of these substances can pass directly and rapidly across the placenta to the developing foetus where they have effects on the developing central nervous system. There is also likely to be an effect on the normal hypothalamic-pituitary-adrenal axis (HPA) functioning. We are now at a stage where it is possible to investigate the ways in which environmental factors act upon the gene to bring about epigenetic changes in both gene expression and behaviour. This will help us to have an increased understanding of the risk factors for ADHD and, in particular, the dynamic nature of the epigenome means that any disruption is potentially reversible. There are a high number of mothers who continue to expose their unborn infants to risk factors for ADHD. Approximately 20% of pregnant women continue to drink moderate amounts of alcohol, and 25% of pregnant women who smoke continue to do so during pregnancy.[13] The risk of developing psychiatric disorders such as ADHD should inform public policy so that mothers are aware of the risk to their unborn babies of exposure to toxins during pregnancy.

IMPACT OF SMOKING IN PREGNANCY IN RELATION TO ADHD

In utero exposure to smoking and alcohol are common risk factors that have been associated in human beings and animal models with ADHD. In addition, many molecular studies have focused on the association between ADHD and abnormalities of dopamine pathway-related genes such as the dopamine transporter gene (DAT1). Neuman and Lobos[14] studied the relationship between ADHD and the DAT1 and dopamine receptor D4 (DRD4) polymorphisms and prenatal substance exposure in a birth record sample of male and female twin pairs aged seven to 19. The interactions between prenatal exposure to smoking with variations in both the DAT1 and DRD4 polymorphisms were observed in children with ADHD. The odds ratio for exposed children with both variants of the dopamine allele was 9.0 indicating that smoking during pregnancy is associated with specific subtypes of ADHD in children who are genetically susceptible. One implication of this is that genetic testing could be done on mothers to advise them of their increased risk of their children developing ADHD if they smoke and have either the DAT1 or the DRD4 polymorphisms in which their risk is substantially increased.

This research builds on the work of Biederman and colleagues,[15] which looked at the association between ADHD and prenatal exposure to maternal cigarette smoking, drug use and alcohol. They also sought to rule out confounding variables such as maternal depression, conduct disorder, and indicators of social diversity in the environment.

Method

This was a retrospective hospital-based case-controlled study conducted with 280 ADHD cases and 242 non-ADHD controls of both genders. ADHD cases were shown to be 2.1 times more likely to be exposed to cigarettes and 2.5 times more likely to be exposed to alcohol *in utero* than were the non-ADHD controlled subjects. Following adjustment by psychopathology, Rutter's indicators[15] of social diversity and comorbid conduct disorder did not count for any prenatal exposure to alcohol or cigarettes. Thus, these researchers were able to conclude that ADHD was likely to be an additional deleterious outcome associated with prenatal exposure to alcohol that is independent of the risk between prenatal exposure to nicotine and other familiar risks with the disorder.

A further study[16] determined to explore whether there was an association between mothers drinking lightly during pregnancy and the risk of behavioural problems and the cognitive deficits in their children at three years of age. Drinking patterns during pregnancy and behavioural and cognitive outcomes were assessed during both interviews and home visits. Behavioural problems were indicated by scores above cut-off points on the parent report version of the Strength and Difficulties Questionnaire (SDQ).[17] Cognitive ability was assessed using the naming vocabulary subscale from the British Ability Scale (BAS)[18] and the Bracken School Readiness Assessment (BSRA).[19] The results of this large representative study showed that at three years of age, children born to mothers who drank not more than one to two drinks per occasion during their pregnancy were not at increased risk of clinically relevant behavioural problems or cognitive deficits compared with children whose mothers did not drink. Boys born to light drinking mothers were less likely to have conduct and hyperactivity problems and these differences remained after statistical adjustment. Boys born to light drinking mothers had higher scores on cognitive ability assessments and for the test on colours, shapes, numbers and letters.

The results of this detailed analysis suggests that there is no risk of behavioural problems or cognitive deficits at three years of age for children whose mothers drank not more than one or two (UK) units of alcohol per week or on any given occasion. It is important to recognise that problem behaviours or cognitive deficits may become apparent in these children of older ages but the evidence presented should be used to guide future research and inform governmental policy.

Future work on the effects of low levels of drinking during pregnancy should consider longer-term developments on behavioural problems and cognitive development. This study used the Millennium Cohort Study,[20] which is funded by grants from the Economic and Social Research Council (ESRC).

FOETAL ALCOHOL SPECTRUM DISORDERS (FASD)

Foetal alcohol spectrum disorders describe a range of conditions in affected foetuses caused by alcohol ingestion in the mother. It is difficult to diagnose the disorder. The effects can depend on the amount of alcohol consumed at specific points in the pregnancy. Broad structures, such as the face, develop early in pregnancy (first trimester) whereas in the third trimester the brain undergoes rapid expansion in terms of white matter gliosis and cell migration. Further research is needed to elucidate the prevalence and characteristic features at different rates of foetal exposure to alcohol during each of the three trimesters.

FASD – the geneticist's view

Dr Shane McKee, clinical geneticist, Northern Ireland, states that, '*alcohol ingested during pregnancy is a proven morphological and neurological teratogen*'.[21]

A child with FASD will show:

➤ developmental delay/learning disability
➤ disruptive behaviour disorders, e.g. autism spectrum disorder (ASD), ADHD, oppositional defiance disorder (ODD), and conduct disorder
➤ microcephaly due to alcohol-induced neuronal cell loss
➤ shortened stature
➤ dysmorphic facial features, e.g. thin upper lip, long smooth philtrum, arched eyebrows and a small nose
➤ jitteriness in neonatal period, unstable temperature and low blood glucose.

The commonest clinical presentation of FASD is ADHD or hyperkinetic disorder. These children show a mixture of hyperactivity, impulsivity and inattention. They may also have specific learning difficulties, e.g. dyscalculia, dyslexia and disorders of written expression. Further clinical characteristics include:
➤ increased suicide risk in adolescents with FASD due to poor tolerance of frustration rather than depression
➤ evidence of deficits in executive function coincided with damage to corpus callosum, hippocampus and cerebellum
➤ a greater history of alcohol craving in those children with antenatal exposure compared to children with a family history of alcoholism.

FASD has been associated with a range of neurological deficits. Green and colleagues[22] showed that children with FASD have deficits in sensory, motor and cognitive processing as evidenced by a developmental delay in oculomotor control. Of note, this would leave this cohort of children potentially less responsive to a new therapeutic paradigm this author has developed: affect regulation therapy (ART). Affect regulation therapy reprocesses memories at a somatosensory, motor, emotional and intercerebral level. Bilateral brainstem activation stimulates oculomotor nerves and cerebellar activity leading to desensitisation and reprocessing of the event. This helps the child to better regulate their emotions and avoid going into a state of either hyper or hypo-arousal.

Treatment options for individuals with FASD
There are a range of interventions, as follows.

Educational
Educational approaches can be tailored to the individual's deficits such as working memory. Santosefano and colleagues, describe cognitive control therapy (CCT),[23] which aims to progressively build cognitive skills. Children with FASD can have their needs met within the Special Education Needs (SEN) system. Adults with FASD also require education-based interventions; however, these are rarely provided.

Psychological
Wide ranges of disorders are comorbid with FASD and can require input from a multidisciplinary team experienced in dealing with child and adolescent mental health problems. Profiles of the individual's strengths and weaknesses can enable

a tailored package of care. Educating the carers, i.e. parents or guardians on the suspected neurodevelopmental trajectory of the disorder, can prepare them for future difficulties. Early intervention for prevention of secondary disabilities has not yet been researched.

Psychosocial

In terms of psychosocial interventions, one study[24] reported on outcomes of 100 children aged six to 12 with FASD who were given Child Friendship Training (CFT). Clinical psychology trainees delivered the programme and showed improvements in social behaviour at three months follow-up.

Pharmacological

There is no specific drug treatment for FASD. If comorbid with ADHD it is likely that stimulants will have an unpredictable response due to the brain abnormalities in FASD. If features of ADHD are present, medication should be part of a comprehensive plan including parent management training and liaison with education.

Nutritional

Newer nutritional approaches have been tried. Choline is an essential nutrient present in beef, liver, egg yolks and soya beans. It is part of the neurotransmitter acetylcholine needed for learning and memory. Benefits may be as a result of increasing the levels of nerve growth factor (NGF). At present research has been on animals and clinical trials are awaited.

Behavioural

Behavioural interventions such as bimanual coordination have been suggested.[25] Tests of bimanual coordination show that this is decreased in patients with FASD compared to controls. Thus, there is the potential for bimanual exercises commenced in early childhood to be a potential treatment for FASD. The theory is that children with FASD would be able to complete more complex tasks progressively, demanding greater inter-hemispheric information transfer. The downstream effects would be less disruptive behaviour and improved executive control. Clinical trials are necessary to prove efficacy of this approach. The author's novel affect regulation therapy approach could also be tested out on this clinical population.

Despite the lack of treatment, FASD is a common preventable cause of learning disability and all professionals coming into contact with children must strive to diagnose the condition in infancy and immediately commence the most appropriate intervention.

SUMMARY

There has been increased interest in the developmental origins of substance use disorders in children and adolescents. Because of its early onset, high prevalence and known risk for substance use disorders (SUDs), ADHD is a developmental disorder which is ideally placed to evaluate the interrelationship with SUDs. In this selective review of the literature, ADHD and comorbid psychopathology have been found to increase the risk for smoking cigarettes and substance use disorders.

However, the treatment of ADHD appears to decrease the risk of cigarette smoking and substance use disorders. Early treatment of ADHD can help to prevent further associated comorbidity.

The chapter now progresses to discuss early associations of ADHD with emotional dysregulation and what can be done to treat this disorder in the context of maternal–infant relationship. As mentioned in the introduction, it is likely that epigenetic factors, i.e. heritable but reversible changes to genomic function that are independent of deoxyribonucleic acid (DNA) sequence, are also important. These processes can be induced following exposure to a range of external factors. It is possible that understanding the processes involved in linking specific environmental factors to an increased risk of ADHD will offer new possibilities for prevention or therapeutic intervention.

The following case study illustrates some of the comorbidity between emotional dysregulation ADHD and substance misuse. In addition, it outlines the principles of the new theoretical paradigm (developed by the author) called affect regulation therapy.[26] This is an amalgamation of information processing from a top-down and bottom-up perspective.

Case study 10.1: Anthony

Anthony (19) was having major issues with his girlfriend during the summer and he had been having arguments recently with his mum. The incident with Anthony's girlfriend Sue happened when they were on holiday. Anthony started drinking and being sick. He remembers blacking out. Only bits of the assault have come into his head. At one point, he remembers Sue saying, 'Get off me'; at that point, he was trying to strangle her. He felt bad about this and ran out of the hotel but was brought back by the manager. We processed the fragmented memory through the therapeutic technique ART. We continued to process this event and linked it to an episode when Anthony was five. He was thrown round the room by his father (when visiting him), and remembers feeling his head as it was sore from the incident.

Anthony described the trauma narrative. Anthony's mother had told him that his father was on drugs. When he repeated this to his father, his father came into the room and threw him towards the bed. He hit his head on the wall. Anthony bit his dad's finger, and was then punched by his father, and left on his own in the room. At the time, Anthony thought his father was going to kill him. His main feelings were of upset and anger towards his mother, and believing that it was his own fault. Once this had been processed, this linked to another memory he had at the age of four, when his father put handcuffs on Anthony and went out. He slept on the bed – he felt abandoned and lonely – no one cared when he shouted for help. He described how his father came back and gave him a yoyo and sweets. However, this had a significant impact on Anthony, particularly the thought of abandonment and being left alone. This was reprocessed until he was able to experience a sense of relief as the anger that was previously in his body dissipated and he felt a lot lighter in himself. This was a good example of the linked processing between anger and substance use and ADHD using an affect reprocessing therapy technique.

Anthony had been attending the service for several years and had been treated mainly with methylphenidate medication which had been increased to 90 mg of Concerta XL mane. Although he was responding to this dose of medication, episodes of anger outbursts were starting to happen on an increased basis. We became confident that this anger had started to diffuse and that Anthony would be better able to choose his behaviour rather than as if he was re-experiencing traumatic events from his past.

Often after the first session of ART, issues can arise that have previously been stored unconsciously. During our next session, Anthony described feelings of depression. However, his mother reported that there were significant unresolved issues of anger. Anthony remained upset by the fact that he had hurt Sue during their row. We started to locate this feeling of upset and anger and his pains in his chest and head area. It then extended to cover all of his body with repeated bilateral stimulation during the process of affect reprocessing therapy.

As Anthony had previously no conscious memory of the attack, Sue reported this. As this process started, he became aware of a twitchy feeling in his right leg. Anthony reported that the evening had started with him pushing Sue onto the bed. He was acting as if in a rage and Sue stated that for a few moments she was unable to breathe and she could not get the key to escape from the room. Sue spent some time unsuccessfully calling for help – and was unable to get out. When Anthony had calmed down, Sue was able to retrieve the key from his pocket. Eventually, she got to a phone and rang her sister. However, a further argument ensued as Anthony ran off after her. Anthony only remembered meeting up with her and discussing the incident from this point on. The opportunity to reprocess this information, while being activated with bilateral auditory stimulation, gave Anthony the chance to develop remorse for his actions.

We were then able to reprocess a more recent argument with his mum. This had started with his mum asking Anthony to do 'lots of jobs'. Anthony believes he is never directly thanked for the work that he does. He had gone out to get some material for a DIY (do-it-yourself) task. When he returned home, there had been an argument over the family pets. The situation would quickly escalate with both Anthony and his mum shouting at each other with increasing ferocity. Anthony stated that he feels that he has to shoulder the burden of task in the house as his mum has physical ill health and claims to be unable to do these tasks.

Of interest during the processing of this memory, Anthony was able to access an early episode of being exposed to drugs when he was only aged four. Anthony described how, at that stage of his childhood, his father was a heroin addict. He would often 'shoot up' in front of him. This was often in the company of several of his drug addict friends. Anthony could clearly remember seeing these people smoke heroin and cocaine and, for amusement, they starting hitting him – they thought it was funny. Anthony was now able to realise how damaging this behaviour was towards him. He described how eventually his mum and uncle rescued him.

As we accessed the feelings that needed to be reprocessed these were strongly located in his gut and were associated with a feeling of disgust and wanting to be sick. Anthony had a very strong feeling of hate towards his dad, which was located in his arms. This then was transformed into a light-headed feeling. He felt as if everything was swaying from side to side. Anthony was encouraged to stick with his feeling and to track and process it until it would resolve. Eventually, Anthony pointed to the back of his neck, i.e. the brainstem, where he could feel the pain disappearing and transforming into a sense of healing and recovery. Eventually, Anthony pointed to his left cerebral cortex. Here he could feel resolution of the experience and complete transformation of the difficult feelings. We discussed how Anthony would now deal with any difficult situations in the future, and we agreed that he would let it all pass. Anthony wants to improve his relationship with Sue and now could accept that those difficult childhood experiences were over. We also agreed that we would have an appointment for family therapy to discuss ongoing family issues.

CONCLUSION

Reprocessing these traumatic memories can activate repressed memories associated with the original event. In this case, the symptoms of ADHD are now much more manageable as the underlying emotional dysregulation has been reprocessed effectively. As we gain a greater understanding of affective neuroscience and the regulation of emotion in infancy, approaches such as ART, which access early somatosensory experiences, could become a cornerstone of future therapy.

In the author's clinical practice, a complete developmental history includes any toxins, e.g. drugs (prescribed or illicit), nicotine, or alcohol exposure in pregnancy. In addition, a modified attachment interview of the child,[27] to draw out the parental–infant relationship in the first five years, is applied. This author is especially interested to see if the Erikson stages of childhood development[28] have been negotiated. In the first 18 months, the infant hopes to seek out a trusting relationship with a primary caregiver. If this does not occur, the basis for mistrust in relationships is laid down. From 18 months to three years, the role of will in identifying autonomy takes precedence. If this is not successfully negotiated, shame and relentless self-doubt can occur. Early evaluation of attachment relationships can help with the formulation and development of an effective care plan.

In summary, the author has discussed the factors in pregnancy associated with the development of ADHD and hyperkinetic disorders. The effect of substance use disorders in pregnancy was illustrated with reference to the relevant literature. Each substance from alcohol to methamphetamine to cocaine has selective impairments on the attention system. The precursor of ADHD is often emotional regulation. There is an increased incidence of traumatic stress in the author's clinical experience often due to impaired attachments and parent–child relationships.

This was illustrated via Anthony's case history. The therapeutic approach, ART, was used to help Anthony develop a state of emotional regulation from his previous state of dysregulation. He was subsequently able to engage in family therapy and became sufficiently motivated to improve his significant interpersonal relationships.

There is a need for continued research into the links between substance use disorders and ADHD so that the professional can improve the treatment options for these individuals experiencing complex mental health needs.

REFERENCES

1 Geva R, Feldman RA. A neurobiological model for the effects of early brainstem functioning on the development of behaviour and emotion regulation in infants: implications for prenatal and perinatal risk. *Journal of Child Psychology and Psychiatry.* 2008; **49**: 1031–41.

2 Chang L, Smith LM, Lo Presti C, *et al.* Smaller subcortical volumes and cognitive deficits in children with methamphetamine exposure. *Psychiatry Research.* 2002; **132**: 95–106.

3 Noland JS, Singer LT, Short EJ, *et al.* Prenatal drug exposure and selective attention in pre-schoolers: *Neurotoxicology and Teratology.* 2005; **27**: 429–38.

4 Linnet KM, Dalsgaard S, Obel C, *et al.* Maternal lifestyle factors in pregnancy, risk of attention deficit hyperactivity disorder and associated behaviours: review of the current evidence. *American Journal of Psychiatry.* 2003; **160**: 1028–40.

5 Mick E, Biederman J, Faraone SV, *et al.* Case-control study of attention-deficit hyperactivity disorder and maternal smoking, alcohol use and drug use during pregnancy. *Journal of the American Academy of Child and Adolescent Psychiatry.* 2002; **41**: 378–85.

6 Accornero VH, Amado AJ, Morrow CE, *et al.* Impact of prenatal cocaine exposure on attention and response inhibitions assessed by continuous performance tests. *Journal of Developmental and Behavioural Paediatrics.* 2007; **28**: 195–205.

7 Jacobson JL, Jacobsen SW, *et al.* Prenatal exposure to polychlorinated biphenyls and attention at school age. *Journal of Paediatrics.* 2003; **143**: 780–8.

8 Ribas-Fito N, Torrent M, Carrizo D, *et al.* Exposure to hexachlorobenzene during pregnancy and children's social behaviour at 4 years of age. *Environmental Health Perspectives.* 2007; **115**: 447–50.

9 French NP, Hagen R, Evans SF, *et al.* Repeated antenatal corticosteroids: effects on cerebral palsy and childhood behaviour. *American Journal of Obstetrics and Gynaecology.* 2004; **190**: 588–95.

10 O'Connor TG, Heron J, Glover V, *et al.* Maternal antenatal anxiety and children's behavioural/emotional problems at 4 years. Report from the Avon longitudinal study of Parents and Children. *British Journal of Psychiatry.* 2002; **180**: 502–8.

11 Neugebauer R, Hoek H, Susser E. Prenatal exposure to wartime famine and development of antisocial personality disorder. *Journal of American Medical Association.* 1999; **282**: 455–62.

12 Bhutta AT, Cleves MA, Casey PH, *et al.* Cognitive and behavioural outcomes of school aged children who were born pre term: a meta analysis. *Journal of the American Medical Association.* 2002; **288**: 728–37.

13 Coleman T. Special groups of smokers. *British Medical Journal.* 2004; **328**: 575–7.

14 Neuman R, Lobos E, Reich W, *et al.* Prenatal smoking exposure and dopaminergic genotypes interact to cause a severe ADHD subtype. *Biological Psychiatry.* 2007; **61**: 1320–8.

15 Biederman J, Faraone SV, Monuteaux MC. Differential effect of environmental adversity by gender: Rutter's Index of Adversity in a group of boys and girls with and without ADHD. *American Journal of Psychiatry.* **159**: 1556–62.

16 Kelly Y, Sacker A, Gray R, *et al.* Light drinking in pregnancy, a risk for behavioural problems and cognitive deficits at 3 years of age? *International Journal of Epidemiology.* 2009; **38**: 129–40.

17 Strengths and Difficulties Questionnaire. Available at: www.sdqinfo.org/ (accessed 11 November 2010).

18 British Ability Scale. Available at: www.gl-assessment.co.uk/health_and_psychology/

resources/british_ability_scales/british_ability_scales.asp?css=1 (accessed 11 November 2010).

19 Bracken School Readiness Assessment. Available at: www.pearsonassessments.com/HAIWEB/Cultures/en-us/Productdetail.htm?Pid=015–8033–078 (accessed 11 November 2010).

20 Millennium Cohort Study. Available at: www.esds.ac.uk/longitudinal/access/mcs/l33359.asp (accessed 11 November 2010).

21 National Organisation on Foetal Alcohol Syndrome UK. Foetal Alcohol Forum. Available at: www.nofas-uk.org/news.htm# (accessed 11 November 2010).

22 Green CR, Munoz DP, Nikkel SM, *et al.* Deficits in eye movement control in children with Foetal Alcohol Spectrum Disorder. *Alcoholism: clinical and experimental research.* 2007; **31**: 500–11.

23 Santostefano S. *Cognitive Control Therapy with Children and Adolescents: psychology practitioner's guidebook.* Oxford: Pergamon Press; 1985.

24 O'Connor MJ, Frankel F, Paley B, *et al.* A controlled study of social skills training for children with foetal alcohol spectrum disorder; 2006. Available at www.escholarship.org/.uc/item/7vh8wom6 (accessed 12 November 2010).

25 Riley E. Proceedings, parents for children conference. Sheffield, UK. Available at: www.tactcare.org.uk/pages/en/parents_for_children_website_visitors_explanation.html (accessed 11 November 2010).

26 O'Malley A. *Affect Reprocessing Therapy.* Unpublished manual; available from the author.

27 O'Malley A. *Proforma for Comprehensive CAMHS Assessment.* Unpublished: available from the author; 2008.

28 Erikson Eight Stages of Child Development. Available at: www.childdevelopmentinfo.com/development/erickson.shtml (accessed 11 November 2010).

TO LEARN MORE

- Fonagy P, Gergely G, Jurist E, *et al. Affect Regulation, Mentalization and the Development of the Self.* New York: Other Press; 2002.
- Ogden P, Minton K, Pain C. *Trauma and the Body: a sensorimotor approach to psychotherapy.* London: Norton; 2006.
- Van der Kolk BA, MacFarlane AC, Weisaeth L, editors. *Traumatic Stress: the effects of overwhelming experience on mind, body, and society.* New York: Guilford Press; 1996.

CHAPTER 11

The older adult

Marilyn White-Campbell

Case study 11.1: Barbara – part i

Barbara (68) was diagnosed with schizophrenia in her early 40s. She lived with an abusive husband and drank to cope with her feelings of isolation and loneliness, and the stigma of her mental illness. She worked as a librarian for many years. Barbara retired at age 60 and began to increase her alcohol intake. Recently, a doctor noticed that her liver function was poor and she was told her 'liver is decaying'. Barbara admits that she drinks 26 ounces of vodka every day and notices that she is not as steady on her feet, often having to crawl up the stairs by the end of her drinking day. Barbara is referred to a liver clinic. The doctor in the liver clinic states that her liver is sclerotic and she must stop drinking. The doctor suggests she attend Alcoholics Anonymous (AA). Barbara becomes distressed with this news and her psychiatric symptoms increase. She is paranoid and cannot leave her home.

SELF-ASSESSMENT EXERCISE 11.1

Time: 10 minutes
- What are the key issues for Barbara?
- How would you address these?

Case study 11.2: Martin – part i

Martin (57), a lifelong drinker, has lived a transient lifestyle. He was pushed down a set of stairs and suffered a subdural haematoma. Recovery is complicated by a protracted withdrawal from alcohol and benzodiazepines. Martin survives but it is uncertain how much he will recover. He spends three months in a critical care unit of the hospital and is transferred for physical rehabilitation when he is stable. During his course of treatment, Martin regains some of his mobility and his memory improves. He is placed on a waiting list for a long-term care facility. With improved memory, Martin remembers that he had an apartment which he refuses to give up for life in a nursing home. He discharges himself back to the community against medical advice, and is cautioned not to drink again. Martin resumes drinking shortly after leaving hospital. He decompensates (functional deterioration; can occur due to fatigue, stress, illness and/or old age) and is not able to care for himself. Martin is referred to an outreach programme that works specifically with older adults experiencing mental health–substance use problems.

SELF-ASSESSMENT EXERCISE 11.2

Time: 10 minutes
- Identify the key issues for Martin.
- What would be an appropriate and helpful response?

REFLECTIVE PRACTICE EXERCISE 11.1

Time: 45 minutes
- How well is your practice equipped to work with older adults experiencing mental health–substance use problems? List the positives and negatives.
- What are your views on the older adult experiencing mental health–substance use problems?
- Can people be helped? If so, how?
- Do you believe it is too late? Why?
- Do you think that drinking is the person's last remaining pleasure, so why bother? If so, why?
- What experiences do you have in working alongside older adults in general?
- Are there barriers in your practice which make it difficult to access services? What are these?
- Are you aware of any resources in your community that can offer support to the older adult living with mental health–substance use issues? What and where are these?
- What supports would you offer Barbara?
- What supports would you offer Martin?

INTRODUCTION

With the 'greying' population of baby boomers, it is not surprising that we begin to notice that there is a 'greying elephant' in clinical practice such as medicine, psychiatry, social work and psychology. The elephant we describe is the problem with mental health–substance use issues experienced by the older person. These are people that live with the stigma of being old, and experiencing mental health–substance use concerns and dilemmas. Many are reluctant to seek help, while professionals and services have no specialised resources to help them.

The metaphor of the 'elephant in the living room', a seminal teaching resource,[1] illustrates for children the existence of addiction in families. The resource's authors[1] found that children easily identify the problems, whereas it is largely ignored, minimised or missed, by the adults of the family or friends, and/or undetected by health and social care professionals. The elephant is the metaphor for the addiction problem which causes a great deal of chaos and instability to the family; breaking furniture, taking up all the space, energy, and the emotional resources of the family. In the story, it is the children that notice the problem of substance use and how it impacts their lives, while the adults ignore the fact that the animal exists in the first place. In the older adult experiencing mental health–substance use problems, we may use the same metaphor in the context of services to older adults. We must, however, call upon ourselves to perceive the elephant, if we intend to address the problem of the elephant in the room, and firstly we have to acknowledge its existence.

ASSESSMENT

Older adults with mental health issues often have complex and ongoing physical problems which are further exacerbated by problematic substance use. The greying elephant in this instance is a common occurrence in our community practice, emergency departments, acute care and psychiatric hospitals. However, the elephant is often ignored or remains undetected because we do not ask the right questions about substance use. We need to examine our sensitivity to screening for mental health–substance use in the older adult population. Ask the questions: Do you drink? How many drinks in the last week have you had? How many drinks per day do you have? Older adult specific tools can help – though we must remember that tools are an aid and will not replace a thorough clinical assessment (*see* Book 5, Chapters 7–9) – such as the:

➤ Geriatric Michigan Alcohol Screening Test (GMAST) short version[2]
➤ Senior Alcohol Misuse Indicator tool (SAMI) developed at the Center for Addiction and Mental Health (CAMH)[3]
➤ Geriatric Depression Scale (GDS) short version[4]
➤ Cognitive screening tools
　— Folstein Mini Mental Status Inventory (FMMSI)[5]
　— Montreal Cognitive Assessment (MoCA).[6]

Such tools can help detect a problem that is hidden or minimised with appropriate probing questions. When screening older adults with substance use problems it is more often the rule than the exception that a co-occurring depression exists.[7]

> **KEY POINT 11.1**
>
> Of all the mental health problems experienced by older adults (e.g. bipolar disorder, schizophrenia, anxiety disorders, Alzheimer's disease and other dementias), depression is the most common – and the most treatable.

The detection of the 'greying elephant' requires the professionals involved looking through different lenses to:

➤ determine the existence of the problem
➤ set out a course of action to provide concurrent care for the person.

WORKING TOGETHER

In care for older adults experiencing mental health–substance use problems, who also experience age-related illness and infirmity, there may be multiple caregivers involved. Comorbidities are more common in older adults, and caregivers must be cognisant of drug–drug interactions and further potential adverse effects.

All professionals and services need to collaborate in their approach in order to provide comprehensive care. This collaboration will help the care team develop a clearer vision of the person and how to provide guidance in setting treatment goals.

TREATMENT APPROACHES

Treatment approaches can vary from one programme to another. However, the Canadian model at the Community Outreach Programs in Addictions (COPA) is an older-person specific treatment approach for the person who is 'precontemplative' or denies and/or minimises their substance use problems[8] (*see* Book 4, Chapter 6). The COPA programme uses a person-centred approach to address mental health–substance use in the context of a case management model. It is non-confrontational, and uses a multi-modality treatment approach. The assessment tool used in the COPA programme is one example of a person-centred assessment that allows the clinical interview to be conducted in the comfort of the person's home, at their pace, and without confrontation.[9]

Assessment areas

To facilitate a complete assessment the following are included:

➤ presenting problem
➤ substance use
➤ quantity and frequency of use
➤ age of onset
➤ treatment history
➤ physical, mental, emotional health
➤ prescription medications including over-the-counter (OTC) and homeopathic or herbal medicines
➤ nutritional status
➤ activities of daily living
➤ family social supports
➤ accommodation
➤ finances
➤ legal
➤ education/vocation
➤ spiritual
➤ leisure activities
➤ sexuality

➤ gender identity
➤ elder abuse
➤ crisis issues
➤ clinical impressions and treatment recommendations
➤ patient treatment goals.

Using a solution focused approach[10] (*see* Book 5, Chapter 10) can be a respectful way of counselling in a way which is congruent with the person's readiness to change. Not admitting there is a problem often precludes the person from accessing mainstream or traditional treatment programmes.

An older adult experiencing mental health–substance use problems may be refused admission to treatment for several reasons:
➤ denial
➤ unwillingness to abstain
➤ unable to physically participate in the programme
➤ generational differences.

This can lead to minimisation of problems, i.e. 'I only drink beer', 'I don't touch the hard stuff', 'I don't touch drugs'. For this reason, the treatment practice for older adults needs to be different in several ways:
➤ least intrusive approach using harm-reduction strategies
➤ home visiting
➤ working alongside the person at varying stages of change
➤ working at a slower pace than mainstream abstinence-based programmes.

SELF-ASSESSMENT EXERCISE 11.3

Time: 10 minutes
How can you help the person who is in denial?

Denial/pre-contemplative
How do you help a person who is in denial/pre-contemplative?
➤ Establish a rapport with the person.
➤ Identify and deal with crisis issues on admission to programme.
➤ Use a non-confrontational approach: motivational interviewing[11] (*see* Book 4, Chapter 7) or solution focused counselling[10].
➤ Encourage the person to identify their view of the problem (goal setting).
➤ Address issues that the person is willing to work on – use motivational interviewing/solution focused counselling.
➤ Make appropriate **but not confrontational** associations between the substance use and the impact on the person's life (i.e. spending money on alcohol only; not paying rent = eviction [crisis]).
➤ Identify and work with the individual's strengths.
➤ Acknowledge and complement the individual's efforts.
➤ Assist follow through on goals in practical ways (i.e. escort to medical or legal appointments, advocacy re-rent arrears . . .).

Helpful tips

Helpful tips when trying to engage with the older person include the following.

➤ It is not important that the person admits that they have a problem with substance use but rather they are willing to accept your initial support on areas which they identify as crisis issues.

➤ Use the phrase 'alcohol use' instead of 'alcohol addiction' or 'alcoholism'.

➤ Generalise/normalise – 'Some people like to take a drink to relax or help them sleep. Does this apply to you?'

➤ Mainstream screening tools may not always apply. The CAGE tool can produce a negative response if asked up front while the GMAST may be less threatening. Generationally, older adults are reluctant to expose a substance use problem as it would be seen as a weakness and cause of shame. Particularly among older women, problem alcohol use can be a hidden problem, whereas prescription misuse among women may be less stigmatising. Non-confrontational approaches in screening can pick up on substance use problems, such as using alcohol to help with sleep or coping with loss, where mainstream tools such as the CAGE can produce negative results and can create discomfort with the older person. The SAMI tool[3] is another tool that is senior specific and addresses the age-related impact of substance use on the older adult.

➤ Harm reduction may be a means to help the older adult reduce the harm of substance use on the body and its impact on their mental health issues.

> ### KEY POINT 11.2
>
> Adopt low-risk drinking guidelines for older adults after age 65. No more than (Canadian standard) one standard drink per day for women and no more than 1.5 standard drinks per day to a maximum of nine per week for men.

Late life depression and alcohol use

Depression affects one in four older adults who have alcohol problems.[12] Depression often occurs with other serious illnesses such as heart disease, stroke, diabetes, cancer and Parkinson's disease. As many older adults face these illnesses, as well as various social and economic difficulties, health and social care professionals may mistakenly conclude that depression is a normal consequence of these problems, an attitude often shared by the person. With complex medical issues in the older adult, alcohol problem use is easily missed, dismissed or goes undetected. Depression can and should be treated when it occurs with other illnesses, as untreated depression can delay recovery or worsen the outcome of other illnesses. Similarly, when alcohol is added to the equation the problems can be amplified. It is important to remember that in Canada and the US risk for suicide in older adults is higher than the general population. In particular older men are at increased risk of suicide.[13]

Case study 11.3: Jill

Depression/alcohol use: which came first?

Jill (72), a diabetic, was referred to addictions treatment by the social worker from the emergency department. She was brought in by ambulance for 'failure to thrive'. On assessment, Jill was cachexic (had muscle wasting), and unable to walk. Her apartment was reported to be squalid. Family members reported that this year Jill started drinking heavily after the death of her husband of 48 years. Jill adamantly denied that the drinking was a problem and that it was only a bit of brandy to help her sleep. She was stabilised in the hospital and returned home against medical advice. Her mobility remained poor and she used a walker to get around the home. However, the home was untidy and Jill was limited in what she could do. Jill agreed to meet with the COPA worker to talk about her situation.

Intervention: On assessment Jill admitted that she started to have problems sleeping after her husband died. Prior to his death, she drank only socially and this was corroborated by family. Jill admitted that she initially started drinking about 3 oz of brandy to help her to sleep. She admitted that she started to wake in the middle of the night and she increased her 'night cap' by another 3 oz and a subsequent 'drink in the morning to get her self-going' and, lastly, 'a glass of wine with her meals'. When it was pointed out to her that she was consuming five standard drinks per day (Canadian measure) at a total of 35 standard drinks per week, she agreed that it was a bit more than she realised. The professional discussed the sugar content of alcohol and how this interacted with her diabetes and possibly her mood. Jill admitted that she let herself go since her husband died and that she too wished she were dead. Jill denies suicidal ideation but admits feeling hopeless and helpless.

Jill was agreeable to the following recommendations:

- Assistance with cleaning her home on a weekly basis. Jill was required to have a 'big clean' prior to agency involvement. Her children agreed to help out.
- Referral to a specialist psychiatrist for assessment of depression.
- Counselling and support to address bereavement issues.
- Medical support for safe withdrawal from alcohol including a medication to ease the withdrawal symptoms (this was done on an outpatient basis).
- Referral to Meals on Wheels to ensure adequate nutritional intake.
- Referral to a geriatric day hospital programme to receive medical support, physiotherapy and occupational therapy to improve her mobility and diabetes monitoring and education.
- Weekly meetings in her home with the COPA worker for counselling.
- COPA volunteer to escort her to medical appointments.
- Attendance in COPA groups.
- Attendance at a seniors social group.

Jill was safely medically withdrawn from alcohol and set goals around safe drinking levels which included social drinking only. She met with the psychiatrist who was able to treat her depression with antidepressant medication. Her depression lifted and she attended day hospital. With physiotherapy and occupational therapy Jill's mobility improved to the point that she no longer needed a walker. She received diabetes education and stabilised her weight. Oral medication used to control her diabetes was reduced. She participated in leisure programmes after discharge from day hospital programmes and COPA group therapy to prevent relapse. She attended a bereavement group for 10 weeks. Jill remains abstinent from alcohol and is managing independently in the community. She started to go back to her previous activities of playing bridge and volunteering with the local hospital. Jill's depression medication was tapered and she began to appreciate the role that alcohol played in her downward spiral. Jill admits that she does not want to go down that road again.

Analysis: Jill is a late onset drinker who drank to cope with the loss of her husband. In this instance the depression came first and the alcohol made it worse. As the bereavement was protracted and complicated by her alcohol use, medication was necessary to help Jill stabilise and as her alcohol use did not cause permanent damage she can now manage independently. There were no lasting effects on her mobility as she received appropriate medical attention and physiotherapy to improve her mobility.

DEMENTIA AND ITS IMPACT ON OLDER ADULTS EXPERIENCING MENTAL HEALTH–SUBSTANCE USE PROBLEMS

Cognitive impairment and problem substance use can further complicate an already complex set of problems in the older adult. The three Ds:
1 Delirium
2 Depression
3 Dementia

. . . may be present at any time and need further investigation.
1 **Delirium:** When an older adult experiences delirium there may be acute infection present or other pathology. The person could be in withdrawal from drugs or alcohol. Acute confusion may be present and will generally resolve with medical intervention; in the latter case, when an older adult is pathologically dependant on alcohol, withdrawal can be more difficult and it is more protracted than in the general population. Medical supervision may be necessary to support the safe withdrawal from alcohol.
2 **Depression:** When depression is present in the older person and there is active substance use, the person can present as confused. Clinical indicators may include poor memory and concentration. These symptoms may be mistaken for dementia.

   Antidepressant medication usually improves depressive symptoms and cognitive performance. Individuals should be encouraged to abstain from alcohol when taking antidepressant medication and cautioned about the depressant effect of alcohol on their condition.

3 **Dementia:** In older persons experiencing alcohol dependence and a diagnosis of dementia there are several risk factors which may be present:
  ➤ human immunodeficiency virus (HIV)/acquired immunodeficiency syndrome (AIDS), where the person has been in treatment with highly active antiretroviral therapy (HAART) and has reduced hepatic or renal insufficiency[14]
  ➤ a history of acquired brain injuries – usually as a result of alcohol-related falls
  ➤ an alcohol associated dementia – Wernicke-Korsakoff syndrome is the most common, with thiamine deficiency an important factor.

For the older adult experiencing substance use problems, and any of the above-mentioned dementias, complete abstinence is highly recommended.[15] Withdrawal from alcohol in individuals with dementia is complicated and requires medical supervision.[16]

CONTINUING CARE

When an older adult experiencing problematic mental health–substance use issues has problems with activities of daily living (ADL), and they have decompensated in areas such as:
➤ poor hygiene
➤ poor nutrition
➤ neglect of self and surroundings
➤ managing finances

. . . the ability to remain in the community may need to be considered as part of continuing care. If the older adult requires admission to long-term care, we need to examine the rationale for the admission:
➤ Is the choice being made on behalf of an incapable person?
➤ Or is this a geographical cure for an out-of-control substance use problem when there is mental instability?

Problem relocation from the community to long-term care can be a temporary solution. However, an older adult experiencing mental health–substance use problems can remain in the community while their substance use and mental health problems are active. Mental health–substance use problems are not a sufficient diagnosis to warrant admission to long-term care. However, there are some instances when it is no longer possible for the person to remain independent. Older adults with severe alcohol-related dementia that requires constant nursing care fit this category. Keep in mind that the older person who is capable may not consent to being institutionalised, and evidence of a single area of concern may not be sufficient to warrant such drastic measures.

KEY POINT 11.3

In these situations, explore all possible solutions to the problems and, as a last resort, recommend admission to long-term care.

Long-term care is a decision not to be taken lightly but may be considered in the following situations.

➤ There are ongoing medical/mental health problems that cannot reasonably be managed by home visiting healthcare agencies.

➤ There is severe cognitive impairment.

➤ The person is unable to care for self, i.e. forgets to eat, cannot remember to take medications, gets lost in the community even in familiar surroundings.

➤ The older person experiencing mental health–substance use problems is no longer capable of making personal care decisions and is a danger to self or others, i.e. harm to self or other behavioural disturbances.

➤ The older person is at risk of neglect and/or abuse in a setting where there is caregiver burnout, or a reluctance to care for the older adult, and there are no community-based home support programmes available.

➤ The older person with problem substance use is a dangerous smoker. Question – is there a history of smoking that has caused a fire? Are multiple burn marks evident on furniture and clothing? There is high risk for fire due to unsafe smoking habits or leaving the stove on (*see* Chapter 6). Check for cognitive impairment and if appropriate arrange for nicotine replacement therapy (*see* Chapter 6).

➤ The older person's mobility is impaired and there is no wheelchair access in their building.

➤ The person is frail and unable to access medical care and meet activities of daily living.

➤ The older person has multiple falls (often alcohol related) and multiple subsequent admissions to hospital as a result of falls, accidents and injuries which are clearly alcohol related.

➤ There is evidence of severe neglect to self and surroundings and an inability or reluctance to resolve these problems independently or with the help of community support services.

Case study 11.4: Hanna (Wernicke-Korsakoff syndrome) and Kathleen (non-alcohol-related delirium)

Two elderly sisters, Hannah and Kathleen, live in a large home. Kathleen, a recent widow, is the owner of the home and suffers from depression and alcohol use problems. Her sister Hanna has moved in and has part of the second floor apartment. She suffers from Wernicke-Korsakoff syndrome which is characterised by the Wernicke's triad (global confusional state, ophthalmoplegia and nystagmus, and ataxia), and Korsakoff's psychosis (severe recent memory impairment associated with confabulation). Kathleen has rented out some rooms in the house to young people who abuse solvents and marijuana. Within the past two years the condition of the home has become squalid and the tenants are known to steal the meals brought to Kathleen, as well as Hannah's pension checks. Hannah has evidence of memory impairment and she has been financially exploited by the tenants and family members. Kathleen is mentally capable of managing her personal care and finances. She responds well to supportive counselling from the COPA professional and reduces and eventually abstains from alcohol. Her bizarre behaviours, which present in the form of acute confusion, including hoarding paranoia and auditory hallucinations, are resolved with abstinence. Kathleen was also diagnosed and treated for a bladder infection and upon treatment with antibiotics, the confusion has resolved. Kathleen is able to manage independently.

Hannah suffered an alcohol-related fall in her home and was hospitalised for a broken hip and jaw. In hospital, Hannah decompensated and it became evident that she was at risk should she return to her home in the community. Admission to a long-term care facility was considered as a discharge plan. Hannah remained in the hospital for three months and made a full recovery from her broken hip and fractured jaw. In her care plan, it was important to ensure that she had access to:

- physiotherapy
- occupational therapy
- home support services
- social activities
- adequate nutrition
- medical care.

Upon discharge from hospital, Hannah's memory is sufficiently intact after three months of abstinence and with proper nutrition and medical care she is deemed capable to make personal care decisions.

Hannah elects to return home. Upon her return she accepts home support services including home making, supportive counselling from COPA to address her substance use problems and encouraged continued abstinence. She accepts an assessment for capacity to manage finances and is found to be incapable of managing finances. She has a trustee and, with careful management of her finances, she is able to remain in her home and out of an institution.

SELF-ASSESSMENT EXERCISE 11.4

Time: 30 minutes
Consider the key issues for Hannah. List those that you find.

Key issues to be considered and for action include:
➤ Poor physical and mental health – poor balance/falls/memory impairment.
➤ Reversibility in Wernicke-Korsakoff syndrome? How much will Hannah

recover? This can be full recovery, or the long-term memory remains intact while the short-term memory is not, or there is no recovery, requiring full nursing care.

➤ Poor nutrition – contributes to poor mobility and memory.
➤ Elder abuse – family and tenants exploiting.
➤ Capacity to make financial decisions.
➤ Capacity to make personal care decisions – should Hannah be moved to a nursing home?
➤ Safety in the home.
➤ Does Hannah intend to drink again?

PHARMACOTHERAPY

Use of medications to deter the older adult from drinking can be prescribed but require caution. An older adult with memory problems generally should never be prescribed disulfiram, as they cannot appreciate the deterrent effect of the treatment.

Naltrexone

Naltrexone can be useful for people who have difficulty cutting down alcohol consumption. Naltrexone is an opiate antagonist which can help prevent relapse if taken regularly, and there is sufficient research to suggest the benefit of prescribing naltrexone in older adults experiencing schizophrenia.[17] Individuals prescribed naltrexone are reported to have fewer drinking days and cravings for alcohol.[17] Older adults with memory problems may also benefit as long as they are medically supervised. However, family members and caregivers need to be aware of the risks. Naltrexone needs to be discontinued if the person requires anaesthesia or dental surgery. It should be noted that naltrexone is not a stand-alone therapy and counselling is required in conjunction with this therapy. Naltrexone can also affect the liver and evaluation is required around the advantages and disadvantages of using this treatment for those with advanced liver disease.

OTHER SYNDROMES
Pseudo Parkinsonism

Older adults experiencing mental health–substance use problems can experience symptoms which may be alcohol or drug induced. These mimic Parkinson's disease which is generally associated with onset in later life. In heavy alcohol users, this medical condition can present in the same manner as a person experiencing advanced Parkinson's disease; namely:

➤ shuffling gait
➤ mask-like facial features
➤ intention tremor
➤ problems with swallowing.

Unlike Parkinson's, people experiencing alcohol-induced Parkinsonism can recover if they receive medical attention, good nutrition and remain abstinent.

Wernicke–Korsakoff syndrome

This is characterised by the Wernicke's triad (global confusional state, ophthalmo-plegia and nystagmus, and ataxia) and Korsakoff's psychosis (severe impairment of recent memory associated with confabulation). More simply put, this syndrome is an alcohol-induced neurological syndrome which affects memory, mood and mobility. These symptoms can present with poor nutrition and engagement in heavy drinking. The memory and balance problems can become permanent, without medical treatment. Thiamine therapy is an important and urgent part of the treatment. People exhibiting these symptoms should be counselled to abstain and to maintain optimal medical and nutritional health.

With all these complex syndromes it is advised that the individual be supported to maintain abstinence. The person who is abstinent for a year should reach their optimal function if there is optimism for physical and cognitive recovery. Intensive physiotherapy to regain mobility, proper nutrition and optimal medical care will help in this process and the person may or may not recover full function.

OUTCOMES FOR MENTAL HEALTH–SUBSTANCE USE PROBLEMS AND OLDER ADULTS

Case study 11.5: Barbara – part ii

Barbara stopped drinking while using disulfiram. She had one episode where she required hospitalisation and stabilisation. Barbara continued to use disulfiram for a year in conjunction with regular weekly home visits for counselling, geriatric psychiatry every six weeks, and other medical appointments as needed. Within the year her mood improved; liver function returned to normal, and Barbara began to address some of her relationship issues. Barbara had a friendly visitor from a senior's agency to meet with her on a weekly basis. She began to volunteer in the community and participate in groups for her particular ethnic group. Her self-esteem improved dramatically and she acknowledged that she had been in a loveless marriage. The focus in counselling was on making healthy choices and positive change. Barbara divorced her husband and moved into an apartment in a seniors building. She self-reports 'that is the best part of my life, and it's never too late to make changes'.

Case study 11.6: Martin – part ii

Martin received one-to-one counselling in his home and later attended group therapy using a solution-focused approach. He identified goals to become abstinent, return to his post-hospital discharge status, and to have meaningful activities. He stopped all substance use abruptly and was admitted to hospital on an emergency basis for medical withdrawal and stabilised. Martin was referred to geriatric day hospital to improve his mobility. He started volunteering with an agency that served the homeless. Martin became a steady and valued volunteer. He was able to save money for the first time in many years and was able to take a trip to see family members he had not seen in two decades. Martin remains abstinent, stating he has won the battle and has purpose to give back to the community of which he was once a recipient of services.

CONCLUSION

The successful outcomes in working with the older adult experiencing very different mental health issues and substance use problems are largely resolved using an intensive community case management model in collaboration with primary outreach services. The focus is harm reduction, supported by optimal psychiatric and medical care that is older-adult focused. The community-based approach to treating the individual and not the illness is the link that helps the care-giving team. While individual professionals may view the 'elephant' through their lenses of expertise and experience, when all the lenses are combined the elephant becomes clearly illuminated.

Treatment outcomes for older adults in the COPA programme have demonstrated excellent outcomes,[19] and age of onset made no difference.[20] In fact, many older adults experiencing mental illness, such as bipolar disorder and schizophrenia, experience reduced psychiatric symptoms and often reach stability as a result of ageing.[21] This bodes well for older adults experiencing mental health–substance use problems as they do as well as, if not better than, younger people. This alone should be enough reason to address the 'greying elephant' in the room because it is never too late to make changes in the way of life and living.

REFERENCES

1 Hastings J, Typpo M. *An Elephant in the Living Room.* Minneapolis, MN: Hazleton Press; 1994.

2 Blow FC, Brower KJ, Schulenberg JE, *et al.* The Michigan Alcohol Screening Test – Geriatric Version (MAST-G). A new elderly-specific screening instrument. *Alcoholism: Clinical and Experimental Research.* 1992; **16**: 372.

3 Busto U, Lum B, Flower M, Center for Addiction and Mental Health. Identifying substance use, mental health and gambling problems in older adults. In: Center for Mental Health and Addiction, Health Aging Project. *Improving our Response to Older Adults with Substance Use, Mental Health and Gambling Problems.* Toronto, Ontario: Center for Mental Health and Addiction; 2008. pp. 44–5.

4 Sheikh JI, Yesavage JA. Geriatric Depression Scale (GDS): recent evidence and development of a shorter version. *Clinical Gerontology: a guide to assessment and intervention.* New York: The Haworth Press; 1986. pp. 165–73.

5 Folstein MF, Folstein SE, McHugh PR. 'Mini Mental State', a practical method for grading the cognitive state of patients for the clinician. *Journal of Psychiatric Research.* 1975; **12**: 189–98.

6 Nasreddine ZS, Collin I, Chertkow H, *et al.* Sensitivity and specificity of the Montreal Cognitive Assessment (MoCA) for detection of mild cognitive deficits. *Canadian Journal of Neurological Science.* 1003; **30**: 30.

7 Minkoff K. An integrated model for the management of co-occurring psychiatric and

substance disorders in managed cares systems. *Disease Management and Health Outcomes.* 2000; **8**: 250–7.

8 Prochaska J, DiClemente C. *The Transtheoretical Approach: crossing the traditional boundaries of therapy.* Homewood, IL: Dow Jones/Irwin; 1994.

9 Graham K, Saunders SJ, Flower M, *et al. Addictions Treatment for Older Adults: evaluation of an innovative client-centered approach.* New York: The Haworth Press Inc.; 1995.

10 De Jong P, Berg IK. *Interviewing for Solutions.* 3rd ed. Florence, KY: Hadsworth; 2007.

11 Millar W, Rollnick S. *Motivational Interviewing: preparing people to change addictive behavior.* New York: Guilford Press; 1991.

12 Spencer C. *Older Adults Alcohol and Depression*; 2005. Available at: www.agingincanada.ca/alcohol_and_depression.htm (accessed 2 December 2010).

13 Canadian Coalition for Seniors Mental Health. *National Guidelines for Seniors Mental Health: the assessment of suicide risk and prevention of suicide*; 2006. Available at: www.ccsmh.ca/en/natlGuidelines/suicide.cfm (accessed 2 December 2010).

14 Gebo KA. HIV and aging implications for patient management, in drugs. Available at: http://blog.utp.edu.co/internaumana/files/2010/10/HIV-and-Aging.pdf (accessed 2 December 2010).

15 Bartsch AJ, Homola G, Biller A, *et al.* Manifestations of early brain recovery associated with abstinence from alcoholism. *Brain.* 2007; **130**: 36–47.

16 White-Campbell M. Addressing Substance Use in Long Term Care and Services. Ontario Association for Non Profit Homes and Services for Seniors Annual General Meeting, Conference proceedings; 7 June 2010; Toronto, Ontario.

17 Batiki S, Dimmock J, Gately P, *et al.* Monitored naltrexone without counselling for alcohol abuse/dependence in schizophrenia-spectrum disorders. *American Journal on Addictions.* 2008; **16**: 253–9.

18 Quyen Q, Mausbach B. Treatments for patients with dual diagnosis: a review. *Alcoholism: clinical and experimental research.* 2007; **31**: 513–6.

19 White-Campbell M, Saunders SJ. The community older persons alcohol program: a community based treatment approach to alcoholism in the elderly. La Sociedad Ante El Envejecimentio y La minusvalia. In: *Proceedings of SYSTED Science & Health: social services for the elderly and disabled.* Barcelona, Spain; 1992; **II**: 1067–72.

20 Saunders G, White-Campbell M. A typology of elderly persons who have alcohol problems. *Alcoholism Treatment Quarterly.* 1992; **9**: 3–4.

21 Howard R, Rabins P, Seeman M, *et al.* Late-onset schizophrenia and very-late onset schizophrenia-like psychosis: an international consensus. *American Journal of Psychiatry.* 2000; **157**: 172–8.

TO LEARN MORE

- Aging in Canada: Available at: www/agingincanada.ca
- Benzodiazepines: how they work and how to withdraw. Available at: www.benzo.org.uk/manual/. This website has withdrawal protocols for benzodiazepines. There is a section specifically dedicated to older adults and how to taper benzodiazepines and the withdrawal symptoms. All withdrawal protocols need to be supervised by a medical professional.
- Community Outreach Programs In Addictions, Toronto, Ontario, Canada. Available at: www.copacommunity.ca
- Geriatric Depression scale. Available at: www.stanford.edu/~yesavage/GDS.html
- Improving our response to older adults with mental health substance use and gambling

problems. Center for Mental Health and Addiction, Toronto, Canada. Available at: www.camh.net/Publications/Resources_for_Professionals/index.html

- National Guidelines for seniors. *Mental Health: the assessment and treatment of depression, delirium, suicide risk/prevention, and mental health issues in long term care.* Available at: www.ccsmh.ca/en/guidelinesUsers.cfm

CHAPTER 12

The young person

Christina KME Sonneborn

PRE-READING EXERCISE 12.1 (ANSWERS ON P. 168)

> **Time: 30 minutes**
> 1 Are motivational interviewing strategies restricted to individual counselling or can they be used in a group or family setting?
> 2 Name specific interventions for young adults with borderline personality disorder and cocaine dependence.
> 3 In which stage of treatment do you offer psychoeducation for young adults experiencing schizophrenia and cannabis use problems?
> 4 What are the possible negative side-effects of residential treatment for young adults experiencing combined severe personality disorders and alcohol dependence?

INTRODUCTION

Young adults experiencing mental health–substance use problems tend to have quite an extensive treatment history, starting with substance use at a young age and experiencing mental health problems in their youth. They often have a history of insecure attachments, abuse, traumatic experiences, constitutional problems such as attention deficit hyperactivity disorder (ADHD – *see* Chapter 10), first psychotic experiences in adolescence, and/or autistic spectrum disorders. In many countries services are fragmented, with little expertise in the treatment of substance use disorders in mental health facilities, and vice versa. There is often extensive use of hospital and crisis facilities but little engagement in long-term treatment, reflecting the combined detrimental effect of mental health–substance use problems on forming meaningful relationships with others, formulating treatment goals and maintaining motivation for change despite setbacks.

This stresses the need to organise services for people with severe mental health–substance use problems in an integrated fashion, using a consistent approach and thereby creating a therapeutic environment where people regain hope. Other goals include the improvement of physical and emotional well-being and better relationships with families (*see* Book 5, Chapter 7), partners and broader social network.

A common goal for many young adults experiencing mental health–substance use problems is to learn to adopt healthier coping strategies, not involving substance use to block out painful emotions, to help with difficulties in complex social situations or to fill in boredom and emptiness.

Case study 12.1: Thomas

Thomas (24) is a single man, admitted for the second time to an integrated programme for mental health–substance use problems. He has been known to mental health services since his adolescence, being treated for ADHD and conduct disorder.[1] Between the ages of 18 and 22 he was admitted to the local psychiatric clinic six times following episodes of self-harm and brief psychotic episodes precipitated by excessive use of cocaine and amphetamines. At the age of 23, he was admitted for the first time to an integrated programme following referral from the local mental health team after he had been thrown out of supported housing due to excessive use of alcohol and cocaine. During his first stay at the integrated programme he was diagnosed with alcohol dependence, cocaine abuse, borderline personality disorder and ADHD. Thomas made a successful recovery, was treated with short-acting methylphenidate and risperidone and was discharged back to the local mental health team and supported housing. After relapses (*see* Chapters 15 and 16; Book 4, Chapter 13) in cocaine abuse he stopped his medication, had several crisis admissions for detoxification but was not able to stabilise again. At readmission, his crisis plan is actualised, he is starting to take long-acting methylphenidate and during the assessment the additional diagnosis of post-traumatic stress disorder[1] is made. Thomas attends the twice-weekly group session aimed at teaching people with ADHD to structure their day, to manage their finances, to remember to take medication and to handle impulsiveness. As his emotion regulation appears satisfactory and Thomas is still applying skills learned during his earlier stay, he formulates new treatment goals aimed at reducing his symptoms of post-traumatic stress disorder.

STABILISATION AND ASSESSMENT

The assessment process usually involves a functional analysis of the problematic behaviour, systematically examining its positive and negative consequences. Functional analyses are most effective when they lead to treatment plans aimed at helping people develop new and more effective behavioural strategies for achieving their goals, rather than treatment plans that focus on eliminating maladaptive behaviours.[2] Additionally, there are often questions about the exact nature of the mental health problems, including validating earlier diagnoses, assessing reflective function/mentalising and exploring protective contextual factors. At this stage it is also important to engage family members by visiting them at home and listening to their view on the problem (*see* Book 3, Chapter 2), letting them express their frustration and engaging them in treatment (*see* Book 5, Chapter 7) by focusing on practical issues (*see* Table 12.1). It is often not feasible to conduct this assessment prior to detoxification.

TABLE 12.1 Treatment stages: stabilisation and assessment

Mental health	Substance use
• Interpersonal functioning	• Safe, drug-free milieu
• Assess mentalisation	• Support
• Crisis plan	• Detoxification
• Medication review	• Functional assessment: addiction severity index (ASI)
• Diagnostic assessment: (brief psychiatric rating scale: severity psychiatric symptoms) – (structured interview for the diagnosis of Personality Disorder-IV: diagnosis personality disorder)	• Motivational stage: persuasion
	• Contact family/network

Case study 12.2: Mary – part i

Mary (23) presents to the local substance use clinic. She is accompanied by her girlfriend who has looked after her at her own flat for a couple of weeks, trying to prevent Mary from using 3–4 grams of cocaine daily. During the initial assessment interview an immediate admission is arranged due to acute suicidal risk and a preliminary diagnosis of borderline personality disorder, post-traumatic stress disorder and cocaine dependence is made. The admission is not a success: Mary reports daily intrusive suicidal thoughts and the nurses are afraid she will throw herself under a train. An urgent psychiatric assessment is arranged at the nearby psychiatric hospital. The diagnosis of borderline personality disorder is confirmed. Due to the cocaine dependence she is deemed not to be a suitable candidate for the day care treatment and is referred back to the substance use clinic. Following reports from fellow inpatients that she is threatening and manipulative, she is discharged from the substance use clinic the next day without aftercare.

After a series of comparable crisis interventions she keeps in touch with a member of the crisis team who refers her to an integrated programme for people experiencing mental health–substance use problems. Following a couple of assessment interviews it is decided that Mary will start her integrated treatment trajectory with a residential stay in order to break the destructive cycle of daily drug use, escalating conflicts with her parents and repeated suicidal acts and self-mutilation. Several weeks prior to her admission she ends her relationship of two years and moves back to live with her parents. She still has a job as a car technician but is finding it increasingly difficult to hide her daily cocaine habit. After a period of detoxification and stabilisation lasting three weeks, a care planning meeting is arranged with Mary and members of the multidisciplinary team.

The following diagnoses have been recorded in a semi-structured interview with the addiction specialist:
• dysthymia
• post-traumatic stress disorder
• social phobia

- cocaine dependence
- alcohol abuse
- borderline personality disorder.[1]

In the assessment interview with the psychiatrist/psychotherapist, Mary seems to have a fragmented sense of self, reports feeling extremely guilt-ridden about the death of a boyfriend when she was 16 and being tormented by daily intrusive images of his dead body following a motorcycle accident which might have been suicide. She also reports having been raped at the age of six, which she is unable to talk about. Mary seems detached from her parents, has never been able to talk to them about traumatic events and her relationship problems, or her feelings of extreme despair prompting self-mutilating acts. Her parents were unsupportive when she disclosed being lesbian in her late teens. Mary has been using cocaine since the age of 16 with gradually increasing use. She wants help with her problems with emotional regulation, relationships and intrusive memories and nightmares connected with the death of her first boyfriend.

At the care planning meeting the following treatment goals are agreed between Mary and the team:

- Stop using all substances for the time being.
- Find words for what is happening inside me.
- Learn to cope with emotions.
- Improve my negative self-image.
- Cope with the death of my friend.

It is further agreed that Mary will have:

- weekly individual psychotherapy using a mentalisation-based treatment approach[3]
- twice weekly group skills training (STEPPS training[4])
- music therapy in group to improve emotion regulation
- social skills training
- psychoeducation
- specific substance use counselling in group.

Her parents will be invited in order to provide psychoeducation and information about the treatment plan.

USING A MENTALISATION-BASED TREATMENT APPROACH FOR YOUNG ADULTS WITH BORDERLINE PERSONALITY DISORDER AND SUBSTANCE USE

The key deficits associated with borderline personality disorder are normally thought to include impulsiveness, difficulty managing emotions and relationship problems. At least the last of these key deficits could be associated with a limited ability to perceive mental states in self and others accurately.[5] The use of substances can be understood as a conscious effort to regulate emotions, an impulsive act or an example of acting out. The overall aim in treatment is to enable consciousness of one's affects while remaining in that emotional state and understanding that state as meaningful.

The reduction of non-mentalising modes of thinking, which have been described as concreteness, impulsivity, affect dysregulation and propensity for acting out, seems likely to be a relevant treatment goal for many people with borderline personality disorder and substance use.

In young adults with poor mentalising capacities due to traumatic experiences in combination with constitutional factors and a poor quality of primary attachment relationships, the engaging in a therapeutic relationship (*see* Book 4, Chapter 2) can lead to an intensification of related problems, such as the return to modes of subjective experience that antedate mentalisation. These have been described as the 'psychic equivalence mode' and the 'pretend mode'.[6] In the psychic equivalence mode the mental reality is perceived to have the same quality as the outer reality. This can lead to a terrifying subjective experience as frightening thoughts such as flashbacks are felt as real. In this mode of experience it is almost impossible for the people to consider alternative perspectives. In the pretend mode people often talk endlessly of thoughts and feelings but the affects frequently do not match the content of the thoughts. This mode has been linked with emptiness, meaninglessness and dissociation following trauma.

THE ROLE OF ATTACHMENT WITHIN A DEVELOPMENTAL MODEL OF BORDERLINE PERSONALITY DISORDER

According to attachment theory, the development of the self occurs in the context of early relationships which are necessary to develop affect regulation. It is assumed that to achieve normal self-experience the infant requires his/her emotional signals to be accurately and contingently mirrored by an attachment figure.[6] This mirroring must be 'marked', i.e. exaggerated, if the infant is to understand the caregivers' display as part of his/her emotional experience rather than an expression of his/hers. It is assumed that when a child cannot develop a representation of her/his own experience through mirroring, she/he internalises the image of the caregiver as part of his/her self-representation. While mentalisation has its roots in the sense of being understood by an attachment figure, mentalising is also more challenging to maintain in the context of an attachment relationship, including the relationship with the therapist.[7] In order to engage the individual with borderline personality disorder in treatment, it is important to match the therapeutic interventions to the level of mentalising capacities and keep in mind that the therapeutic relationship in itself can lead to a reactivating of modes of subjective experience antedating mentalisation (*see* Box 12.1).

BOX 12.1

Mentalisation-based interventions:
- take into account that attachment to the therapist can lead to a breakdown in mentalising
- are based on a 'not knowing' stance of the therapist
- take into account the level of agitation and emotional distress
- are generally brief and focus on the current situation.

Case study 12.2: Mary – part ii

Mary has a good start in the residential treatment programme, attends all individual and group sessions and manages to remain abstinent for the first three months of her stay. She finds the weekend visits to her parents stressful. In a family session her parents seem helpless to cope with her bouts of anger at home, following which Mary will often run off or lock herself in her room for hours. Mary's parents frequently express their view that this really is her last chance to stop abusing drugs as otherwise they will not support her any longer. The longer she remains abstinent from cocaine and works on her goal of 'finding words for what is happening inside me' in the individual sessions, the more she seems to find it difficult to handle her emotions. Parallel to her behaviour at home she frequently retreats to her room in the unit when emotionally upset or when having traumatic flashbacks. She will then only contact a member of staff after she has already cut herself. A crisis plan is set up, integrating strategies for emotion regulation from the group skills training and supportive interventions from members of staff such as offering to go for a walk. Mary decides to restart on quetiapine, a medication she has used before her admission and which helps her to regulate her anger and self-mutilation. In the individual sessions interpersonal situations on the unit and at home are talked through, using the 'stop and rewind' method, playing back to moments that triggered strong emotional responses. This is done by modelling good mentalising from a 'not knowing stance' and interrupting her when she is describing a situation in the 'pretend mode', whereby there seems to be no connection between her emotion (which is often cynical and detached) and her narrative. After about three months into her admission, Mary develops an affection for a male fellow patient, a married father of two with a diagnosis of cocaine dependence and a personality disorder with narcissistic, antisocial and borderline traits. Both are eventually asked to leave the unit temporarily after being found to use cocaine outside of his room. Mary gets extremely angry, smashing a glass door at the entrance to the unit before heading off.

In the ensuing individual session Mary remains mainly in the 'pretend mode', appears cynical and detached and tells a story of talking to her grandmother, who is the only person in her family she feels attached to. They had been talking about the death of her grandfather and Mary realised that nobody in her family ever talks about how they feel. She has decided that she will continue her treatment as an outpatient, attending the unit three times a week for the group skills training and her individual psychotherapy sessions. She wants to stop with music therapy as she finds that she gets frequently overwhelmed by emotions that she cannot handle after the session. Mary also reports an increase of intrusive flashbacks, seeing her dead boyfriend in the mortuary and asks for additional help to stop these images. Since she has started using cocaine again, albeit less frequently than before her admission, and seems more unstable following her discharge and aggressive outburst, it is agreed to increase the dose of quetiapine and actualise her crisis plan. Once she has managed to use her crisis plan constructively, applying behavioural skills to regulate self-mutilation and substance use and has not used cocaine for a month, she will be referred to another psychotherapist from the same integrated programme for a course of eye movement desensitisation and reprocessing (EMDR – *see* Chapter 8; Book 4, Chapter 12)[8] This eventually helps her to regain stability, the intrusive traumatic images disappear and she is able to continue her treatment as an outpatient.

EARLY ACTIVE TREATMENT

An integrated approach for the treatment of borderline personality disorder and other mental health–substance use problems need to take into account the stages of change which have been described in the transtheoretical model of change[9] (*see* Book 4, Chapter 6), as well as matching psychotherapeutic interventions to the level of mentalising capacity. Both models are more directed towards the process of change instead of being focused on the problematic behaviour in itself and can therefore easily be integrated.

Many young adults experiencing mental health–substance use problems have difficulties engaging in treatment. This can be due to earlier unsuccessful treatment experiences, to general difficulties with relationships or a lack of shared problem definition and related goals.

Table 12.2 lists several strategies used at this stage in order to engage the individual in treatment and enhance motivation for change.

TABLE 12.2 Treatment stages: early active treatment

Mental health	Substance use
• Therapeutic relationship	• Working alliance
• Stabilise symptoms	• Motivational interviewing
• Mentalising interventions	• Advantages/disadvantages
• Psychoeducation	• Psychoeducation
• Medication review	• Functional analysis
• Psychotherapy: cognitive behavioural therapy (CBT), mentalisation-based treatment (MBT), EMDR	• Psychotherapy (CBT)
	• Family support/therapy
• Family support/therapy	
Motivational stage: decide/prepare	

MOTIVATIONAL STRATEGIES

The use of motivational interventions (*see* Book 4, Chapter 7) is important through-out the treatment process but seems especially vital in the early stages of treatment when people often are still regularly using substances but in the process of prepar-ing to stop. In motivational interviewing[10] therapists help the individual to identify personal goals and develop motivation to change their substance use when they perceive it as interfering with achieving those goals. When using a mentalisation-based approach to the treatment of borderline personality disorder, it is equally important to be alert to decreases in motivation and alter the interaction with the person accordingly. In general, the level of motivation seems inversely proportional to the person's degree of agitation and emotional distress. Motivating strategies that have been described within the mentalisation-based approach are:

➤ demonstrate support
➤ reassurance and empathy when exploring the person's mind
➤ reappraise gains and identify continuing problem areas
➤ identify the discrepancy between the experience of the self and the ideal self.[6]

An integrative approach to the treatment of mental health–substance use problems includes the establishment of motivational groups, which apply a stage-wise, non-judgemental, supportive and collaborative approach to group therapy.[11] Typical interventions in motivational groups include eliciting talk about change around a group theme and discussing the stages of change whereby group members are encouraged to identify their own stage of change.

Family interventions at an early stage of the treatment help families to overcome their ambivalence to change, using the same motivational strategies that are used with the individual, avoiding confrontation and argumentation, identifying which factors are interfering with achieving shared family goals and providing psychoedu-cation about substance use and mental health.

The general characteristics of motivational strategies are outlined in Box 12.2.

BOX 12.2

Motivational strategies:
● are related to the stage of change
● are especially important in early stages
● take into account the level of agitation and emotional distress
● can be employed in groups and families.

FUNCTIONAL ANALYSIS OF THE SUBSTANCE USE BEHAVIOUR AND ENSURING INTERVENTIONS

The purpose of a functional analysis is to understand which factors maintain the person's substance use behaviour. This usually involves the following factors:

➤ **social:** social network consisting of people using substances
➤ **affective:** using substances for relief from strong negative emotions or for pleasure

➤ **cognitive:** the belief 'once I have this craving for the drug I cannot stop myself from using it'
➤ **physiological:** withdrawal symptoms
➤ **economic:** money received in exchange for drugs.

One of the strategies that can increase the perceived advantages of not using substances is the decisional balance method; this involves constructing a list, alongside the individual, of the disadvantages of using substances and the advantages of not using substances. Interventions designed to decrease the negative effects of not using substances include social skills training to improve the capacity to develop new relationships with people who do not use substances. People using substances as a way to cope with mental health problems can be taught alternative coping skills to address problems such as the following:
➤ depression
➤ anxiety
➤ sleep problems
➤ hallucinations
➤ affect dysregulation
➤ traumatic flashbacks.

People using substances as one of their only sources of pleasure can be taught recreational skills to help them develop alternative ways of enjoying themselves.

At this stage, it is often helpful to review medication (*see* Book 5, Chapter 13); important principles here are simplification of the medication regime in order to increase medication adherence, reduction of medications that interfere with treatment goals and the management of newly diagnosed conditions.

Case study 12.3: James

James (31), a single man, is referred to an integrated programme for the treatment of substance use and mental health problems by his psychiatrist who has treated him for paranoid schizophrenia[1] for the past seven years. He has also been admitted for detoxification from cannabis at the local addiction clinic two years previously. James became psychotic for the first time as a student in his early 20s. His illness was untreated for more than a year in which he gradually withdrew from his social contacts, started to use increasing amounts of cannabis and eventually dropped out of university and became homeless. He has been treated with a variety of antipsychotic medication, including haloperidol, risperidone, olanzapine and quetiapine. His delusions and hallucinations have not reacted to medication; he hears several voices who comment on his actions almost continuously; he also has delusions about being filmed by a camera throughout the day. He feels regularly very low in mood and occasionally thinks about suicide. James uses cannabis sometimes with the only friend he has left but mostly smokes it on his own, in order to block out his feelings of depression, sometimes when the voices become too much and sometimes because he has nothing else to do. He currently lives with his mother who is often critical and avoids contact with mental health services. James has attended a day care rehabilitation programme in the past, including psych-oeducation about psychotic disorders. In periods when functioning slightly better, James has worked as a freelance photographer and painter. In the beginning, the use of cannabis made him more creative in his painting but more recently he has not been able to produce anything, partly because his whole day is filled with smoking cannabis. The depressive symptoms have been previously treated with lithium carbonate which he is still taking on admission, in combination with a high dose of olanzapine, mirtazapine to help him sleep, and a small dose of diazepam. During detoxification from cannabis the dose of diazepam is increased and he is getting a lot of help from staff and fellow inpatients to help him stabilise his day-night rhythm. His mother is invited to attend in order to provide information about the combination of schizophrenia and cannabis dependence but she does not want to have anything to do with mental health services. After a period of detoxi-fication and stabilisation, James eventually agrees to have a trial of clozapine. This has been discussed with him earlier but was not feasible because of his drug use and possible suicidal risk. He is also fearful of possible side-effects.

The switch from olanzapine to clozapine takes several weeks and greatly increases his anxiety; he is also more distressed by the voices and spends days lying on his bed. Nursing staff initially leave him, thinking that he needs the rest, but in regular staff meetings it is stressed that James needs encouragement and support to help him through a difficult period. He also takes himself off a few times and has several slips in cannabis use. Once he returns to the ward obviously under influence of drugs and is asked to remain in his room until the obvious effects of cannabis use have weaned off so that his fellow patients will not suffer negative effects such as an increase in craving. James responds in an angry way, is seem-ingly highly distressed by his voices but at the same time rude and obviously intoxicated. He is then asked to spend the night and next day at his mother's house. Eventually, he manages to persevere with the clozapine trial and a few weeks after the plasma level of clozapine is in the therapeutic range his psychotic symptoms gradually diminish. A period of readjustment follows in which James describes a pervasive feeling of emptiness and loss after both his voices and delusions have disappeared and he has stopped using cannabis for recreational and social rea-sons. The functional analysis of both his psychotic symptoms and the related use of cannabis is used as a guidance for further interventions (*see* Table 12.3).

TABLE 12.3 Functional analysis: James

Prodromal signs		Mental health symptoms
• I can't stop racing thoughts • I feel down because I have this terrible illness • My heart races • I am sweating • I feel restless		• I feel confused and can't differentiate between my experiences and reality • I hear voices • I have the impression that others follow me or keep an eye on me • I don't have any energy to do things • I can't move my body very well • I have the impression that I'm somebody else • I think that I'm the main character in a TV programme
Internal risk factors substance use		**External risk factors substance use**
• I feel low • I am very critical of myself • I am paranoid, especially when on my own • I expect far too much of myself • I feel anxious and doubt my own thoughts and perceptions		• Being alone • Too much leisure time • Others are very authoritarian and keep telling me the rules • Critical comments from my mother • Certain programmes on TV • Money in my pocket • Several conversations at the same time which I can't follow any more
	Protective factors	
Protective skills	**Protective activities**	**Protective contextual factors**
• I'm good at sports • I like studying • I'm creative	• Painting • Taking photographs • Sculpting • Cycling • Walking • Listening to music • Writing down my thoughts	• Being with some (not too many) other people • My best friend phones if he hasn't heard me for 4–7 days. I phone him if I feel OK • Contact with my personal coach, my psychiatrist or my case manager

ACTIVE TREATMENT STAGE

Once people have developed sustained motivation for change they are ready to move into the stage of active treatment. The overall aim of an integrated approach is to achieve sustainable goals by teaching the skills necessary to reduce substance use, combined with increased control over mental health problems. This sometimes involves a change in lifestyle or mental illness management, at other times more internal changes such as an improved ability to mentalise, a more stable self-image and resulting improvements in relational functioning.

The corresponding interventions in this stage include active treatment groups, which follow logically the motivational groups described earlier. In these weekly groups psychoeducation about the specific interactions between substance use and mental illness continues to have an important role, but this is now combined with a focus on skills and behaviours to help achieve the person's goals of reducing substance use or maintaining abstinence. The individual learns to recognise situations that increase the risk for using substances and to apply relapse prevention techniques. Possible skills that can help prevent relapses are relaxation techniques, physical activity such as running, listening to music or contact with members of the social network or helping agencies (*see* functional analysis James – Table 12.3).

Family interventions at this stage aim to modify stressful communication styles that may exacerbate mental health symptoms and increase substance use. Families can also be taught to set limits, to help people cope with persistent symptoms and to structure daily activities such as household chores, finding voluntary work and developing alternative leisure activities.

Case study 12.2: Mary – part iii

After the stabilisation of her post-traumatic stress symptoms using EMDR, Mary continues her weekly psychotherapy sessions in combination with substance use counselling in a group. Following a series of short and rather destructive relationships she falls in love with Jasmine, a 35-year-old woman who also suffers from borderline personality disorder and is dependent on alcohol. Many sessions are used to help her mentalise her feelings for Jasmine and at her request monthly systemic sessions are started, aimed at helping her to apply her improved ability to mentalise within the new attachment relationship with Jasmine. As the intrusive memories of her dead boyfriend gradually disappear, Mary struggles with the fact she has to readjust her life and finally 'let him go' in order to form a new attachment to Jasmine. At the same time she adopts a helping stance in order to stabilise Jasmine's serious and self-destructive drinking. At times the worry about Jasmine's drinking and the effort to obtain help for her seems to help Mary to remain stable and abstinent herself. At other times she relapses into cocaine use, sometimes for recreational reasons, sometimes in order to block everything out and sometimes because Jasmine is also not doing her best to stop. As the therapy progresses Mary manages more often to mentalise successfully when describing interpersonal situations and this is highlighted regularly in the sessions. The focus of therapy remains on her affect and her mind instead of her behaviour. Some affects seem easier to tolerate than others while Mary seems to think more often about the mind of the therapist. In one of these sessions she comes in and says: 'Now the thing has happened what you have been working on for the past nine months: I'm emotionally broken, I feel vulnerable and small and can't pretend any longer.' This seems to be related to feelings of loneliness and dependency, brought on by the need for a brief admission for detoxification. By discussing her assumptions about the mind of the therapist Mary manages to mentalise both her own affect as well as her feelings about the therapy and being in need of help from attachment figures in general. She is able to tolerate her feelings of abandonment and isolation connected to her parents.

RESIDENTIAL TREATMENT VERSUS OUTPATIENT SERVICES/ OUTREACHING

The Yogi and the Commissar and other essays by Arthur Koestler[12] describes two competing views about how to achieve change: the yogi believes that internal changes lead to a transformation of the world whereas the commissar's approach is based on the notion that internal transformation follows changes in outside reality. In the treatment of young adults with complex and challenging mental health–substance use problems health professionals often promote either a 'yogi' or a 'commissar' approach, the 'yogis' advocating the exploration of the subjective functioning and relationship patterns and the 'commissars', in contrast, targeting symptoms and behaviour.[13]

The use of an integrated approach where increased mentalising capacities and improved emotion regulation are equally important as illness management and coping skills to handle craving is advocated. In this context, the question of whether or not to admit people experiencing mental health–substance use problems arises. There is often a need for inpatient treatment in order to get out of a destructive environment, as a first step to changing substance use and in order to achieve diagnostic clarification and engage people in treatment.

As the case study of Mary illustrates, there are also negative aspects of inpatient treatment for people with severe personality disorder and substance use. The constant presence of staff can be very threatening as it activates attachment difficulties. It is therefore not surprising that the mentalisation-based approach for borderline personality disorder has been developed in a day care or outpatient setting. First results in these settings in a Dutch population with high comorbidity of addiction are promising.[14]

Other negative aspects of inpatient treatment can be the rather repressive environment of secure facilities or general psychiatric wards as this is not helpful in early stages of change.

Case study 12.2: Mary – part iv

In the ensuing period Mary establishes a pattern of regular periods of daily cocaine use, short admissions for detoxification and more stable periods. The relapses in cocaine use seem related to the high-risk situation of living with a partner who also has a substance use problem; Jasmine has by now changed her substance of preference from alcohol to cocaine. Mary seems reluctant to make the necessary lifestyle changes to remain abstinent; at the same time it becomes increasingly clear that her cocaine use interferes with progress. Following a relapse, Mary quickly returns to her pattern of daily use which has deleterious effects on her mood, her physical health and her attendance at the individual sessions.

It is decided to continue with the focus on mentalisation in which Mary progresses well and to address the cocaine addiction which is increasingly interfering with her mental health treatment by using the Community Reinforcement Approach, outlined below.

Community Reinforcement Approach (CRA)

The Community Reinforcement Approach is a bio-psychosocial approach to change a lifestyle of substance use. It acknowledges the importance of the social environment and focuses on the development of alternative rewarding social activities that are incompatible with substance use.[15] The CRA integrates cognitive behavioural interventions to change environmental contingencies such as work, leisure and family relations with pharmacological interventions such as disulfiram and naltrexone. CRA encompasses interventions aimed at behaviours that can be strengthened or weakened by their consequences, such as participating in a rewarding activity, and interventions addressing the environment such as an important significant other.[16]

Case study 12.2: Mary – part v

Mary starts on the combination of disulfiram 250 mg and naltrexone 50 mg daily which she tolerates well. She reports that the effect of cocaine is 'less strong'. In periods where she takes the medication she manages to remain abstinent but there are also periods when she decides to stop medication and resumes her cocaine habit. The help of her partner Jasmine and her parents is established to find activities that are incompatible with drug use. These include scheduling daily long walks with their dog during the early evening when craving is at its highest. Her partner is also convinced of the importance of abstinence and progresses herself to accept treatment. With the help of a social worker, Mary manages to find voluntary work after she lost her job as a car technician which was highly stressful due to the condemning attitude of several work colleagues. She also starts attending a weekly self-help group.

REHABILITATION AND CURE

TABLE 12.4 Treatment stage: rehabilitation and cure

Mental health	Substance use
• Responsibility and goals	• Motivational approach
• Stability	• Abstinence
• Adapt crisis plan	• Change of lifestyle
• Work/relationships	• Work/relationship
• Acceptance	• Acceptance
• Self-help groups	• Self-help groups
Motivational phase: persevere/relapse	

The relapse prevention stage of treatment consists of psychiatric follow-up with regular medication reviews, sheltered housing, self-help groups and a reduced frequency of individual psychotherapy sessions. Regular home visits can facilitate the transition from intensive inpatient treatment or day care to less intensive outpatient care, in order to maintain lifestyle changes. Specific interventions include help with structuring daily activities, finding voluntary work, expanding the social network and maintaining medication adherence. There is a shift towards increasing the person's responsibility. They should be allowed to learn from their mistakes. Integrated relapse prevention plans include strategies to prevent a relapse in substance use and mental illness relapses. Individuals experiencing borderline problems learn to recognise warning signs for reduced mentalising capacity and generally learn to apply healthier coping skills to their problems with emotion regulation.

HOW DID THOMAS, MARY AND JAMES PROGRESS IN THE LONG RUN?
Thomas
After a successful inpatient stay Thomas is allowed back into sheltered housing and starts attending the local day care centre. He receives outreach home visits by a member of the nursing staff and attends five sessions of EMDR with the programme's psychotherapist. He maintains abstinence and is referred back to the local mental health team.

Mary
Mary will continue to attend the programme as an outpatient for the individual psychotherapy using a mentalisation-based approach. The frequency of appointments will gradually decrease. Mary has not had any crisis admissions for the past six months.

James
Working alongside the nursing team, James manages to pursue his painting and photography and eventually hires a studio. At discharge he is waiting for a place in supported housing and uses cannabis occasionally. He has made great gains in

accepting his mental illness and uses his relapse prevention plan which is based on the functional analysis on an almost daily basis.

After several home visits his mother eventually agrees to engage in psychoeducation regarding schizophrenia and substance use.

CONCLUSION

Treatment for mental health–substance use problems ideally adopts an eclectic stage-wise approach. One of the most important aspects of the integrated form of treatment outlined above seems to be the provision of care within the same treatment team, including psychotherapy, medication, family interventions and help with the necessary lifestyle changes.

REFERENCES

1 American Psychiatric Association. *Diagnostic and Statistical Manual of Mental Disorders. DSM-IV-TR.* Washington, DC: American Psychiatric Association; 2000.
2 Corrigan PW, McCracken SG, Holmes EP. Motivational interviews as goal assessment for persons with psychiatric disability. *Community Mental Health Journal.* 2001; **37**: 113–22.
3 Bateman AW, Fonagy P. *Psychotherapy for Borderline Personality Disorder: mentalization-based treatment.* Oxford: Oxford University Press; 2004.
4 Van Wel B, Kockmann I, Blum N, *et al.* STEPPS group treatment for borderline personality disorder in the Netherlands. *Annals of Clinical Psychiatry.* 2006; **18**: 63–7.
5 Fonagy P, Target M, Gergely G. Attachment and borderline personality disorder: a theory and some evidence. *Psychiatric Clinics of North America.* 2000; **23**: 103–22.
6 Bateman AW, Fonagy P. *Mentalization-based Treatment for Borderline Personality Disorder: a practical guide.* Oxford: Oxford University Press; 2006.
7 Gunderson JG. The borderline patient's intolerance of aloneness: insecure attachments and therapist availability. *American Journal of Psychiatry.* 1996; **153**: 752–8.
8 Shapiro F. *Eye Movement Desensitization and Reprocessing: basic principles, protocols, and procedures.* New York: Guilford Press; 2001.
9 Prochaska JO, DiClemente CC, Norcross JC. In search of how people change: applications to addictive behaviors. *American Psychologist.* 1992; **47**: 1102–14.
10 Miller WR, Rollnick S. *Motivational Interviewing: preparing people for change.* 2nd ed. New York: Guilford Press; 2002.
11 Velasquez MM, Maurer G, Crouch C, *et al. Group Treatment for Substance Abuse: a stages of change therapy manual.* New York: Guilford Press; 2001.
12 Koestler A. *The Yogi and the Commissar and other essays.* New York: Macmillan; 1945.
13 Bleiberg E. *Treating Personality Disorders in Children and Adolescents: a relational approach.* New York: Guilford Press; 2001.
14 Bales; 2009. Personal communication.
15 Schottenfeld RS, Pantalon MV, Chawarski MC, *et al.* Community reinforcement approach for combined opioid and cocaine dependence: patterns of engagement in alternate activities. *Journal of Substance Abuse Treatment.* 2000; **18**: 255–61.
16 Roozen, HG, Boulogne JJ, Van Tulder MW, *et al.* A systematic review of the effectiveness of the Community Reinforcement Approach in alcohol, cocaine and opioid addiction. *Drug and Alcohol Dependence.* 2004; **74**: 1–13.

TO LEARN MORE

- Allen JG, Fonagy P. *Handbook of Mentalization-based Treatment*. Chichester: John Wiley & Sons Ltd; 2006.
- Arkowitz H, Westra HA, Miller WR, *et al. Motivational Interviewing in the Treatment of Psychological Problems*. New York: Guilford Press; 2008.
- Mueser KT, Noordsy DL, Drake RE, *et al. Integrated Treatment for Dual Disorders: a guide to effective practice*. New York: Guilford Press; 2003.
- Center for Addiction and Mental Health. Available at: www.camh.net/
- UCL Psychoanalysis Unit. Available at: www.ucl.ac.uk/psychoanalysis/

ANSWERS TO PRE-READING EXERCISE 12.1

1 An integrative approach to the treatment of mental health and substance use problems includes the establishment of motivational groups.[11] Family interventions at an early stage of the treatment help families to overcome their ambivalence to change, using the same motivational strategies that are used with the individual, avoiding confrontation and argumentation, identifying which factors are interfering with achieving shared family goals and providing psychoeducation about substance use and mental health.

2 An integrated approach for the treatment of borderline personality disorder and cocaine dependence needs to take into account the stages of change which have been described in the transtheoretical model of change,[9] as well as matching psychotherapeutic interventions to the level of mentalising capacity. This can be combined with group skills training (STEPPS training[4]) and the Community Reinforcement Approach (CRA[15]).

3 Psychoeducation for people experiencing schizophrenia and cannabis use problems is an ongoing part of the integrated treatment and can be used with individuals, groups and families.

4 The constant presence of staff can be very threatening as it activates attachment difficulties. Actually, the mentalisation-based approach for borderline personality disorder has been developed in a day care or outpatient setting. Other negative aspects of inpatient treatment can be the rather repressive environment of secure facilities or general psychiatric wards as this is not helpful in early stages of change.

CHAPTER 13

The young person and dialectical behaviour therapy

Lorne M Korman and Kyle Burns

INTRODUCTION

Young adults frequently present with substance use and other concurrent self-destructive behavioural problems related to impulsivity and deficits in emotion regulation. These concurrent problem behaviours include suicidal and deliberately self-injurious acts including:

➤ cutting
➤ binge eating
➤ intense and inappropriate anger
➤ gambling
➤ risky sex.

Dialectical behaviour therapy (DBT) is a promising treatment to address these concurrent behavioural problems. In this chapter we provide a brief overview of DBT and describe DBT adaptations for use with individuals with substance use disorders. We describe a rationale for the application of DBT with young adults, and highlight some of the adaptations of DBT for treating young adults experiencing mental health–substance use problems and other self-destructive behavioural problems related to impulsivity and deficits in emotion regulation.

WHAT IS DBT?

DBT was developed for and evaluated with individuals diagnosed with borderline personality disorder (BPD).[1] People with BPD frequently present with multiple comorbid problems, including:

➤ chronic suicidality and/or deliberate self-injury
➤ substance use
➤ other impulsive harmful behaviours.

A central tenet of DBT is that BPD is characterised by deficits in the inability to regulate emotions. DBT views these out-of-control, self-destructive behaviours as the sequelae of dysregulated emotions, and/or as behaviours that serve to modulate dysregulated emotions.

KEY POINT 13.1

The treatment focus is on helping people to acquire skills to better regulate their emotions, cope with distress, improve judgement and manage important relationships.

DBT is a comprehensive psychotherapy integrating behaviour therapy with aspects of Zen mindfulness traditions. The approach is informed by a dialectical philosophy, which views reality as consisting of opposite, antithetical truths that are dynamic and transactional. When faced with the tension presented by truths that appear opposite and irreconcilable, a dialectical way of thinking seeks to acknowledge aspects of truth in both opposite perspectives, and in doing so leads to the creation of a new synthesis. This approach is well-suited to people who frequently see the world from a polarised perspective (e.g. idealising and then devaluing others) and who act in similarly extreme ways (e.g. suicide). Dialectics pervades DBT, and this tension between opposites is apparent in the core dialectic of the treatment. On the one hand, DBT focuses on change through behaviour therapy; on the other hand, DBT validation strategies focus on accepting the individual and reality exactly as they are.

The goals and modes of standard DBT
DBT has five clearly articulated goals and the treatment is highly structured. The five goals of DBT are to:
1 Motivate individuals to engage in therapy.
2 Teach individuals new skills.
3 Ensure generalisation of these skills to the individuals' natural environments.
4 Provide support for therapists.
5 Orient the individuals' networks of significant others to support the treatment.

Comprehensive DBT consists of four modes, each of which is designed primarily to achieve one specific goal.

The goal of individual therapy is to increase the person's motivation to participate in therapy. An assumption in DBT is that motivation to engage in therapy is likely to be insufficient. Because of the multitude of problems people currently face in their lives, the traumatic histories reported by the majority of these individuals,[2,3] and their difficulties controlling their emotions and actions, therapy typically represents a daunting and painful task. Therefore, DBT relies on the therapist to establish and maintain strong alliances with the person, and to use specific strategies to establish, strengthen and maintain their commitment to fully engage in all aspects of treatment. Each person in DBT has an individual therapist who acts as a consultant to the person and is responsible for treatment planning and progress, and for helping the individual to integrate and apply the skills they are learning.

Individual DBT psychotherapy sessions typically occur once weekly and last an hour. Sessions typically begin with a review of diary cards that are completed each day and brought to the sessions. On the diary cards, individuals monitor instances of self-harm, substance use, skills use and other behaviours relevant to treatment that have occurred since the last session. DBT therapists use a hierarchy of targets to determine the behaviours that will be addressed in any given session.

KEY POINT 13.2

In DBT, life-threatening behaviours are the highest priority.

In DBT, life-threatening behaviours are the highest priorities (e.g. suicide-related behaviours), followed by behaviours that interfere with therapy (e.g. missing a session), and then behaviours that reduce quality of life (e.g. substance use). The hierarchy is particularly useful in helping therapists prioritise session targets when people present with multiple serious problems. Session targets are explored primarily through interventions like behavioural analysis, insight strategies and solution analyses. Behavioural interventions typically include exposure, contingency management, cognitive restructuring, and skills training. Individual therapists balance this emphasis on change strategies with a dialectically opposite focus on acceptance and validation of the person and their experience.

The goal of skills training groups is for people to acquire new skills. In standard DBT individuals are taught skills from four different modules.[4] The four modules are:
1 Mindfulness.
2 Interpersonal effectiveness.
3 Emotion regulation.
4 Distress tolerance.

These four skills modules focus, respectively, on the following:
➤ being present in the moment and making decisions based on wisdom
➤ identifying interpersonal goals, acting assertively and managing relationships
➤ identifying and regulating emotions
➤ accepting reality and tolerating painful affect without resorting to impulsive self-destructive behaviours.

Additional skills and adaptations have been developed for young adults,[5] anger problems[6] and eating disorders.[7]

Another goal of DBT is to generalise new skills to individuals' natural environments. Skills generalisation primarily is achieved through the use of homework and pager/telephone skills coaching outside of therapy hours.

DBT also recognises that therapists require support to maintain their motivation to work with their individual and to improve their skills in working with people who pose a challenge (*see* Book 2, Chapters 10–12). This is the objective of the consultation team, which routinely meets for two hours each week. The consultation team is made up of all of the therapists on a DBT team, including skills trainers and individual therapists. The functions of the team also include providing validation for the therapists, improving therapists' abilities to treat complex problems, and routinely addressing therapists' behaviours that interfere with therapy.

DBT ADAPTATION FOR MENTAL HEALTH–SUBSTANCE USE DISORDERS

DBT has been adapted for and evaluated with individuals with comorbid borderline personality and substance use disorders.[8,9] This adaptation has been called DBT-S. The treatment is similar in most respects to standard DBT but places more focus on addressing addictive behaviours. Below we describe some of the adaptations for substance use in DBT-S.

Dialectical abstinence

DBT-S recognises that both abstinence-based and harm-reduction approaches are associated with particular benefits, and thus tries to establish a dialectical balance between these approaches.[10,11] On the one hand, approaches like 12-step programmes that emphasise complete abstinence have been associated with longer intervals between substance use episodes.[12,13] On the other hand, relapse prevention strategies based on harm reduction principles have been shown to be effective in reducing the frequency and intensity of substance use after relapses.[14] A major premise of relapse prevention (*see* Chapters 15 and 16; Book 4, Chapter 13) is that substance use relapse or 'slips' are likely to occur among individuals working through addictions problems as individuals learn, practise and acquire new behaviours necessary to support abstinence. In this view, rather than representing a complete treatment failure, relapses pose opportunities to identify gaps in skills and problem solving and are viewed more as part of an often necessary process in working through addictions problems. Throughout there is focus on avoiding blaming or stigmatising individuals for relapsing.

'Dialectical abstinence' tries to adopt the strengths of both abstinence and relapse prevention approaches by focusing on getting commitments from individuals to work completely towards absolute abstinence for a given period of time. This period is negotiated between the individual and therapist, and to some degree depends on how long particular individuals feel they can imagine tolerating being abstinent. The approach is similar to focusing on one day at a time in 12-step programmes. Once the agreed-upon period of abstinence is over, a new period of abstinence is agreed upon. At the same time, individuals and the therapists systematically plan to help limit any damage should a relapse occur, and for a speedy return to abstinence. Relapse is a relatively common phenomenon among individuals working through addictions problems. Marlatt and Donovan[14] observed that once an individual has committed to abstinence, subsequent relapses can lead the individual to make negative internal attributions (e.g. 'I relapsed because I am weak') and engender feelings like shame and guilt. Marlatt and Gordon[15] referred to this as the 'abstinence violation effect' and noted that the phenomenon tended to make individuals vulnerable to continued substance use and further relapse (*see* Chapters 15 and 16). From a behavioural perspective, individuals may be more likely to continue their substance use after a relapse because substance use is negatively reinforced by the reduction of aversive emotions.

The danger of continued use after a relapse can be addressed among young adults by educating the individual and their families about the abstinence violation effect, and reframing relapses as events that are not uncommon during recovery processes. It is also important for therapists to adopt a supportive and non-judgemental stance (*see* Book 4, Chapter 2) when young adults have relapsed, to welcome them back to treatment, and to acknowledge and praise them for stopping their use after relapsing. In working with young adults, it is particularly important to also engage family and significant others in adopting similar approaches to their family members (*see* Book 3, Chapter 2; Book 5, Chapters 4 and 7). Families are encouraged to take a more behavioural approach to their young adults' substance use behaviours, focusing for example on reinforcing the young adults' efforts to stop use rather than imposing punishment *after* the young adult has stopped using, and extinguishing rather than punishing substance use behaviours. While encouraging family members to observe their own limits and to avoid enabling their young adult to continue abusing substances, DBT therapists also try to inoculate families against blaming their young adult for relapsing and/or dismissing the young adult's motivation and efforts to stop using.

DBT-S hierarchy and substance-related targets

DBT-S makes use of a slightly adapted hierarchy of targets, in which substance-related behaviours are considered the priorities among quality-of-life interfering behaviours. These targeted behaviours are not limited solely to the actual consumption of substances. Substance-related behaviours also include the acquisition of illicit drugs, over-the-counter drugs, alcohol and legal substances that are not used in the manner or quantity prescribed. Other substance-related targets that may be monitored on weekly diary cards and addressed in therapy include urges and cravings to use, physical discomfort associated with abstinence and withdrawal, and lying.

DBT-S places considerable emphasis on increasing functional behaviours that are inconsistent with a life of substance use (e.g. going to school, studying, working, developing friendships with individuals who do not use substances, exercise, etc.). These behaviours are particularly critical to developing young adults. Along with skills use, these behaviours may also be monitored on diary cards as significant treatment targets.

DBT-S: engagement

DBT-S recognises that many individuals with substance use problems often are particularly challenging to engage in therapy. Relapse frequently is the norm rather than the exception among individuals struggling with serious substance use problems. In the midst of substance use relapse episodes, many individuals simply disappear from treatment. DBT-S refers to individuals in such situations as 'butterflies'.[10] Re-engaging 'butterflies' in therapy can be challenging. Individuals commonly experience shame, disappointment and anger during and after relapse episodes. Individuals often are more emotionally and physically vulnerable during states of acute intoxication or withdrawal, and commonly face other consequences of relapse (e.g. loss of money and/or housing, damaged relationships, violence victimisation and/or perpetration, sexual exploitation). Psychotherapy after relapse requires individuals to expose themselves to their own and their therapists' scrutiny of their substance use behaviours and the ensuing damage, and not surprisingly many avoid returning to treatment.

DBT-S addresses the problem of individuals as butterflies in a number of ways. First, individual therapists take a detailed history of substance use habits at the beginning of therapy. For example, knowing where and with whom individuals tend to use substances can make it more likely that therapists can find the person in the midst of a relapse. Second, DBT-S emphasises the importance of strategies that increase the attachment of the person to their individual therapists. Early in therapy and during times of high stress and/or relapse, this often involves increasing the frequency of contact between therapists and the young adult.[11] DBT-S also emphasises the importance of improving the valence of treatment by making therapy more inviting. This can involve offering meals or other food to individuals (and families) who attend skills training groups, greeting individuals warmly and offering them coffee or tea, ensuring some time to reconnect in a friendly way in individual sessions, and starting and winding down sessions whenever possible in a friendly and casual manner. At the end of session, this may involve talking about subjects that are pleasant, innocuous and that serve to increase attachment between therapist and individual (e.g. sharing something that they like about each other), and using distress tolerance and emotion regulation skills to reallocate attention and improve affect before leaving therapy sessions.

KEY POINT 13.3

Young adults can be difficult to engage in treatment.

Young adults can be particularly difficult to engage in treatment. This is frequently true in cases when parents or others may appear more invested in the young adult's treatment than the person. Particularly when there is conflict between family members, young adults may perceive therapy and therapists as being aligned with parents 'against' their interests. DBT is well-suited to addressing this common challenge by assigning clinicians from the consultation team other than the individual's therapist to serve as the primary liaisons to family members. These clinicians can receive information from parents and other family members and provide validation and after-hours skills coaching to families. Though individual therapy typically is not provided to family members, family 'liaisons' from DBT consultation teams serve roles similar to the individual therapists by establishing alliances with parents and other family members, coordinating care with the rest of the consultation team, and working to increase and maintain parents' motivation to attend skills training and to otherwise support the treatment.

DBT-S: relapse prevention

In the early stages of treatment, individuals experiencing mental health–substance use problems frequently continue to have strong urges to use substances but have few skills to tolerate these urges or to regulate their emotions and actions. This increases the individuals' susceptibility to relapse. Initially, it is important to help individuals plan to avoid drugs and alcohol as well as the cues or prompts associated with substance use (e.g. places, people and situations). An important feature of relapse prevention involves identifying high-risk situations in which the individual is vulnerable to relapse, and using coping strategies to prevent relapse.[16] Therapy also involves proactively planning with individuals for what to do when they unexpectedly are faced with cues or situations that prompt substance use. These common relapse prevention strategies have been termed 'planning ahead' in DBT.[10]

DBT-S: burning bridges to use

DBT for people experiencing mental health–substance use problems also emphasises 'burning bridges to use' substances. This may involve severing relationships with drug dealers and drug-using acquaintances, deleting drug-related phone and pager numbers, getting rid of drug use paraphernalia, or disclosing one's substance-related habits to parents and/or other significant others to make it more difficult to relapse. These behaviours are also monitored on the weekly diary cards. In addition, therapists and individuals monitor 'apparently irrelevant decisions[15] or behaviours'. These are behaviours that, though seemingly insignificant, may indicate that the individual may be less committed to maintaining abstinence, and can signal imminent relapse. Examples of an apparently unimportant behaviour include individuals taking a different route home that involves walking past a drug dealer's place of business, or re-establishing contact with other young adults or cliques who use substances.

WHY APPLY DBT TO WORKING ALONGSIDE THE YOUNG ADULTS?

DBT is a promising treatment for working alongside the young adult experiencing substance use disorders and concurrent self-destructive behavioural problems related to impulsivity and deficits in emotion regulation. To our knowledge, there are currently no published randomised control studies that have evaluated DBT with young adult populations. Nevertheless, there are numerous randomised trials supporting the efficacy of DBT in the treatment of adults with borderline personality disorders (BPD), including those with substance use disorders. BPD is a disorder in which numerous comorbidities are the norm rather than the exception, and individuals with BPD frequently behave impulsively in ways that are self-destructive.

Personality disorders like BPD are not generally diagnosed before adulthood because these diagnoses require that a long-standing pattern of these behaviours be present. In addition, some degree of exploratory and impulsive behaviours is common during adolescence. To the degree that these behaviours become problematic and impact on the young adults' development, age-appropriate functioning, and safety, DBT is useful because it employs a number of strategies to address multiple behavioural and other problems in an integrated treatment. These strategies include:

➤ an integrated diary card to monitor multiple behaviours simultaneously

➤ a hierarchy of targets to support therapists in prioritising behaviours to address in session
➤ the use of multiple skills modules focusing on reducing impulsivity and increasing emotion and behaviour regulation
➤ a behaviour therapy foundation from which thoughts, actions and emotions can be analysed, understood and targeted for change.

In addition, DBT builds in a number of strategies to address ambivalence and problems of motivation and treatment compliance, issues that are common among young adults experiencing substance use and other behavioural problems. These include commitment strategies, dialectical communication styles, and the monitoring and prioritisation of treatment interfering behaviours. Engaging and retaining people in treatment are a common challenge among both young adults and adults experiencing mental health–substance use problems. With adults, DBT has been shown to be particularly effective in engaging and retaining people in treatment.[8]

ADAPTING DBT FOR YOUNG ADULTS
In this section we will discuss some of the adaptations in DBT we have found helpful in working with young adults experiencing mental health–substance use problems and other concurrent self-destructive behaviours related to impulsivity and deficits in emotion regulation. These changes include involving the family and significant others in therapy, and the addition of new skills for young adults, families and caregivers.

Involving families and significant others in treatment
As mentioned earlier, one of the five main goals of DBT is to orient families and significant others to the therapy in order to foster support for the treatment within the individual's network. By orienting this network, DBT therapists strive to teach and guide the individual's network of family and significant others to behave in ways that foster the generalisation of newly acquired skilful behaviours, avoid reinforcing dysfunctional behaviours and otherwise support the treatment. When working with young adults, this is especially important because parents and significant others often exert significant influence on functioning and development. Once oriented, parents and other caregivers can be enormously effective in identifying and reinforcing the young adults' skilful behaviours outside of sessions. On the other hand, family members may reinforce (usually inadvertently) and maintain maladaptive behaviours, and/or ignore or punish adaptive behaviours.

KEY POINT 13.4

An important part of DBT with young adults is to help family members avoid the common pitfalls of reinforcing maladaptive behaviours.

In addition to helping young adults generalise new skills to their natural environments, involving families and/or other caregivers in DBT also aims to improve family functioning, reduce conflict, promote healthy parenting, and increase the family's ability to validate the young adult.[5,17]

DBT skills training is typically done in a classroom format. Groups last 2–2.5 hours, and often begin with a mindfulness exercise, followed by a review of participants' homework. New skills are taught in the second half of the group, and homework is assigned at the end of the group. Skills groups are usually co-facilitated by two therapists, one of whom is primarily responsible for teaching and leading the group. The co-therapist watches over the group, monitoring the attention and affect of group members, acts a 'model student', and ensures that participants understand the material.

There are a number of ways of involving parents and significant others in DBT skills training groups. One way is to include them with young adults in integrated family skills training groups. There are a number of advantages to this. Doing so provides family members with 'real time' exposure to newly taught skills. Family members are oriented to new skills alongside the young adult, and family members can practise new skills together with individuals in the group, and receive feedback and shaping immediately from therapists. Homework can also be assigned to the entire family unit in order to maximise the generalisation of skills. Young adults can be particularly difficult to get into therapy; they often have undeveloped personal management skills, and may not be optimally motivated to attend therapy sessions. Having parents attend skills training sessions often means that parents bring along their young adult children to skills training, increasing the likelihood that the individual actually makes it to skills training.

Integrating families and significant others in skills groups may also pose challenges. Some young adults baulk at having their families included in groups, and may be less willing or able to participate actively in groups. Families experiencing greater levels of dysfunction may also evidence conflict and expressed hostility in groups. High conflict and the intense negative affect it engenders are likely to interfere with attention and new learning in groups. Because skills acquisition is a prime objective of skills training groups, individuals and families must be able to sufficiently regulate their behaviours and affect sufficiently (with some coaching) in order to process and learn new material. In instances where family units are intensely conflictual, disruptive or otherwise dysregulated, family members may require more intense coaching to benefit from participation in skills groups. In worst-case scenarios, young adults may be less motivated to continue on in treatment, and some adamantly refuse to participate in treatment should their parents be included in groups in which they are expected to participate.

Another method of involving parents and significant others is to provide separate family skills training groups that do not include the young adult. In this approach, young adults participate together in skills training groups, while parents and significant others attend together in a separate group.

> **KEY POINT 13.5**
>
> Offering separate training groups for young adults and their family members may be more tolerable, and sometimes makes groups more viable when working with highly conflictual families.

Separate family groups for family members and significant others also allow for allocating more time to topics like validation and parenting skills that may be particularly beneficial for family members. Finally, family support groups can be added to family skills training groups that do not include the young adult. These support groups provide the opportunity for parents to share their difficulties and provide support to one another. A drawback associated with providing separate training for young adults and parents/significant others is that separate groups do not give parents and young adults the opportunity to learn and practise skills together in a regular weekly format with therapists present to direct and coach families, and provide feedback. In situations where families experience difficulties in generalising effective use of skills at home and other natural environments, additional skills-focused sessions with family/significant others and young adults may be necessary.

Adapted DBT skills for young adults, families and caregivers

In addition to the four skills training modules used in standard DBT, a fifth module has been developed for suicidal young adults and their families.[17] The 'middle path' module addresses the core dialectic of DBT, focusing on skills to help young adults and their families to balance acceptance and change. The middle path module involves teaching young adults and their significant others about dialectics, helping them to recognise that there is an opposite, equally valid perspective for every truth, and suggests adopting a dialectical 'middle path' of thinking and acting. The three major components of the middle path are described below.

1 Dialectical dilemmas

The first component of the middle path[17] focuses on helping individuals and their families to become more balanced and dialectical in their thinking. Three dialectical dilemmas are introduced with which emotionally and behaviourally dysregulated young adults and their families (and their therapists) often struggle. For each of these dialectical dilemmas, 'a middle path' of behaving is suggested. The first dialectic is between being either permissive or authoritarian. In the former, caregivers are overly lenient, make no or few age-appropriate demands and the young adults assume little or no age-appropriate responsibilities. In the latter, caregivers are excessively strict and inflexible, make too many demands and set limits that are overly restrictive. The corresponding middle path is to establish clear reasonable rules that are consistently enforced. The second dilemma is between pathologising normal behaviours and normalising problem behaviours. In the former, typical behaviours that are developmentally appropriate (e.g. sexual experimentation) are punished or treated as bad. In the latter, dangerous and damaging behaviours (e.g. unsafe sex) are minimised. The corresponding middle path involves tolerating age-appropriate experimentation and addressing maladaptive behaviours. The final dialectical dilemma is between prematurely forcing autonomy and fostering dependence. In the former, young adults assume adult responsibilities when they are developmentally unprepared (e.g. moving out on their own). In the latter, young adults do not assume age-appropriate responsibilities and are sheltered from the consequences of their action or inaction. The corresponding middle path involves providing appropriate support and gradually increasing autonomous behaviours and expectations.

2 Learning theory

A second component of the middle path[17] involves teaching learning theory to young adults and their caregivers. The goal is to help young adults and their families become active agents of change outside of therapy to effectively promote more functional behaviours on the part of both the young adults and their family members. In a sense, young adults and their caregivers are deputised as behaviour therapists to help them to modify the behaviours that both young adults and their family members want to change.

KEY POINT 13.6

Behavioural interventions are not intended to be imposed on the individual or their families. The individual, the therapist and families decide together which behaviours to target.

In addition, in keeping with DBT's emphasis on levelling the playing field and encouraging effective behaviour consistent with a life worth living, everyone's behaviour is 'fair game' for change, including young adults, families and therapists.

Targeting behaviours for change first requires operationally defining distinct behaviours that participants want to develop or eliminate. 'Anger', for example, is too general and subjective a construct to serve as a clearly defined behaviour that can be targeted for change. On the other hand, yelling (or speaking more frequently in a lowered tone) and discrete episodes of substance use are clearly defined and observable behaviours that can be readily identified, and which can be monitored and targeted for change.

Learning theory describes how behaviours are acquired, maintained and changed. In operant conditioning, behaviours are more likely to reoccur when reinforcement follows a certain behaviour. Reinforcement can entail either the provision of a reward (positive reinforcement) or the removal of an aversive stimulus (negative reinforcement). Extinction, on the other hand, serves to eliminate previously learned behaviours by eliminating all consequences after similar behaviours occur. Finally, punishment, the provision of an aversive consequence following a certain behaviour, tends to suppress behaviour, at least in the presence of cues associated with the punishment.

A number of key points are emphasised during the learning theory module.

Individuals and their families are taught that, for the most part, behaviours are controlled by factors *outside* of individuals' awareness, rather than being deliberately motivated. The goals are to encourage participants to adopt a compassionate, non-judgemental stance, as well as a scientific, systematic approach to behavioural change. Adopting a non-judgemental stance is a key part of the core mindfulness skills module in DBT. Punishment is generally discouraged as a routine means of changing behaviour, as punishment suppresses rather than eliminates behaviour and does not lead to the development of new behaviours. Worse yet, punishment may inadvertently reinforce dysfunctional behaviours (e.g. angry attention by family members after an individual self-harms), and also sometimes suppresses emerging behaviours that are adaptive (e.g. punishing an individual for misusing a small amount of a drug, after the individual has worked effectively to reduce and discontinue use). Instead, extinction, reinforcement and shaping are encouraged as more effective means of changing behaviours.

Shaping describes a process by which successive approximations of a desired behaviour are systematically reinforced. Families and young adults are taught that shaping is an integral strategy for fostering new and complex behaviours. Imagine, for example, a young adult whose substance use is routinely prompted when he/she gets intensely angry. Targeting substance use may entail addressing numerous micro behaviours, and families are encouraged to be realistic and patient, to be scientific in identifying and reinforcing new behaviours that may be required in order to achieve sobriety. These 'micro behaviours' may include the individual learning to be mindful or aware when she/he is becoming angry or feeling other primary emotions; learning to use distress tolerance strategies to tolerate anger; using emotion regulation and distraction strategies to modulate anger; and learning to use interpersonal effectiveness strategies to effectively communicate anger and needs. In addition, the family would be encouraged to reinforce these new behaviours, and to validate and reinforce more functional expressions of anger from the individual, including 'imperfect' but improved expressions of anger (e.g. yelling less loudly and not swearing).

3 *Validation*

The last component of the middle path in DBT involves teaching validation skills to young adults and their families. Validation refers to the genuine and respectful acknowledgement of another person and often takes the form of communicating that something in another person's feelings, actions, thoughts or beliefs is valid. DBT validation strategies can involve being fully present with another person, accurately reflecting the other's communication, understanding tacit or inchoate aspects of their experience, communicating that some or all of another person's behaviour makes perfect sense, or treating the other person as an equal human being rather than as a fragile person or child.

In standard DBT for adults,[1] therapists validate the individual as well as other clinicians on the DBT consultation team. In the treatment of young adults, validation skills are also taught to young adults and to their families and/or significant others. These skills are taught and practised initially in skills training groups. The goals of teaching validation skills include improving family communication and reducing conflict, increasing accurate reflection and acceptance of young adults' and family members' experience, reducing invalidation/dismissal of young adults' experience with family members, and increasing trust, being radically genuine.

SUMMARY

DBT is a promising treatment for young adults experiencing mental health–substance use disorders and other concurrent self-destructive behaviours related to impulsivity and deficits in emotion regulation. DBT's goals include helping people to learn and generalise new skills to regulate emotions and behaviours, increasing the individuals' and therapists motivation to engage in therapy, and orienting the person's interpersonal network to support therapeutic change. For individuals with multiple problems, DBT uses a foundation of behaviour therapy, from which thoughts, actions and emotions can be analysed, understood and targeted for change.

DBT-S is an adaptation of DBT that has been demonstrated to be effective for individuals experiencing mental health–substance use problems. DBT-S:
➤ balances abstinence and harm reduction strategies
➤ focuses on a comprehensive range of substance-related targets
➤ integrates relapse prevention strategies into treatment
➤ uses additional strategies to engage people using substances
➤ helps the individual to burn bridges to continued substance use.

Adaptations for young adults include:
➤ involving parents and significant others in therapy
➤ teaching young adults and families about dialectical dilemmas and to be more balanced in their behaviours
➤ teaching young adults and families about learning theory/behavioural change strategies, and validation skills.

REFERENCES

1 Linehan MM. *Cognitive Behavioral Treatment for Borderline Personality Disorder.* New York: Guilford Press; 1993.
2 Herman JL, Perry JC, van der Kolk BA. Childhood trauma in borderline personality disorder. *The American Journal of Psychiatry.* 1989; **146**: 490–5.
3 Silk KR, Lee S, Hill EM, *et al.* Borderline personality disorder symptoms and severity of sexual abuse. *The American Journal of Psychiatry.* 1995; **152**: 1059–64.
4 Linehan MM. *Skills Training Manual for Borderline Personality Disorder.* New York: Guilford Press; 1993.
5 Miller AL, Rathus JH, DuBose AP, *et al.* Dialectical behavior therapy for adolescents. In: Dimeff LA, Koerner K, editors. *Dialectical Behavior Therapy in Clinical Practice: applications across disorders and settings.* New York: Guilford Press; 2007. pp. 245–63.
6 Korman LM. Treating anger and addictions concurrently. In: Skinner WJ, editor. *Treating Concurrent Disorders: a handbook for practitioners.* Toronto, Ontario: Centre for Addiction and Mental Health; 2005. pp. 215–33.
7 Safer DL, Telch CF, Chen EY. *Dialectical Behavior Therapy for Binge Eating and Bulimia.* New York: Guilford Press; 2009.

8 Linehan MM, Schmidt H, Dimeff LA, *et al.* Dialectical behavior therapy for patients with borderline personality disorder and drug dependence. *The American Journal on Addictions.* 1999; **8**: 279–92.

9 Linehan MM, Dimeff LA, Reynolds SK, *et al.* Dialectical behavior therapy versus comprehensive validation therapy plus 12-step for the treatment of opioid dependent women meeting criteria for borderline personality disorder. *Drug and Alcohol Dependence.* 2002; **67**: 13–26.

10 Dimeff LA, Linehan MM. Dialectical behavior therapy for substance users. *Addiction Science and Clinical Practice*; 2008. Available at: http://depts.washington.edu/brtc/files/Dimeff,%20L.A.,%20Linehan,%20M.M.%20(2008)%20DBT%20for%20Substance%20Abusers.pdf (accessed 16 November 2010).

11 McMain S, Sayrs JH, Dimeff LA, *et al.* Dialectical behavior therapy for individuals with borderline personality disorder and substance dependence. In: Dimeff LA, Koerner K, editors. *Dialectical Behavior Therapy in Clinical Practice: applications across disorders and settings.* New York: Guilford Press; 2007. pp. 145–73.

12 Hall SM, Havassy BE, Wasserman DA. Commitment to abstinence and acute stress in relapse to alcohol, opiates, and nicotine. *Journal of Consulting and Clinical Psychology.* 1990; **58**: 175–81.

13 Supnick JA, Colletti G. Relapse coping and problem solving training following treatment for smoking. *Addictive Behaviors.* 1984; **9**: 401–4.

14 Marlatt AG, Donovan DM, editors. *Relapse Prevention: maintenance strategies in the treatment of addictive behaviors.* 2nd ed. New York: Guilford Press; 2005.

15 Marlatt AG, Gordon JR, editor. *Relapse Prevention: maintenance strategies in the treatment of addictive behaviors.* New York: Guilford Press; 1985.

16 Marlatt AG, Witkiewitz K. Relapse prevention for alcohol and drug problems. In: Marlatt AG, Donovan DM. *Relapse Prevention: maintenance strategies in the treatment of addictive behaviors.* 2nd ed. New York: Guilford Press; 2005. pp. 1–44.

17 Miller AL, Rathus JH, Linehan MM. *Dialectical Behavior Therapy with suicidal adolescents.* New York: Guilford Press; 2007.

TO LEARN MORE

• Linehan MM. *Cognitive Behavioral Treatment for Borderline Personality Disorder.* New York: Guilford Press; 1993.

• Linehan MM. *Skills Training Manual for Borderline Personality Disorder.* New York: Guilford Press; 1993.

• Miller AL, Rathus JH, Linehan MM. *Dialectical Behavior Therapy with Suicidal Adolescents.* New York: Guilford Press; 2007.

CHAPTER 14

Prison, crime and active intervention

David Marteau

NATURE AND SIZE OF THE PROBLEM

Drug and alcohol problems are far more common among offenders than the wider population: approximately 60% of male prisoners and 80% of female prisoners have a history of problematic use. More than half of these will be dependent on alcohol and/or street drugs on the day of their arrival in prison.[1]

A survey conducted in 16 large city police custody suites in England and Wales[2] found that almost 70% of arrestees tested positive for one or more illicit drugs. Nearly 40% tested positive for opiates and/or cocaine. Almost 80% of those arrested for acquisitive crimes (such as theft, fraud and burglary) tested positive for at least one illicit drug.[2] The survey excluded any arrestees who were unfit due to intoxication. Despite this criterion, almost a half of all suspected cases of criminal damage, and 37% of those arrested in connection with a violent offence, tested positive for alcohol consumption. Due to the exclusion of intoxicated arrestees, the true figure may be substantially higher. Research has found, for instance, that alcohol had been consumed prior to the offence in nearly three-quarters (73%) of domestic violence cases, and was a 'feature' in almost two-thirds (62%). Furthermore, almost half of these convicted domestic violence offenders (48%) were found to be alcohol dependent.[3,4]

People with offending problems tend to have poor health: 90% of prisoners have a mental health problem (including personality disorder) and/or substance use problem. More than 80% of prisoners smoke, and 24% report having injected drugs.[5]

Studies indicate that around 38% of male prisoners with a substance use problem enter custody as regular injectors.[5,6] Many of these severely dependent men have other complex physical, psychological and social needs, ranging across:

➤ deep vein thrombosis
➤ depression
➤ type 1 diabetes
➤ learning needs
➤ homelessness
➤ self-harm
➤ withdrawal seizures.

Blood-borne viruses are also a substantial problem among injecting drug users, particularly those who have been to prison (*see* Table 14.1)

TABLE 14.1 Prevalence of hepatitis B and C and self-report injecting drug use in England and Wales

N = 2839	Been to prison 1740 (61%)	Not been to prison 1099 (39%)
Hepatitis B positive	24%	17%
Hepatitis C positive	39%	28%
Injected while in prison (self-report)	17%	N/A

Source: Department of Health. Prevalence of HIV and hepatitis infections in the United Kingdom 2001: annual report of the Unlinked Anonymous Prevalence Monitoring Programme 2001. Available at: www.dh.gov.uk/en/Publicationsandstatistics/Publications/PublicationsStatistics/ DH_4006493 (accessed 16 November 2010).

The higher rate of hepatitis infection among injecting drug users who have been to prison cannot necessarily be attributed to needle sharing while in prison. Prisoners tend to be more severely dependent drug users. Additionally, offenders are also more prone to risk taking. It is plausible, therefore, that a sizeable proportion of these additional infections were contracted outside of prison. In response to the high prevalence, disinfecting tablets are now available in adult prisons in England, to facilitate the cleansing by prisoners of illicit injecting equipment. To take best advantage of the personal and public health opportunity that a stay in prison represents for a drug user, the largest national programme of hepatitis B vaccination has been set up in prisons across the UK. As an apparent consequence, reports of new cases of hepatitis B have declined recently.[7]

In considering the effectiveness of any treatment system, it is important to keep sight of the ability of that system to serve the whole population. More than 20% of prisoners are from black and minority ethnic backgrounds[8] but the prevalence of mental health problems in black and minority ethnic prisoners appears to be significantly lower than the white population.[9] Services need to audit themselves and survey people who use substances to see that their service is equally open to all.

PATTERNS OF OFFENDING

The association between offending and substance use is well-established and takes on several guises. The first type is the most direct – an offence that relates to the consumption of a substance: driving while drunk, drunk and disorderliness, and – under the UK Drugs Act[10] 2005 – consumption of an illicit substance such as cannabis or cocaine.

The second category deals with procurement or supply of substances. These may be either substances banned by the Misuse of Drugs Act, or illicit (such as supplying contraband alcohol or tobacco).

The third type of offence is the one that concerns the treatment services most: the crimes committed as an indirect but genuine consequence of substance use.

These include acts related to intoxication, where a loss of inhibition may result in destructive behaviour (criminal damage, assault), or acquisitive crimes such as shoplifting or burglary, which can be fuelled by an imperative to secure funds to attain intoxication or ward off withdrawal.

LEGAL AND CLINICAL FRAMEWORK

The recognition by, among others, the World Health Organization[11] that drug dependence is a condition that can distort the motivations and behaviours of an individual to the point where he/she becomes more prone to offending led the UK government to construct a legal and clinical framework for the treatment of drug dependence. In the first instance, these took the form of Drug Treatment and Testing Orders and, with the passing of the 2005 Drugs Act,[10] Drug Rehabilitation Requirements and Alcohol Treatment Requirements. Because the relationship between drug dependence and acquisitive crime is so strong,[12] there was a very clear case for an investment in drug treatment for people involved in contact with the justice system. This is reflected by an increase in the number of drug treatment orders made by the courts of England and Wales, from 4854 in 2001/02 to 16 607 in 2007/08.[13]

IMPRISONMENT: RISKS AND REMEDIES

For those offenders unable to benefit from a community substance use treatment programme (such as the Drug Rehabilitation Requirement, mentioned above), prison can afford a chance to address a substance use problem. There are currently 114 treatment programmes of differing levels of intensity operating across 99 prisons in England and Wales. These range from low-threshold four-week courses, through more intensive cognitive behavioural and 12-step programmes to five long-term therapeutic communities (TCs).

Imprisonment has also presented three particular risks for drug users:
1   A heightened rate of suicide among prisoners with drug problems in the early days of custody, associated with drug withdrawal.
2   Drug overdose in the first few days that follow release from prison.
3   The premature breaking of community drug treatment in prison, leading to increased rates of relapse and attendant re-offending after release.

Regarding the vulnerability of drug users in prison to suicide in prison and to death on release, an enquiry into 172 suicides in prisons in England and Wales[14] found that drug-dependent individuals entering prison had double the risk of suicide in the first week of custody compared with all prisoners.

Although no detailed UK data is currently available in relation to its effectiveness, a sense of greater stability with a consequent reduction in self-harm has been reported by prisons that have introduced methadone programmes. The introduction of these programmes across all women's prisons from 2005 coincided with a fall in self-inflicted deaths in women's prisons from a total of 36 in the preceding three full years (2002–4) to 15 in the three years 2005–7.

There is an increased risk of fatal opioid overdoses among drug users leaving prisons both here and abroad.[15,16] A study of more than 48 000 prison releases[17] found that injecting drug users were eight times more likely to die in the two weeks that followed release from prison than at any other point. Ninety-seven per cent of these deaths involved opioid drugs. Loss of tolerance to the effects of opioids during imprisonment appeared to be the most likely explanation for these tragedies.

A randomised controlled trial of methadone maintenance in prisons in New South Wales, Australia[18] found evidence that methadone maintenance treatment could reduce rates of re-offending and, at four-year follow-up,[19] the rate of death among released prisoners. A similar US prisons randomised trial[20] found evidence for lower levels of drug use and re-offending among a prison-initiated methadone maintenance treatment cohort compared with two other groups (counselling only and counselling plus methadone post-release). A meta-analysis of the impact of methadone maintenance[21] found a consistent, statistically significant reduction in illicit opiate use, HIV risk behaviours and drug and property-related criminal behaviours. Methadone maintenance was most effective in its ability to reduce drug-related offending.

In the light of the available research evidence, new clinical substance misuse guidance for UK prisons was published in 2006.[22] The guidance recommended very early (i.e. first night) intervention in remand prisons for the treatment of drug withdrawal. It also emphasised the need to consider methadone programmes that extended beyond release, to retain the person's tolerance to opiate-based drugs, and thereby provide some protection from heroin overdose and to re-offending following a relapse.

CONTINUITY OF TREATMENT
Research into drug treatment results in the consistent finding that retention in treatment, particularly over the course of several months, is associated with good outcomes.[12,23] Two studies[24,25] reported evidence to support intensive supervision following release.

The prospect for people receiving drug treatment who are sent to prison is that they are most likely to require that treatment to continue across a number of settings as their case progresses. An offender may be moved from police custody to a court, then a remand prison, back to the court, on to a different remand prison, then into a secondary 'trainer' prison, and finally be released to the community. The continuation of care (including mental health–substance use treatments), across all these thresholds requires a large amount of time from professionals based across these settings. In view of the advantages that such continuity brings, this concentration of effort is justified on both ethical and economic grounds.

Continuity of care for drug users is secured across justice sectors in England and Wales via the Drug Interventions Programme (DIP). DIP case managers provide a link between the community and prison, and from prison to the community. The avenue for continuity of care for drug users who need help with significant mental health problems is the care programme approach, which is overseen by the statutory mental health services. For drug users with less severe mental health problems, a coordinated approach between substance use and primary care services is seen by many as the best model of care.[26,27]

The Drug Interventions Programme does not extend to Scotland or Northern Ireland, although similar work linking criminal justice and treatment agencies aims to reduce drug-related crime.

TREATMENT MODALITIES

Therapeutic communities

Wexler[28] studied the effectiveness of a Californian prison Therapeutic Community (TC) drug treatment programme. There were three study groups: no treatment; TC only; TC plus aftercare programme following release. At three-year follow-up, only 27% of prison programme graduates who also completed community aftercare were re-incarcerated compared with around 75% of the subjects in the other study groups. There had been a lower level of return to prison among TC-only attendees versus non-treatment at two-year follow-up, but this effect had eroded by the end of year 3. A study of a Texas prison TC[29] reported similar findings.

Another study[30] followed up individuals who had been randomly assigned to either a modified therapeutic community (MTC), or mental health (MH) treatment programme. Of the 75 entrants to the MTC programme, 43 also entered an aftercare programme. The results at 12-month follow-up favoured strongly MTC plus aftercare (5% re-incarceration) over MTC only (16%) and MH (33% return to custody). As with Wexler[28] and Knight[29] prison TC studies, voluntary entry to aftercare represents a potential selection bias. One author[30] commented that fewer of the mental health intervention group had reported drugs as the principal reason for their offending.

The National Institute for Health and Clinical Excellence (NICE)[32] agreed with the conclusion reached by Smith and colleagues,[31] in their systematic review of TCs, that there is a lack of research assessing the effectiveness of therapeutic communities, or whether one type of therapeutic community is superior to another. They also concluded, however, that: 'Prison TC may be better than prison on its own or Mental Health Treatment Programmes to prevent re-offending post-release for inmates.'[32]

Drug-focused counselling

In a review of more than 1600 studies of prison-based drug treatment programmes, it was concluded that drug-focused counselling was largely ineffective.[33]

12-step meetings

Attendance at 12-step meetings has been found to reduce both alcohol and illicit drug use.[12,34–38] Attendance does not, however, necessarily improve other outcomes such as quality of life and psychosocial functioning,[39] nor impact significantly on some types of offending. Twelve-step meeting attendance ranked as the best single predictor of positive outcome following treatment for substance use disorders.[34] Tonigan[40] found this association held true and strengthened with increased severity of dependence.

Cognitive behavioural therapy (CBT)

One controlled study[41] measured the impact of a prison CBT drug treatment programme. Relapse was reported among 42% of completers compared with 48.8% in the non-treatment group. The study did not feature outcome data for all course participants versus the non-treatment group.

A combined analysis of two high-rigour studies[42,43] by NICE produced a net zero effect from CBT versus standard care. As a principle consequence of this result, NICE[32] recommended: '*Cognitive behavioural therapy and psychodynamic therapy focused on the treatment of drug misuse should not be offered routinely to people presenting for treatment of cannabis or stimulant misuse [or those receiving opioid maintenance treatment].*'

Three separate trial results[44-46] indicate that active treatment of mental health–substance use problems, principally via CBT, may improve substance misuse outcomes.

Behavioural couples therapy: couples-based interventions

Behavioural couples therapy has been found to help reduce the use of illicit opioids or cocaine among individuals undergoing methadone maintenance,[47,48] and to reduce offending among a similar client group.[49]

Contingency management

This intervention features the offer of incentives (usually vouchers that can be exchanged for a range of goods or services of the person's choice, or other privileges), contingent on the production of a drug-negative test.

One study[50] found that contingency management was superior to standard treatment in reduction of drug use (largely cocaine) over the first three months of treatment, but found no difference in abstinence rates (CM vs. standard treatment) at six- and nine-month follow-ups. Epstein[51] reported a similar diminishing of beneficial effect over time, in a study of cocaine use by methadone-maintained patients.

There is one robust study[52] that indicates the efficacy of contingency management in managing substance (cocaine) use over the course of a full year.

A systematic review of 52 studies of drug interventions for offenders, concluded that '*The evidence for treating dependence on substances other than opioids shows very limited success to date in community settings, and is non-existent in offender settings*.'[53] The report added that 'Higher-intensity programmes were more likely to result in reduction of criminal behaviour than low intensity equivalents', estimating a potential 50% differential.

Other therapeutic factors: person–therapist relationship

There is evidence from the UK Alcohol Treatment Trial (UKATT) research team,[54] Project MATCH,[55] and from other psychotherapy studies,[56,57] that better treatment outcomes are associated with the rating of a more positive 'working alliance' by both the individual and the therapists.

Other therapeutic factors: life skills

Moos and Moos[58] calculated that the odds of sustaining abstinence was positively associated with 'self-efficacy', approach coping styles, vocational engagement, income, having clean and sober friends, and having 'social and spiritual support'.

FAMILIES AND CARERS

Where they are willing to become involved in helping, families and carers may provide valuable effective support to an offender. Prisoners who received at least one visit during their imprisonment were found to be more likely to have accommodation and employment arranged upon release; the frequency of visits increased the likelihood of engagement in employment, training or education.[59]

Findings from three similar studies[60-62] demonstrate that self-help interventions appear to be as effective as more intensive psychological interventions in reducing stress and improving psychological functioning for carers and families of problem drug users.

A NICE[32] meta-analysis of the effect of 'boot camps' found no net reduction in substance use or offending at follow-up.

THE FUTURE OF SUBSTANCE USE TREATMENT

Take-home naloxone as an emergency means to reverse overdose may become a more common intervention for problematic drug users leaving prison or other residential settings.[63]

Two promising treatment models may gain favour in the years to come. The first is the International Treatment Effectiveness Project (ITEP).[64] ITEP is essentially a cognitive behavioural approach that seeks to concentrate the individual on routes to recovery via graphic representation (i.e. maps).

Bob Johnson's cognitive-emotional therapy (CET) combines Freudian unconscious processes with a singular distorted construct: that we are in grave danger. Johnson asserts that emotions serve one vital function – the assurance of our survival.[65] To ensure survival, our sense of fear must be very powerful in childhood, to alert both ourselves and our parents of dangers we encounter. With maturity comes self-security and our emotions ease, but for some of us a dreadful childhood event has never been resolved. This absolute fear of non-survival, because it could not be set to rest, lives on into our adult selves, but concealed from ourselves by the unconscious process of repression. This hidden fear then becomes the engine that drives all mental suffering, including substance use problems. Only the exposure, confronting and reasoning out of the fear can diminish its influence and emasculate dependence.

CONCLUSION

Policy and practice for managing offenders experiencing mental health–substance use problems are under continual development. We are entering a new outcome-focused era with a concentration on recovery. The coming years will provide some fascinating insights into what may be gleaned from this new approach.

REFERENCES

1 Stewart D. *The Problems and Needs of Newly Sentenced Prisoners: results from a national survey.* London: Ministry of Justice Research Series 16/08; 2008.

2 Holloway K, Bennet T. The results of the first two years of the NEW-ADAM programme, Home Office Online Report 19/04; 2004. Available at: www.scan.uk.net/docstore/HO_-_The_results_of_the_first_two_years_NEW-ADAM_(rdsolr1904).pdf (accessed 16 November 2010).

3 Gilchrist E, Johnson R, Takriti R, *et al.* Domestic Violence Offenders: characteristics and offending related needs. *Findings 217.* London: Home Office; 2003.

4 Mirrlees-Black C. *Domestic Violence: findings from a new British Crime Survey self-completion questionnaire. Home Office Research Study no. 191.* London: Home Office; 1999.

5 Singleton N, Farrell M, Meltzer H. *Substance Misuse among Prisoners in England and Wales: further analysis of data from the ONS survey of psychiatric morbidity among prisoners in England and Wales carried out in 1997 on behalf of the Department of Health.* London: Office for National Statistics; 1998.

6 Home Office. *An Analysis of CARAT Research Data as at 3 December 2002.* London: Research Development and Statistics Directorate, Home Office; 2003.

7 Health Protection Agency. *Success in Vaccination Programme for Preventing Hepatitis B.* 2010. Available at: www.hpa.org.uk/NewsCentre/NationalPressReleases/2010Press Releases/100803hepatitisBvaccsuccessmixed/ (accessed 26 November 2010), and Health Protection Agency. *Prison Hepatitis B Vaccination Monitoring Programme*; 2009. Available at: www.hpa.org.uk/Topics/InfectiousDiseases/InfectionsAZ/PrisonInfectionPrevention Team/PrisonHepatitisBVaccinationProgramme/ (accessed 26 November 2010).

8 Rickford D, Edgar K. *Troubled Inside: responding to the mental health needs of men in prison.* London: Prison Reform Trust; 2005.

9 Coid J, Bebbington P, Brugha T, *et al.* Ethnic differences in prisoners 1: criminality and psychiatric morbidity. *British Journal of Psychiatry.* 2002; **181**: 473–80.

10 The Drugs Act 2005. Available at: www.banksr.com/statutes/Drugs_Act_2005.pdf (accessed 16 November 2010).

11 World Health Organization. *International Classification of Diseases and Related Health Problems, 10th Revision*; 2007. Available at: http://apps.who.int/classifications/apps/icd/icd10online/ (accessed 16 November 2010).

12 Gossop M, Marsden J, Stewart D, *et al.* The National Treatment Outcome Research Study (NTORS): 4–5 year follow-up results. *Addiction.* 2003; **98**: 291–303.

13 National Offender Management Service. *The National Offender Management Service Drug Strategy*; 2008–2011. Available at: www.justice.gov.uk/noms-drugs-action-plan.pdf (accessed 16 November 2010).

14 Shaw J, Appleby L, Baker D. *Safer Prisons: a national study of prison suicides 1999–2000 by the National Confidential Inquiry into Suicides and Homicides by People with Mental Illness.* London: Department of Health; 2003.

15 Seaman SR, Brettle RP, Gore SM. Mortality from overdose among injecting drug users recently released from prison: database linkage study. *British Medical Journal.* 1998; **7**: 426–8.

16 Darke S. From the can to the coffin: deaths among recently released prisoners. *Addiction.* 2008; **3**: 256–7.

17 Farrell M, Marsden J. *Drug-related Mortality among Newly Released Offenders 1998 to 2000.* Home Office Online Report 40/05; 2005. Available at: http://rds.homeoffice.gov.uk/rds/pdfs05/rdsolr4005.pdf (accessed 26 November 2010).

18 Dolan KA, Shearer J, MacDonald M, *et al.* A randomised controlled trial of methadone maintenance treatment versus wait list control in an Australian prison system. *Drug and Alcohol Dependence.* 2003; **72**: 59–65.

19 Dolan KA, Shearer J, White B, *et al.* Four-year follow-up of imprisoned male heroin users and methadone treatment: mortality, re-incarceration and hepatitis C infection. *Addiction.* 2005; **100**: 820–8.

20 Gordon M, Kinlock T, Schwartz R, *et al.* A randomized clinical trial of methadone maintenance for prisoners: findings at 6 months post-release. *Addiction.* 2008; **103**: 1333–42.

21 Marsch L. The efficacy of methadone maintenance interventions in reducing illicit opiate use, HIV risk behaviour and criminality: a meta-analysis. *Addiction.* 1998; **93**: 515–32.

22 Department of Health, National Treatment Agency for Substance Misuse, Royal College of General Practitioners, Royal College of Psychiatrists and Royal Pharmaceutical Society of Great Britain. *Clinical Management of Drug Dependence in the Adult Prison Setting, including psychosocial treatment as a core part.* London: Department of Health; 2006. Available at: www.dh.gov.uk/en/Publicationsandstatistics/Publications/PublicationsPolicyAndGuidance/DH_063064 (accessed 16 November 2010).

23 Simpson D, Joe G, Brown B. Treatment retention and follow-up outcomes in the Drug Abuse Treatment Outcome Study (DATOS). *Psychology of Addictive Behaviors.* 1997; **11**: 294–307.

24 Martin SS, Scarpitti FR. An intensive case management approach for paroled IV drug users. *The Journal of Drug Issues.* 1993; **23**: 43–59.

25 Deschenes EP, Turner S, Petersilia J. A dual experiment in intensive community supervision: Minnesota's prison diversion and enhanced supervised release programs. *The Prison Journal.* 1995; **75**: 330–56.

26 Department of Health, Ministry of Justice. *A Guide for the Management of Dual Diagnosis for Prisons;* 2009. Available at: www.dh.gov.uk/en/Publicationsandstatistics/Publications/PublicationsPolicyAndGuidance/DH_097695 (accessed 16 November 2010).

27 Drummond C, Phillips T, Boland W. *Substance Misusing Clients with Mental Health Problems: a brief practitioner's guide for Criminal Justice Integrated Teams.* London: Specialist Clinical Addiction Network; 2008. Available at: www.dualdiagnosis.co.uk/uploads/documents/originals/Substance%20misusing%20clients%20with%20mental%20problems.pdf (accessed 16 November 2010).

28 Wexler H, De Leon G, Thomas G, *et al.* The Amity Prison TC Evaluation: reincarceration outcomes. *Criminal Justice and Behaviour.* 1999; **26**: 147–67.

29 Knight JR, Shrier LA, Bravender TD, *et al.* A new brief screen for adolescent substance abuse. *Archives of Pediatrics and Adolescent Medicine.* 1999; **153**: 591–6.

30 Sacks S, Sack J, McKendrick K, *et al.* Modified TC for MICA Offenders: crime outcomes. *Behavioural Sciences and the Law.* 2004; **22**: 477–501.

31 Smith LA, Gates S, Foxcroft D. Therapeutic communities for substance related disorder. *Cochrane Database of Systematic Reviews.* 2006; **1**: CD005338. Available at: www.cochrane.org/reviews/en/ab005338.html (accessed 3 December 2010).

32 National Institute for Health and Clinical Excellence (NICE). *Drug Misuse Psychosocial Interventions: National Clinical Practice Guideline Number 51.* London: The British Psychological Society and the Royal College of Psychiatrists; 2007. Available at: www.nice.org.uk/nicemedia/pdf/CG51FullGuideline.pdf (accessed 16 November 2010).

33 Pearson F, Lipton D. A meta-analytic review of the effectiveness of corrections-based treatments for drug abuse. *Prison Journal.* 1999; **79**: 384–410.

34 Morgenstern JD, Bux E, Labouvie T, *et al.* Examining mechanisms of action in 12-step community outpatient treatment. *Drug and Alcohol Dependence.* 2003; **72**: 237–47.

35 Humphreys K, Moos R. Can encouraging substance abuse patients to participate in self-help groups reduce demand for health care? A quasi-experimental study. *Alcoholism: clinical and experimental research.* 2001; **255**: 711–6.

36 Moos R, Schaefer J, Andrassy J, *et al.* Outpatient mental health care, self-help groups, and patients' one-year treatment outcomes. *Journal of Clinical Psychology.* 2001; **573**: 273–87.

37 Fiorentine R. After drug treatment: are 12-step programs effective in maintaining abstinence? *American Journal of Drug and Alcohol Abuse.* 1999; **25**: 93–116.

38 Project MATCH Research Group. Matching alcoholism treatments to client heterogeneity: Project MATCH Post-treatment drinking outcomes. *Journal of Studies on Alcohol.* 1997: **58**: 7–29.

39 Humphreys K. *Circles of Recovery: self-help organizations for addictions.* Cambridge University Press; 2004.

40 Tonigan JS, Toscova R, Miller WR. Meta-analysis of the literature on Alcoholics Anonymous: sample and study characteristics moderate findings. *Journal Studies on Alcohol.* 1996; **57**: 65–72.

41 Porporino FJ, Robinson D, Millson B, *et al.* An outcome evaluation of prison-based treatment programming for substance users. *Substance Use and Misuse.* 2002; **37**: 1047–77.

42 Crits-Christoph P, Siqueland L, Blaine J, *et al.* Psychosocial treatments for cocaine dependence. *Archives of General Psychiatry.* 1999; **56**: 493–502.

43 Maude-Griffin PM, Hohenstein JM, Humfleet GL, *et al.* Superior efficacy of cognitive-behavioural therapy for urban crack cocaine abusers: main and matching effects. *Journal of Consulting and Clinical Psychology.* 1998; **66**: 832–7.

44 Charney DA, Paraherakis AM, Gill KJ. Integrated treatment of comorbid depression and substance use disorders. *Journal of Clinical Psychiatry.* 2001; **62**: 672–7.

45 Hesse M. Achieving abstinence by treating depression in the presence of substance-use disorders. *Addictive Behaviors.* 2004; **29**: 1137–41.

46 Watkins KE, Paddock SM, Zhang L, *et al.* Improving care for depression in patients with comorbid substance misuse. *American Journal of Psychiatry.* 2006; **163**: 125–32.

47 Kelley ML, Fals-Stewart W. Couples- versus individual-based therapy for alcohol and drug abuse: effects on children's psychosocial functioning. *Journal of Consulting and Clinical Psychology.* 2002; **70**: 417–27.

48 Winters J, Fals-Stewart W, O'Farrell TJ, *et al.* Behavioral couples therapy for female substance-abusing patients: effects on substance use and relationship adjustment. *Journal of Consulting and Clinical Psychology.* 2002; **70**: 344–55.

49 Fals-Stewart W, O'Farrell TJ, Bircher GR. Behavioral couples therapy for male substance-abusing patients: a cost outcomes analysis. *Journal of Consulting and Clinical Psychology.* 1997; **65**: 789–802.

50 Petry NM, Alessi SM, Carroll KM, *et al.* Contingency management treatments: reinforcing abstinence versus adherence with goal related activities. *Journal of Consulting and Clinical Psychology.* 2006: **74**: 592–601.

51 Epstein DH, Hawkins WE, Covi L, *et al.* Cognitive-behavioral therapy plus contingency management for cocaine use: findings during treatment and across 12-month follow-up. *Psychology of Addictive Behaviors.* 2003; **17**: 73–82.

52 Higgins ST, Budney AJ, Bickel WK, *et al.* Incentives improve outcome in outpatient behavioral treatment of cocaine dependence. *Archives of General Psychiatry.* 1994: **51**: 568–76.

53 Holloway K, Bennett T, Farrington D. *The Effectiveness of Criminal Justice and Treatment Programmes in Reducing Drug-Related Crime: a systematic review. Home Office Online Report 26/05.* Home Office: London; 2005.

54 UK Alcohol Treatment Trial Research Team. Cost-effectiveness of treatment for alcohol problems: findings of the UK Alcohol Treatment Trial. *British Medical Journal.* 2005; **331**: 544–7.

55 Connors GJ, DiClemente CC, Dermen KH, *et al.* Predicting the therapeutic alliance in alcoholism treatment. *Journal of Studies on Alcohol and Other Drugs.* 2000; **61**: 139–49.

56 Hanson WE, Curry KT, Bandalos DL. Reliability generalization of working alliance inventory scale scores. *Educational and Psychological Measurements.* 2002; **62**: 659–73.

57 Martin DJ, Garske JP, Davis MK. Relation of the therapeutic alliance with outcome and other variables: a meta analytic review. *Journal of Consulting and Clinical Psychology.* 2000; **68**: 438–50.

58 Moos RH, Moos BS. Treated and untreated alcohol use disorders: course and predictors of remission and relapse. *Evaluation Review.* 2007; **31**: 564–84.

59 Niven S, Stewart D. *Resettlement Outcomes on Release from Prison in 2003: Home Office research findings 248.* London: Home Office; 2005.

60 Copello A, Templeton L, Orford J, *et al.* The relative efficacy of two levels of a primary care intervention for family members affected by the addiction problem of a close relative: a randomised trial. *Addiction.* 2009; **104**: 49–58.

61 Meyers RJ, Miller WR, Smith JE, *et al.* A randomized trial of two methods for engaging treatment-refusing drug users through concerned significant others. *Journal of Consulting and Clinical Psychology.* 2002; **70**: 1182–5.

62 Kirby KC, Marlowe DB, Festinger DS, *et al.* Community reinforcement training for family and significant others of drug abusers: a unilateral intervention to increase treatment entry of drug users. *Drug and Alcohol Dependence.* 1999; **56**: 85–96.

63 Strang J, Manning V, Mayet S. Family carers and the prevention of heroin overdose deaths: unmet training need and overlooked intervention opportunity. *Drugs: education prevention and policy.* 2008; **15**: 211–8.

64 Joe G, Dansereau D, Pitre U, *et al.* Effectiveness of node-link mapping-enhanced counselling for opiate addicts: a 12 month post treatment follow-up. *Journal of Nervous and Mental Diseases.* 1997; **185**: 306–13.

65 Johnson R. *Emotional Health: what emotions are and how they cause social and mental diseases.* Ventnor, Isle of Wight: Truth, Trust Consent Publishing; 2005.

TO LEARN MORE

- Holloway K, Bennett T, Farrington D. Effectiveness of Treatment in Reducing Drug-Related Crime. Report for Bra. Sweden: brotlsförebyggande rädet, Swedish National Council for Crime Prevention; 2008. Available at: www.bra.se/extra/measurepoint/?module_instance=4&name=Drugs_webb.pdf&url=/dynamaster/file_archive/081023/0983648516b5240635413 5728071ea66/Drugs%255fwebb.pdf
- Marteau D. *Addiction.* Wiltshire: Quay Books; 2001.
- Orford J. *Excessive Appetites: a social-behavioural-cognitive-moral model*, Chichester: Wiley; 2001.
- Patel K. *Reducing Drug-Related Crime and Rehabilitating Offenders*; 2010. Available at: www.dh.gov.uk/prod_consum_dh/groups/dh_digitalassets/@dh/@en/@ps/documents/digitalasset/dh_119850.pdf
- Book 3, Chapter 14.

CHAPTER 15

Relapse prevention in mental health

Rami T Jumnoodoo and Patrick Coyne

INTRODUCTION

It is reported that health and social care professionals use a variety of treatment interventions to aid the individual to reduce relapse rates and prevent hospital readmissions.[1] However, a structured model of relapse prevention (RP) to influence those outcomes is not undertaken systematically. Such structure is needed if we are to enable and restore hope, and empower the individual and family to receive an evidence-based relapse prevention approach to mental healthcare.

SELF-ASSESSMENT EXERCISE 15.1

Time: 5 minutes
What does the term relapse prevention mean to you and your practice?

The UK Government has produced many documents that discuss relapse prevention in the treatment of those with a serious and enduring mental illness. However, despite this, there is little evidence that describes a well-developed and tested model of relapse prevention for the field of mental health. Consequently, Brent Rehabilitation and Supporting Services are using a well developed and tested model of relapse prevention originating from the substance use field[2–4] and transferring and testing this model within a psychiatric setting.[5,6]

Marlatt and Gordon's model[2] is based on a combination of two sets of theories:
1 Cognitive-behavioural.[7]
2 Social learning.[8]

They define relapse prevention as a '*self-management program designed to enhance the maintenance stage of the habit-change process*'.[2]

This new technology (relapse prevention – RP) offers the ability to use skills systematically that aid the individual to:
➤ develop self-efficacy
➤ maintain his/her overall well-being
➤ recover in her/his community.

Moreover, it has benefit for the family in adjusting and enhancing their RP skills to offer care and to manage the resulting change in their relationships. The RP programme is structured, person-centred and proactive and addresses the needs of the individual and family. This programme involves a series of group or individual therapy sessions – counselling and knowledge and skills training – where the individual learns how to manage his/her illness and prevent relapse.

THE LOCAL CONTEXT AND NEED

It has been observed that individuals using the service are frequently admitted to hospital with varied lengths of stay,[9] and often complain of the unsettling and traumatic process of readmission to hospital. This is costly to the individual and services, and causes disruption, distress, despair and distrust.[10] The concept of a relapse prevention programme is to optimise the chances of recovery within the community. In addition, it seeks to promote a reduction in hospital admissions, with the concomitant benefits of also reducing the financial burden which can be redirected to improve services in the community, and access for the individual who needs inpatient care and treatment.

THE RELAPSE PREVENTION MODEL AND DEVELOPMENT

Over the past 10 years, the aim has been to maximise quality of life in the community through recovery, and to maintain wellness, thus minimising relapse rates. The model developed from frustration among individuals, families and professionals at the regular reoccurrence of preventable relapses and lengthy periods of hospitalisation.

SELF-ASSESSMENT EXERCISE 15.2

Time: 5 minutes
Reflect on the following. How should 'quality of life' be determined?

It was identified that community support reduces the isolation felt by many individuals experiencing mental health disorders, and often minimises the need for hospital admissions. However, this is often prevented by the stigma (*see* Book 1, Chapters 5, 6, 7 and 8) attached to the diagnosis. Relapse prevention strategies were developed as powerful tools that can be used by the individual and family to break down such barriers and inspire society.

KEY POINT 15.1

Relapse prevention programmes provide a realistic method of ensuring social inclusion within mental health.

RP was designed to remove the traditional stereotypes associated with mental health treatment, as it is a model that can be applied to everyday lifestyle issues. The RP programme is simple to understand and use. Many individuals within Central and North West London NHS Foundation Trust (UK) have employed relapse prevention strategies to achieve their goals and objectives. Individuals have access to opportunities that they did not feel they had before, and have gone on to access training and employment within the community.

DEFINITIONS

The following terms are used within treatment intervention for people experiencing mental health problems.

➤ **Affect:** expression through feelings and emotions.
➤ **Attribution:** the process of assigning causality to events around us.
➤ **Cognitive behavioural:** psychological interventions, which target specific thoughts, images, beliefs and behaviour.
➤ **Cognitive reframing/restructuring:** the process of positively challenging and modifying thinking errors in a non-threatening way.
➤ **Cognitive:** a human response to thinking, images and beliefs.
➤ **Craving:** a recurrence of a thought process, which may lead to desirable but unhealthy behaviour.
➤ **Cue:** anything in the environment that triggers urges and craving and leads to potential.
➤ **High-risk situation:** the breaking down of a resolution or a control situation, due to inter- or intra-personal relationships or other factors in a person's life.
➤ **Lapse:** a slight error or a slip, a single re-emergence of previous habits that may or may not lead to a relapse.
➤ **Lapse and relapse plan:** having a lapse and relapse plan in place helps to prevent admission and readmission.
➤ **Lifestyle balance:** maintaining healthy behaviours.
➤ **Lifestyle interventions:** interventions or activities needed in correcting an imbalance in lifestyle.
➤ **Positive outcome expectancies:** the anticipation of feeling better due to the result of a particular course of action.
➤ **Rule violation effect:** a breaking down of a set resolution the individual has made to himself.
➤ **Seemingly irrelevant decisions:** a precursor to a high-risk situation. At the time the decision in itself does not seem harmful, and can be defended, rationally or irrationally. It may signal a change away from a healthy behavioural pattern.
➤ **Self-efficacy:** a person's beliefs in his or her ability to succeed with a specific task.
➤ **Self-monitoring:** after developing relapse prevention skills individuals can identify high-risk situations and their antecedents.
➤ **Social learning theory:** assumes that a new behaviour can be learned simply by exposure to another person modelling that behaviour.

> **Thinking errors:** any irrational thinking or belief not supported by evidence that is unhelpful to a person managing their mental health.
> **Urge:** a strong impulse to suddenly act without careful thinking.

THE RELAPSE PREVENTION TEN SESSION MODEL

Relapse prevention can be undertaken as a general approach to include:
> open exploratory sessions
> individual sessions
> close group structured sessions
> homework.

SELF-ASSESSMENT EXERCISE 15.3

Time: 15 minutes
What might be helpful for the individual and family to know prior to course commencement?

Education and training in the therapeutic sessions covers the following 10 areas:

1 **Engagement:** The primary consideration is for the individual and family to engage on a relapse prevention programme. It may be necessary to involve other individuals in the initial stages of engagement to highlight the benefits of RP, and the feeling of community within a group setting. Thus, involving other individuals, families and the professional within the process can be beneficial to all.

KEY POINT 15.2

Group interactions between course participants are vital in ensuring friendly and productive participation and mutual support.

The individual is required to agree to the second session. This offers exploration of what is on offer in the relapse prevention programme. This provides a chance for a conscious decision to make a change through contracting, and provides the professional with a chance to enhance individual and family motivation.

2 **Introduction to the model:** An initial session explains the RP model to clarify how this simple but useful model can help the individual and family. It covers expectations of the individual and family and the professional delivering the education and training. At this point a signed agreement of willingness to participate in the RP programme is required to formalise commitment of all parties involved in the process.

3 **Understanding the ideas of lapse and relapse:** This session clarifies that deterioration in mental health is usually a staged process where rarely are people simply 'well' and then 'unwell'. It is a pivotal session in the exploration of the

process from good to bad health. The stages are opportunities for action – to reverse, where possible, trends towards a return to illness or to undesired states. Moreover, it offers the opportunity to explore previous relapse and the precursor lapses, and begins to put together the relapse repertoire.

SELF-ASSESSMENT EXERCISE 15.4

Time: 5 minutes

How might you identify individuals and families who are at high risk of lapse or relapse?

4 **Identifying high-risk situations:** Identifying those circumstances that stress the individual and family that may be associated with a recurrence of an illness process or which may initiate such a process is pivotal. Education and training looks at what these are and how meaningful they may be to the individual and family. Mapping these, making a list, raising an awareness of them and keeping a diary is helpful. The individual and family are encouraged to gain an insight of these precursors and to develop a relapse prevention plan to minimise risks, and develop confidence to avoid those situations. It is an opportunity to continue with the previous exploration to further identifying the 'lapse and relapse history' of the individual, including issues such as:
   ➤ What is the pattern of relapse from the past?
   ➤ What can be learned from that?

With this knowledge, actions and strategies can be planned and practised to reduce the risk of relapse.

SELF-ASSESSMENT EXERCISE 15.5

Time: 10 minutes

What warning signs could you identify that might aid the individual and family?

5 **Identifying warning signs:** It is essential to explore what the individual and family believe to be the earliest warning signs. From this, an understanding that these are not psychotic symptoms can be developed. These may include:
   ➤ withdrawal from help
   ➤ reluctance to take medication
   ➤ desire to take alcohol and/or other drugs
   ➤ sleeplessness
   ➤ restlessness
   ➤ increased agitation or irritability.
6 **Identifying stress and stress management:** At this point there is a need to have an appreciation of how the person experiencing mental health problems copes when in stressful situations, and how this might contribute to increased risk of

relapse. At this point, effective (adaptive) coping strategies can be put in place to deal with stressful events. The individual and family are able to make plans for dealing with stressful situations. For the family, the plan will also contain information about coping strategies and how they cope in such situations.

SELF-ASSESSMENT EXERCISE 15.6

Time: 10 minutes
Consider what coping strategies might be used by the individual and the professional. Make a list and add/review this with experience.

7 **Identifying thinking errors/faulty thoughts and management:** Here we examine thinking errors adopted by the individual, looking for statements such as: 'If I cut myself I will feel better.' It is important to collect a list of thinking errors and encourage the individual and family to gather the evidence to support their thinking. Encouraging the use of a 'thought diary' that invites the recording of their thoughts and feelings and resultant behaviour is helpful. From this, the professional, alongside individual and family, can introduce new ways of thinking about given situations.

8 **Identifying and exploring rule violation effect – emotions and management:** Rule violation requires vigorous exploration and examination of how the individual (and family) feels when she/he has not continued with a health plan, e.g. with their medication regime. The rule violation effect is about helping the individual explore their feelings of, for example, guilt or blame, when they have lapsed or relapsed. This enables plan development that the individual and family can use so as not to distract from further developing their relapse plan, thus encouraging a successful outcome.

9 **Identifying and exploring lifestyle balance:** This session is about education related to lifestyle choices that maintain a good balanced lifestyle.

SELF-ASSESSMENT EXERCISE 15.7

Time: 10 minutes
- Consider the lifestyle components you embrace in your own life. Note them down.
- Remember, what applies to you will also apply to those individuals and families you work alongside.

The notion of lifestyle has many components including:
➤ nutrition
➤ diet
➤ exercise
➤ friends
➤ family

> ➤ education and training
> ➤ recreation
> ➤ occupation
> ➤ holidays
> ➤ spiritual beliefs
> ➤ sexual beliefs
> ➤ accommodation
> ➤ finances
> ➤ spouse or partners.

Lifestyle choices cover practical issues ensuring that the individual has some activity in each field, and is specifically aimed at education around choice and empowerment (*see* Book 4, Chapter 15).

10 **Devising a lapse and relapse plan:** This session (one or two sessions may be needed) looks at problem-solving techniques – with the aim of educating and reminding the individual and family of problem-solving techniques that can be drawn upon prior to or during lapse or relapse (*see* Chapter 16; Book 4, Chapter 13). This session pulls together all the information gathered in the previous sessions and draws up a plan for managing high-risk situations, such that the plans will reduce the risk of lapse, or if one occurs, the chance of continuation to the state of full relapse is reduced. Each plan is person-centred as relapse in each individual can be triggered by different factors.

REVIEW AND PROGRESS EVALUATION

The final session includes a review of the work undertaken by the individual and family and how they feel they have progressed. This should also include identification of areas and strategies that require additional work from the individual, family and/or professional. From the above, booster sessions can be organised, for the individual requiring additional support, education and/or training. Here, a period of reflection – for the individual, family and professional – is of value.

RP TECHNIQUES

The model proposed provides a comprehensive list of interventions for the individual, family and professional to work alongside, rather than a selective aspect of relapse prevention.

Techniques commonly used in RP include:
> ➤ recovery approach
> ➤ cognitive behavioural therapy
> ➤ social learning theories
> ➤ motivational interviewing techniques
> ➤ family intervention
> ➤ role play
> ➤ visualisation
> ➤ relaxation techniques
> ➤ complementary therapy
> ➤ solution-focused therapy

> harm minimisation
> medication compliance
> planning
> network development
> group therapy.

ENGAGEMENT

Engagement with the individual and family is vital to enhance motivation and enable conscious personal health decisions as part of an ongoing learning process (*see* Book 5, Chapter 7).

The core conditions of genuineness, empathy, respect and warmth are essential to begin the development of an engaging and trusting relationship.[11] Initial meetings should indicate the common issues existent between the professional, the individual and family. Common interests and values stimulate conversation and in doing so create a platform of reciprocal learning.

CONCLUSION

In lapse and relapse prevention, individuals, families and professionals work in partnership to determine the achievements of person-centred goals. Empowerment is the ultimate aim. Relapse prevention is a simple model to understand and practise. Advanced competencies for the individual, family and professional are achievable on completion of the advanced training in relapse prevention.

Relapse prevention programmes target the individual and family and aim to reduce readmissions. Often readmission is prevented by the early identification of changes to health status or health behaviours by non-health and social careworkers, for example community police, local shop personnel or work colleagues. Small changes may be noticed early and if invited to be part of the relapse prevention plan, could inform the family and care coordinators of possible concerns and dilemmas needing careful follow-up.

Prevention of return to illness and readmission has enormous health benefits. We have found that a group approach to RP can be supportive to the individuals and family, and aids mutual identification of early warning signs ensuring careful management, and intervention when required. Such information and resultant support at key points is pivotal, as this can be introduced at any stage when such intervention will be most effective and outcomes positive.

REFERENCES

1 Department of Health. National service framework for mental health services: modern standards and service models. London: HMSO; 1999. Available at: www.dh.gov.uk/en/Publicationsandstatistics/Publications/PublicationsPolicyAndGuidance/DH_4009598 (accessed 17 November 2010).

2 Marlatt GA, Gordon JR. *Relapse Prevention: maintenance strategies in the development of addictive behaviours.* New York: Guilford Press; 1985.

3 Bowers E, Dunn ME, Wang MC. Efficacy of relapse prevention: a meta-analytic review. *Journal of Consulting and Clinical Psychology.* 1999; **67**: 563–57.

4 Carroll KM. Relapse prevention as a psychological treatment. A review of controlled clinical trials. *Experimental and Clinical Psychopharmacology.* 1996; **4**: 46–54.

5 Jumnoodoo R, Coyne P, Singaram E. Preventing readmission in mental health. *Nursing Times.* 2001; **97**: 48.

6 Foster JH, Jumnoodoo R. Relapse prevention in serious and enduring mental illness. A pilot study. *Journal of Psychiatric and Mental Health Nursing.* 2008; **15**: 552–61.

7 Beck A, Rush A, Shaw B, *et al. Cognitive Therapy of Depression.* New York: Guilford Press; 1977.

8 Bandura A. Self-efficacy: towards a unifying theory of behavioural change. *Psychological Review.* 1979: **84**: 191–215.

9 Appleby L. Defining the needs of patients with intellectual disabilities in high security psychiatric hospitals in England. *Journal of Intellectual Disability Research.* 2004; **48**: 603–10.

10 Jumnoodoo R, Marlatt A, Coyne P, *et al.* Development of a 'whole system approach' to relapse prevention in Brent mental health services. *Nurse 2 Nurse.* 2002; **2**: 46–9.

11 Coffey M. Psychosis and medication: strategies for improving adherence. *British Medical Journal.* 1999; **8**: 225–30.

TO LEARN MORE

• Beck-Sander A. Relapse prevention: a model for psychosis? *Behaviour Change.* 1999; **16**: 191–202.

• Brooker C, Repper J, editors. *Serious Mental Health Problems in the Community: policy, practice and research.* London: Balliere Tindall; 1999.

• Folkman S, Lazarus RS. Coping and emotion. In: Monat A, Lazarus RS, editors. *Stress and Coping: an anthology.* New York: Columbia University Press; 1991. pp. 207–27.

• Marlatt GA. Models of relapse and relapse prevention: a commentary. *Experimental and Clinical Pharmacology.* 1996; **4**: 55–60.

• Meichenbaum D. *Cognitive-Behaviour Modification: an integrative approach.* New York: Plenum; 1977.

• Padesky CA, Greenberger D. *A Clinician's Guide to Mind over Mood.* New York: Guilford Press; 1995.

CHAPTER 16

Relapse prevention in substance use

Sharon H Hsu and G Alan Marlatt

INTRODUCTION

Relapse, defined as the returning to symptomatic behaviour after a period of remission, is a common outcome following treatment of substance use and other psychological problems.[1] Most people who try to change a behaviour (e.g. quit smoking) will likely experience setbacks (lapses) that often lead to a return to problematic behaviour (relapses).[2] Since the term relapse prevention was coined, it has established a significant role in the field of psychological research and clinical practice in the past 30 years. In this chapter, we will discuss:

➤ the theoretical and empirical background for relapse and relapse prevention
➤ a new dynamic model of relapse
➤ relapse prevention for treating psychological disorders
➤ the theoretical and empirical background for mindfulness-based relapse prevention
➤ clinical strategies to reduce the risk of relapse
➤ a case study.

RELAPSE

The challenge of defining relapse given the inherent complexity of behavioural change process is well documented.[1,2] In Marlatt and colleagues' model,[3-5] relapse has been viewed as both an event and a process of behavioural change. While there is a consensus that relapse should be conceptualised as a recovery process, it is almost always assessed as a discrete event.[2] This may be attributed to the difficulty in accurately assessing relapse and the cause of relapse.[2] For example, to assess relapse as a process, dynamic repeated assessment of factors, such as the frequency and quantity of the target behaviour (e.g. number of drinks/day), cognitive and affective indices, level of functioning and consequences of the behaviour change are needed.[6] Relapse and cause of relapse are mostly commonly assessed by retrospective recall, although some recent studies have utilised real-time techniques (e.g. ecological momentary assessment).[7] In addition to relapse, *lapse* and *prolapse* have been described as two possible outcomes in Marlatt and Gordon's model. A *lapse* refs to the initial setback of a previously changed behaviour, and a *prolapse* refers to the process of returning to positive behavioural change.

RELAPSE PREVENTION (RP)

Relapse prevention has been used to describe a theoretical framework and to offer an umbrella term for a collection of cognitive behavioural intervention strategies designed to prevent lapse and relapse among individuals with addictive behaviour problems.[4] RP is based on the bio-psychosocial model of addiction. According to this model, addictive behaviours are conceptualised as acquired, over-learned habits, with biological, psychological and social determinants and biological, psychological and social consequences.[4a]

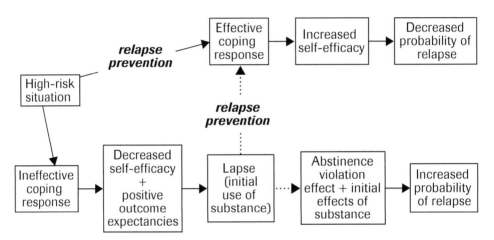

FIGURE 16.1 Cognitive behavioural model of relapse

As outlined in Figure 16.1, a key concept in this model is *high-risk situation*, defined as any experience, emotion, setting, thought or context that introduces an increased risk for one to engage in some transgressive behaviour.[4] Attending a company party that serves alcohol is an example of a high-risk situation for individuals whose treatment goal is to be abstinent from alcohol. More examples of *high-risk situation* are provided in the case study.

Based on this model, if an ineffective coping response is utilised, the individual's confidence for dealing with high-risk situations may be reduced. This is referred to as a decrease in self-efficacy.[8] Individuals' beliefs about positive effects of using the substance may also increase. This is referred to as high positive outcome expectancy.[9] Individuals with high positive outcomes expectancies generally believe that ingesting substances may result in an increase in positive consequences (e.g. euphoria) and/or reduction of negative consequences (e.g. withdrawal symptoms). As indicated in Figure 16.1, the risk for lapse is increased if the individual experiences low self-efficacy and positive outcome expectancies. Following a lapse, the individual may experience the *abstinence violation effect* (AVE), which is defined as a loss of perceived control after the defiance of self-imposed rules.[10] Once a lapse has occurred, experiencing AVE and the initial positive effects of using a substance may increase the probability of a full-blown relapse. Conversely, as indicated in Figure 16.1, if an individual utilises effective coping strategies in the face of a high-risk situations, he/she is more likely to experience an increase in self-efficacy, which in turn may reduce the risk of relapse.

Given the development of an addictive behaviour is a learned process, building a new behaviour repertoire to manage high-risk situations is especially important for individuals. The overall goal of RP is to teach individuals to replace ineffective coping behaviour, which generally focuses on obtaining immediate rewards, with effective coping behaviour that typically provides long-term benefits (e.g. increased coping capacity and greater lifestyle balance).

A number of studies have evaluated the efficacy of RP as a comprehensive treatment of substance use problems.[11-13] For instance, Caroll[11] reviewed randomised-controlled trial studies of RP and found that, across substance use treatment, there is evidence for the effectiveness of RP relative to no-treatment control conditions. The effectiveness is especially strong for smoking cessation. However, evidence with regard to its superiority compared to control conditions or other active treatments (e.g. supportive therapy) has been less consistent. What could be concluded from this review is that RP is at least as effective as other active treatments. Irvin and colleagues[12] conducted a meta-analysis on the efficacy of RP techniques in treating alcohol use, smoking, cocaine use and polysubstance use. Twenty-six studies (n = 9504) were included in this review. Three main findings emerged:

1   RP was effective in the reduction of substance use, with an overall effect size of r = 0.14, and the improvement of psychosocial adjustment, with an overall effect of r = 0.48
2   RP was most effective in treatment of alcohol use (r = 0.37).
3   RP was equally effective across treatment modalities (e.g. individual, group).

Following the wide application of RP, the National Institute on Alcohol Abuse and Alcoholism initiated the Relapse Replication and Extension Project (RREP) to evaluate the cognitive behavioural model of relapse developed by Marlatt and Gordon.[4] Five hundred and sixty-three individuals entering treatment for alcohol problems were interviewed every two months for one year in three study sites.[14] Results indicate that while levels of stressful situations to which participants were exposed were not predictive of relapse, coping style for such situations did predict outcomes. Specifically, avoidant coping patterns were associated with relapse. When coping skills were controlled, cognitive factors (e.g. self-efficacy, alcohol expectancies), craving and mood states did not contribute unique variance in predicting subsequent relapse. Additionally, as Marlatt and Gordon[4] predicted, endorsement of the disease model beliefs was positively associated with increased likelihood of an incoming relapse. This finding provided evidence for Marlatt's abstinence violation effect. Currently, RP has been credited as an evidence-based treatment programme by the Substance Abuse and Mental Health Services Administration. For more information, please visit www.nrepp.samhsa.gov/.

DYNAMIC MODEL OF RELAPSE

To capture the complexity of behavioural change as a phenomenon and to incorporate new research evidence in the conceptualisation of relapse, Witkiewitz and Marlatt[5] reformulated Marlatt's original relapse model. As shown in Figure 16.2, high-risk situations remain to be the central feature in the dynamic model of relapse. The other important feature of the model is the introduction of distal and proximal relapse risks. *Distal risks* (solid lines) are depicted as stable predispositions, which raise an individual's vulnerability to lapse. *Proximal risks* (dotted lines) refer to immediate precipitants, indicating the statistical probability of a lapse.[15] The connected boxes are hypothesised to have a reciprocal causation between them. For example, Gossop and colleagues[16] suggested that coping skills influence drinking behaviour, and, similarly, drinking influences coping.

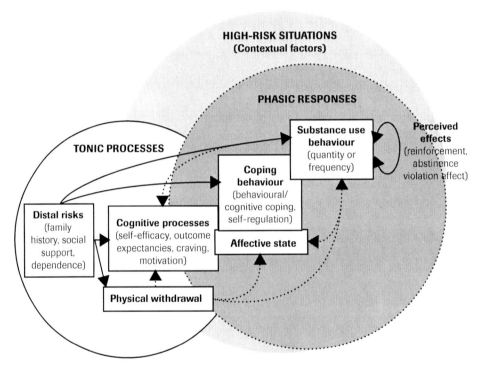

FIGURE 16.2 Dynamic model of relapse proposed by Witkiewitz and Marlatt[5]

Another important feature of the model is its emphasis on the temporal relationship between proximal and distal risk factors. As illustrated in Figure 16.2, the *tonic processes* refer to a person's chronic susceptibility for relapse. This susceptibility may accumulate and initiate a high-risk situation, which in turn may increase the possibility of a lapse. The *phasic responses* refer to situational cognitive, affective and physical states, and coping skills utilisation. In this model, phasic responses are conceptualised as the turning point, such that change in these states may result in abrupt change in substance use behaviour. As Witkiewitz and Marlatt[4] have suggested, a number of studies examining outcomes following treatment have demonstrated the interrelationship between tonic processes and phasic responses in the prediction of lapses and relapse.[10,17–23]

INCORPORATING RP WHEN TREATING OTHER PSYCHOLOGICAL DISORDERS

RP can be incorporated as part of a cognitive behavioural-based treatment for individuals with psychological disorders such as generalised anxiety disorder (GAD).[1] For example, in treating individuals with GAD, RP can easily be used to identify potential warning signs or cues for worry and to generate problem-solving strategies to prevent pathological worry and avoidance.[24] Additionally, it is often commonly employed as part of the treatment for those with co-occurring addiction and mental illness (e.g. schizophrenia). The treatment of co-occurring disorders has been mostly effectively enhanced through combining traditional mental health and addiction psychological treatment.[25] Dual recovery therapy[26] is an example of such an approach. Targeting individuals with schizophrenia and substance use problems, it blends elements of traditional substance abuse relapse prevention and motivational enhancement therapy with traditional mental health treatments of social skills training/psychosis relapse prevention. Relapse prevention skills include teaching individuals how to identify and manage external (e.g. people, places and things) and internal triggers (e.g. anger, depression and anxiety). Additionally, functional analyses of recent relapses for substance use can help connect medication non-compliance and psychotic symptoms to the relapse, which in turn will aid professionals to formulate strategies to avoid future relapses to substances.[25]

MINDFULNESS-BASED RELAPSE PREVENTION

Bowen and colleagues[27] have developed and evaluated the mindfulness-based relapse prevention (MBRP), a manual-guided and group-based aftercare programme for individuals with substance use disorders. Modelled after empirically supported mindfulness-based interventions for managing stress and depression,[28,29] MBRP integrates traditional cognitive behavioural relapse prevention techniques[4,30] with mindfulness meditation. MBRP is designed to help individuals cultivate awareness and acceptance of thoughts, emotions and bodily sensations, specifically those that are central to relapse.[31] The practice of meditation serves as a viable method for monitoring reaction to environmental (e.g. social pressure) and internal triggers (e.g. negative emotions). Mindfulness meditation may serve as an alternative coping strategy to manage high-risk situations for relapse.[31] The programme teaches individuals to 'pause' and respond to urges and cravings with awareness, rather than reacting impulsively. The practice of mindfulness meditation may offer positive consequences, such as tension reduction and relaxation. It may also offer long-term rewards such as greater lifestyle balance and emotional well-being.[32]

To evaluate the efficacy and feasibility of MBRP, Bowen and colleagues[33] conducted an initial randomised-controlled trial at a non-profit community-based outpatient treatment centre to evaluate an eight-week outpatient MBRP programme as compared to treatment as usual (TAU). In this study, the TAU condition is a process-oriented treatment programme based on the disease model of addiction and the 12-step approach. One hundred and sixty-eight individuals with substance use disorders who had recently completed intensive inpatient or outpatient treatment participated in the study. Assessments were administered prior to intervention, immediately after intervention, and at two and four months after intervention. With regard to efficacy, results indicated that MBRP participants exhibited significantly lower rates of substance use relative to those in TAU over the four-month post-intervention period. MBRP participants also reported positive outcomes, such as higher deduction in craving and higher increases in acceptance and acting with awareness, as compared to TAU. With regard to feasibility, results indicated that MBRP participants demonstrated consistent homework compliance and attendance, as well as high satisfaction. For instance, 86% of MBRP participants reported practising meditation immediately after completing the intervention, and over half of the participants reported continued practice four months after receiving treatment. On average, these participants practised close to five days per week and about 30 minutes per occasion. Taken together, these findings demonstrate the feasibility and initial efficacy of MBRP as an aftercare programme for substance use disorders.

Using the data collected for the clinical trial, a follow-up study examined the relations among language use, mindfulness and substance-use treatment outcomes.[34] A research team composed of expert mindfulness practitioners generated two categories of mindfulness language (ML), describing the mindfulness state and the more encompassing 'mindfulness journey', including words describing challenges with regard to developing a mindfulness practice. Examples of words describing mindfulness state include: accept, balance and calm. Examples of words describing mindfulness journey include: sober, react and struggle. Analysis was based on 48 MBRP participants. A word count programme[35] was used to assess frequency of ML in participants' responses to open-ended questions about their impressions of mindfulness practice and MBRP immediately following intervention. Increased use of ML was associated with fewer alcohol and drug use days in the four-month follow-up period.

To illuminate how and for whom MBRP works, two additional follow-up studies have investigated potential mediators and moderators of this novel intervention.[36,37] The first study examined the relations among depressive symptoms, craving and substance use using data collected for the clinical trial.[37] An association between negative affect and craving has been demonstrated in laboratory and clinical studies.[38-43] For instance, individuals with depressive symptomatology tend to exhibit particularly strong links to craving and relapse.[44,45] It was hypothesised that in utilising mindfulness-based practices, MBRP may teach individuals to respond to emotional discomfort with acceptance and non-judgemental awareness and this in turn may reduce the over-learned, habitual response of craving in the face of depressive symptoms. Consistent with prediction, Witkiewitz and Bowen[37] found that while craving accounted for the association between depressive symptoms and substance use among TAU participants, it did not account for this relation among MBRP participants. This suggests that MBRP attenuated the relation between depressive symptoms and craving. Such effect was predictive of substance use four months following intervention. Taken together, this study offers preliminary evidence that MBRP seems to alter individuals' cognitive and behavioural responses to depressive symptoms, which in turn accounts for reduction in substance use after intervention.

The second study examined the role of distress tolerance using the same data-set.[36] In this study, distress tolerance refers to the degree to which an individual is able to withstand negative psychological states.[46] Empirical literature has indicated that lower distress tolerance is associated with a number of negative substance use treatment outcomes and psychopathology.[46-51] As indicated earlier, mindful-ness meditation can be considered as a training of affect regulation, and it may be particularly beneficial for individuals with lower distress tolerance. Thus, we inves-tigated whether distress tolerance moderated the relationship between treatment assignment and outcomes.[36] We hypothesised that MBRP participants with lower distress tolerance would report better outcomes than TAU participants with lower distress tolerance. Results indicated that, as hypothesised, distress tolerance signifi-cantly moderated treatment effects on days of substance use. Specifically, among individuals with low distress tolerance, those who received MBRP had fewer days of alcohol and other drug use than those who received TAU immediately after treat-ment and two months following treatment. Overall, these two studies demonstrate that MBRP may be particularly helpful for individuals with low distress tolerance or those experiencing co-occurring substance abuse and depressive symptoms.

SUMMARY

The classic RP model has gone through some major revision in the past decade. While the dynamic model and the MBRP approach are still in their infancy, the initial evidence is encouraging. With regard to the dynamic model, future research focusing on better assessment of the dynamic interplay of relapse factors will add to the understanding of the process of relapse.[52] With regard to the MBRP approach, many questions await to be answered. For example, in addition to studies mentioned above, what are other potential mediators and moderators for MBRP? Do MBRP and RP share similar mechanisms of action? The investigation of these important empirical questions will enhance our understanding of the key ingredients of these treatments and offer implications for treatment matching.

CLINICAL STRATEGIES TO REDUCE THE RISK OF RELAPSE

Based on reviewing evidence in the RP literature, Douaiht and colleagues[52] rec-ommended seven clinical strategies for implementing relapse prevention. These strategies involve helping individuals:

➤ understand relapse as a process and an event, and learn to recognise early warning signs
➤ identify personal high-risk situations and learn effective cognitive and behavioural coping responses
➤ improve communication skills and interpersonal relationships, and establish social networks for recovery
➤ manage negative affect (e.g. anxious mood, depressed mood, anger, boredom)
➤ identify and manage cravings and conditioned cues that precede cravings
➤ recognise and challenge cognitive distortions (e.g. catastrophising, jumping to conclusions, overgeneralising)
➤ consider the use of medications to treat withdrawal syndromes and to assist individuals with relapse prevention.

Some of these strategies will be discussed in the case study.

The following section will be dedicated to introducing important constructs in the RP model and clinical strategies implemented in a case study. This case study is extracted from the *Relapse Prevention over Time* DVD produced by the American Psychological Association. Please refer to www.apa.org/videos/4310805.html for details of the DVD.

Case study 16.1

Kevin (35) is an African American male who has a bachelor's degree and works full time for a publishing company. Kevin was living with his sister when therapy began but moved to several different locations (e.g. recovery housing) throughout the course of the therapy. Kevin and the therapist met for six one-hour sessions during a nine-month period.

The main objective of the initial session was to gather Kevin's bio-psychosocial history and history of drug use. This is imperative, given that RP is grounded on the bio-psychosocial model of addictive behaviours.[4] A second goal of the session is to identify Kevin's goals for recovery.

Bio-psychosocial history: Kevin had a complicated family history. Kevin's father abandoned the family when he was very young. Kevin's mother was a chronic drug user, who relied on him to take care of his younger sibling. At the age of 16, Kevin filed for emancipation and started living by himself. Kevin's relationship with his former partner ended due to his substance use issues. They had a three-year-old daughter, and Kevin reported having a very close relationship with her.

Kevin had a long history of using alcohol and drugs. He experimented with alcohol at the age of 14 and tried marijuana at the age of 15. As an adult, he continued to use alcohol and marijuana and experimented with powder cocaine. Prior to entering therapy, Kevin has been using crack cocaine for two and a half years. Kevin stated that while alcohol and marijuana are no longer problems for him, he continued to struggle with crack cocaine. Kevin reported that he started using crack cocaine for social reasons (i.e. a way to spend time with his brother, whom he tried to please). Then the use of crack cocaine gradually became a means to cope with emotions. To Kevin, crack cocaine seems very appealing: relative to other substances, crack is cheaper and easier to hide from others, and it gave him a quicker intoxication. Kevin received inpatient treatment for his crack cocaine use and experienced a brief lapse episode (i.e. only used once on one occasion) three weeks prior to working with the therapist. Utilising the dynamic model of relapse to conceptualise Kevin's case, maternal drug use, lack of social support, history of and early initiation of drug use serve as distal risks of relapse.

Goals: The goals for therapy were established. Kevin expressed desire to maintain complete abstinence from crack cocaine, his primary drug of choice. To achieve this goal, several clinical strategies consistent with those recommended by Douaiht and colleagues were utilised.[52] These skills were aimed to help Kevin reduce the risk of, as well as the harm of, relapse.

Clinical strategies: The most common clinical strategy used in the course of therapy was to help Kevin identify personal high-risk situations and develop cognitive and behavioural coping responses. This strategy was implemented as early as the first session by conducting a *lapse debriefing*, which elucidated the cognitive and behavioural factors leading to lapse and relapse in a temporal fashion. For instance, Kevin reported that payday was a significant high-risk situation for him, as he described, '*I found the cheque that come in the mail to me. Oh, I can go cash this and maybe go grab something to eat. Left the cash and cheque place, money in hand. My head was saying, walk this way. My feet walked somewhere else. Maybe I'll just see who is in the neighbourhood. Maybe I'll just turn around and go back to the store to get a pack of cigarettes. I made the turn to turn around and there was the dealer.'*

Kevin's description is an example of *apparently irrelevant decision.*[4] While Kevin's initial plan did not involve using drugs, a series of seemingly unimportant decisions (e.g. 'see who is in the neighbourhood') led him to use. Additionally, Kevin reported that feelings of shame and guilt of use were major internal triggers that led him to use. As described earlier in the RP section, this is an example of abstinence violation effect (AVE), a significant internal reaction hypothesised in the original RP model.

During the course of therapy, another lapse debriefing was conducted in order to understand the cognitive and behavioural factors associated with Kevin's most recent relapse episode. Kevin experienced interpersonal conflicts with his former partner. Feelings of loneliness and isolation served as internal triggers. When a high-risk situation (the Christmas holiday) occurred, these internal triggers were intensified and Kevin chose to use substance in order to ease his emotional pain. Contributing to this lapse is another internal trigger – memory of his mother, which evoked intense feelings of resentment and anger.

A second clinical strategy aimed to help Kevin understand relapse as a process and an event, and learn to recognise early warning signs. This strategy is grounded on the belief that education about the relapse *process* and the likelihood of a lapse occurring may prepare individuals to manage the challenging journey of cessation attempts more effectively. To implement this clinical strategy, a lapse debriefing was conducted every time Kevin experienced a lapse or relapse, thereby helping him restructure negative thoughts about lapses. Rather than responding to relapses with a judgemental attitude and viewing those as a failure, the therapist treated them as mistakes that Kevin could learn from. Here is an example. During the course of therapy, Kevin reported that a major relapse episode occurred over a three-day period. The high-risk situation identified was social pressure – Kevin's housemates asked him for money to buy drugs and invited him to use together. Unable to resist temptation, Kevin caved in and had a lapse. This lapse turned into relapse when he experienced another personal high-risk situation, a payday. Kevin used his pay cheque to purchase more drugs and continued to use for the next two days. When Kevin discovered that a dealer, to whom he owed money, threatened to hurt his family, he considered the consequences of his action and decided to stop using. Kevin reported that facing severe negative consequences was a turning point for him and he has not used since this relapse episode. To turn relapse into *prolapse*, the therapist and Kevin worked together to develop alternative coping strategies to manage 'payday', a reoccurring high-risk situation. One useful strategy for Kevin was to ask his sister to manage pay cheques for him and restrict the amount of cash he could carry on a daily basis.

To help Kevin recognise the warning signs of relapse, the therapist discussed a potential high-risk situation with him.

Kevin: My birthday is coming up. It's expected that I am going to, or that I already have, relapsed. I am angry that there's some behaviours that precludes relapse that takes more than just six to eight weeks of clean time to get rid of . . . I am emotionally pretty close to a pre-lapse right now . . .

The therapist: So how does it feel or how do you feel that this could be coming towards a pre-lapse?

Kevin: I feel lonely. I feel disappointed in myself. I feel like turning 36 was not where I want it to be as a father and as someone who can give love, not having someone around . . .

Another clinical strategy implemented was to help Kevin identify and manage cravings and cues that precede cravings. For instance, the therapist alongside Kevin identified an important environmental trigger; that is, the neighbourhood he lived in. Kevin reported 'being approached by dealers outside of the recovery house' and struggling with rejecting the dealer. In Kevin's case, this environmental cue triggered cravings which became apparent in cognitive (thoughts of using) as well as physiological changes (increased anxiety).[53] To effectively manage this environmental cue, Kevin chose to move out of the neighbourhood to be with his sister, who provided better support for his recovery.

An additional strategy was to help Kevin enhance interpersonal communication skills. This was achieved by encouraging Kevin to discuss difficult emotions in sessions. For example, Kevin realised that he used drugs for coping with negative affect, as he reported: 'I am using because I am hurt, I am using because I don't know how to express something. I am using to run away from something.' Kevin also pointed out that he had trouble maintaining relationships: 'Intimacy around other people may be what I am running from in my life.' Given that Kevin had trouble expressing emotions, allowing him to discuss feelings and thoughts in the therapeutic setting may in turn improve his ability to communicate in intimate relationships occurring outside of therapy.

Two additional clinical strategies were used to help Kevin reduce the risk of relapse: managing negative affect and identifying and challenging cognitive distortions. Since Kevin reported that he used substance for the purpose of coping emotions, the therapist worked on helping him manage negative emotional states more effectively. For example, Kevin was encouraged to accept his feelings and share his feelings with someone he could trust. The therapist recommended Kevin practise meditation as a way to gain acceptance towards negative emotions and to achieve lifestyle balance. Throughout the course of therapy, Kevin's cognitive distortions were noticed, which indicated that he was extremely self-critical. For example, rather than viewing relapse episodes as opportunities for learning, Kevin felt deeply ashamed and expressed desire to discontinue therapy. Kevin rarely acknowledged his education and career achievement. Instead, he tended to focus on his identity as a 'drug addict'. To challenge these cognitive distortions, the therapist used various cognitive and behavioural strategies in session (e.g. gathering evidence of strength rather than weaknesses).

Overwhelmed by guilt and shame as a result of experiencing relapse episodes, Kevin's motivation to return to therapy decreased. To enhance Kevin's motivation to change, he was encouraged to identify several interpersonal recovery goals and negative consequences of substance use. With regard to the goals, Kevin stated that he would like to reunite with his daughter and former partner. With regard to negative consequences, Kevin reported that over-inflated self-esteem, homelessness and losing his family were the most important consequences to him.

Conclusions: In the course of therapy, it was acknowledged that Kevin's presenting problems were substance abuse, symptoms of depression and issues related to family conflicts. Kevin's case, presenting a complex set of problems, is not rare among individuals with substance use issues. Empirical literature has indicated that negative affect (i.e. depression and anxiety) as well as interpersonal conflicts represent two of the most common triggers for individuals with substance abuse problems.[30] Based on Kevin's self-report, symptoms of depression should be further assessed for a mood or an anxiety disorder.[54,55] Once diagnoses are formulated, psychologists should work collaboratively with other providers (e.g. psychiatrists or medical doctors) to formulate a comprehensive treatment plan.

Surviving a difficult childhood, Kevin has developed maladaptive ways of coping, most notably his tendency to use substances as a way to cope with negative emotions (e.g. symptoms of depression, feelings of loneliness, anger, etc.). Kevin's case demonstrated that addictive behaviour is a learned process. Despite experiencing multiple negative consequences, Kevin found it difficult to maintain abstinence due to the immediate rewards offered by using drugs (e.g. alleviation of negative emotions). The establishment of effective cognitive and behavioural coping response in the face of high-risk situation was extremely important in helping Kevin achieve his recovery goals. In the case study, we demonstrated clinical strategies that can be implemented to prevent relapse.

CONCLUSION

As demonstrated in the case study, it is imperative for professionals to help the individual understand that relapse could be a valuable learning experience in recovery. This in turn will normalise the relapse experience, reduce guilt and shame elicited by relapse, and allow the individual to begin exploring high-risk situations associated with a particular relapse episode. The risk of future relapse can be reduced once personal high-risk situations are identified and effective coping strategies are formulated.

Continued practice of RP or MBRP skills is an important part of the treatment that must be conveyed to the individual. With RP, individuals are encouraged to practise skills designing to identify internal and external triggers and challenge cognitive distortions. More detail on how to implement these cognitive behavioural skills can be found in Daley and Marlatt's workbook.[30] Additionally, adapting Marlatt and colleagues' work, a protocol for treating cocaine-dependent individuals is available online (*see* To Learn More). With MBRP, individuals are encouraged to practise meditation daily. Regular meditation practice may increase awareness for triggers. Learning how to *respond* with acceptance and non-judgemental attitude, rather than *react*, will in turn reduce the risk of relapse. For professionals who are interested in implementing MBRP, Bowen and colleagues' book[27] is an excellent resource. The guided meditation CDs produced by Dr Jon Kabat-Zinn may be helpful for professionals and individuals to establish regular meditation practice. We also recommend professionals to become familiar with different models of relapse. Although Marlatt and colleagues' models of relapse have been influential, they are not the only approach in conceptualising relapse. We recommend Brandon and colleagues' article,[2] which summarised different models of relapse, and other relapse prevention approaches that have received empirical support. Understanding various relapse models and the menu of options available for prevention will help professionals choose the treatment approach that may be most appropriate for a particular individual.

REFERENCES

1 Witkiewitz KA, Marlatt GA. *Therapist's Guide to Evidence-based Relapse Prevention.* Amsterdam: Elsevier; 2007.

2 Brandon TH, Vidrine JI, Litvin EB. Relapse and relapse prevention. *Annual Review of Clinical Psychology.* 2007; **3**: 257–84.

3 Marlatt GA, Donovan DM. *Relapse Prevention: maintenance strategies in the treatment of addictive behaviors.* 2nd ed. New York: Guilford; 2005.

4 Marlatt GA, Gordon JR. *Relapse Prevention: maintenance strategies in the treatment of addictive behaviors.* 1st ed. New York: Guilford; 1985.

5 Witkiewitz K, Marlatt GA. Relapse prevention for alcohol and drug problems: that was Zen, this is Tao. *American Psychologist.* 2004; **59**: 224–35.

6 Donovan DM. Marlatt's classification of relapse precipitants: is the Emperor still wearing clothes? *Addiction.* 1996; **91**: 131–7.

7 Shiffman S, Hufford M, Hickcox M, *et al.* Remember that? A comparison of real-time versus retrospective recall of smoking lapses. *Journal of Consulting and Clinical Psychology.* 1997; **65**: 292–300.

8 Bandura A. Self-efficacy: toward a unifying theory of behavioral change. *Psychological Review.* 1977; **84**: 191–215.

9 Brown SA, Goldman MS, Christiansen BA. Do alcohol expectancies mediate drinking patterns of adults? *Journal of Consulting and Clinical Psychology.* 1985; **53**: 512–19.

10 Curry S, Marlatt GA, Gordon JR. Abstinence violation effect: validation of an attributional construct with smoking cessation. *Journal of Consulting and Clinical Psychology.* 1987; **55**: 145–9.

11 Carroll KM. Relapse prevention as a psychosocial treatment: a review of controlled clinical trials. *Experimental and Clinical Psychopharmacology.* 1996: **4**: 46–54.

12 Irvin JE, Bowers CA, Dunn ME, *et al.* Efficacy of relapse prevention: a meta-analytic review. *Journal of Consulting and Clinical Psychology.* 1999; **67**: 563–70.

13 Lancaster T, Hajek P, Stead LF, *et al.* Prevention of relapse after quitting smoking: a systematic review of trials. *Archives of Internal Medicine.* 2006; **166**: 828–35.

14 Lowman C, Allen J, Stout RL, *et al.* Replication and extension of Marlatt's taxonomy of relapse precipitants: overview of procedures and results. *Addiction.* 1996; **91**: 51–71.

15 Shiffman S. Conceptual issues in the study of relapse. In: Gossop M, editor. *Relapse and Addictive Behavior.* London: Routledge; 1989. pp. 149–79.

16 Gossop M, Stewart D, Browne N, *et al.* Factors associated with abstinence, lapse or relapse to heroin use after residential treatment: protective effect of coping responses. *Addiction.* 2002; **97**: 1259–67.

17 Burgess ES, Brown RA, Kahler CW, *et al.* Patterns of change in depressive symptoms during smoking cessation: who's at risk for relapse? *Journal of Consulting and Clinical Psychology.* 2002; **70**: 356–61.

18 Cinciripini PM, Wetter DW, Fouladi RT, *et al.* The effects of depressed mood on smoking cessation: mediation by postcessation self-efficacy. *Journal of Consulting and Clinical Psychology.* 2003; **71**: 292–301.

19 Cohen LM, McCarthy DM, Brown SA, *et al.* Negative affect combines with smoking outcome expectancies to predict smoking behavior over time. *Psychology of Addictive Behaviors.* 2002; **16**: 91–7.

20 Hedeker D, Mermelstein R. Random-effects regression models in relapse research. *Addictions.* 1996; **91**: S211–S29.

21 Litt MD, Kadden RM, Cooney NL, *et al.* Coping skills and treatment outcomes in cognitive-behavioral and interactional group therapy for alcoholism. *Journal of Consulting and Clinical Psychology.* 2003; **71**: 118–28.

22 Rohsenow DJ, Monti PM. Does urge to drink predict relapse after treatment? *Alcohol Research and Health.* 1999; **23**: 199–202, 225–32.

23 Shiffman S, Balabanis M, Paty J, *et al.* Dynamic effects of self-efficacy relapse. *Health Psychology.* 2000; **19**: 315–23.

24 Whiteside U, Nguyen T, Logan D, *et al.* In: Witkiewitz K, Marlatt GA, editors. *Therapist's Guide to Evidence-based Relapse Prevention.* Amsterdam: Elsevier Academic Press; 2007. pp. 91–116.

25 Ziedonis D, Yanos P, Silverstein SM. In: Witkiewitz K, Marlatt GA, editors. *Therapist's Guide to Evidence-based Relapse Prevention.* Amsterdam: Elsevier Academic Press; 2007. pp. 117–140.

26 Ziedonis D, Stern R. Dual recovery therapy for schizophrenia and substance abuse. *Psychiatric Annual.* 2001; **31**: 255–64.

27 Bowen S, Chawla N, Marlatt GA. *Mindfulness-Based Relapse Prevention for Addictive Behaviors: a clinician's guide.* New York: Guilford; 2010.

28 Kabat-Zinn J, Massion A, Kristeller J, *et al.* Effectiveness of a meditation-based stress reduction intervention in the treatment of anxiety disorders. *American Journal of Psychiatry.* 1992; **149**: 936–43.

29 Teasdale JD, Segal ZV, Williams JM, *et al.* Prevention of relapse/recurrence in major depression by mindfulness-based cognitive therapy. *Journal of Consulting and Clinical Psychology.* 2000; **68**: 615–23.

30 Daley DC, Marlatt GA. *Overcoming your Alcohol or Drug Problem: effective recovery strategies – therapist guide.* Oxford: Oxford University Press; 2006.

31 Witkiewitz K, Marlatt GA, Walker D. Mindfulness-based relapse prevention for alcohol and substance use disorders. *Journal of Cognitive Psychotherapy.* 2005; **19**: 211–18.

32 Marlatt GA, Chawla N. Meditation and alcohol use. *Southern Medical Journal.* 2007; **100**: 451–3.

33 Bowen S, Chawla N, Collins SE, *et al.* Mindfulness-Based Relapse Prevention for substance use disorders: a pilot efficacy trial. *Substance Abuse.* 2009; **30**(4): 295–305.

34 Collins SE, Chawla N, Hsu SH, *et al.* Language-based measures of mindfulness: initial validity and clinical utility. *Psychology of Addictive Behaviors.* 2009; **23**: 743–9.

35 Pennebaker JW, Booth RJ, Francis ME. *Linguistic Inquiry and Word Count (LIWC): LIWC 2007.* Austin, TX: LIWC Inc.; 2007.

36 Hsu SH, Collins S, Marlatt GA. The role distress tolerance in Mindfulness-Based Relapse Prevention. New York: Poster presented at Association for Behavioral and Cognitive Therapies; 2009.

37 Witkiewitz K, Bowen S. Depression, craving, and substance use following a randomized trial of mindfulness-based relapse prevention. *Journal of Consulting and Clinical Psychology.* 2010; **78**: 362–74.

38 Cooney NL, Litt MD, Morse PA, *et al.* Alcohol cue reactivity, negative-mood reactivity, and relapse in treated alcoholic men. *Journal of Abnormal Psychology.* 1997; **106**: 243–50.

39 Perkins KA, Grobe JE. Increased desire to smoke during acute stress. *British Journal of Addiction.* 1992; **87**: 1037–40.

40 Shiffman S, Waters AJ. Negative affect and smoking lapses: a prospective analysis. *Journal of Consulting and Clinical Psychology.* 2004; **72**: 192–201.

41 Sinha R, O'Malley SS. Craving for alcohol: findings from the clinic and the laboratory. *Alcohol and Alcoholism.* 1999; **34**: 223–30.

42 Stewart J. Pathways to relapse: the neurobiology of drug- and stress-induced relapse to drug-taking. *Journal of Psychiatry and Neuroscience.* 2000; **25**: 125–36.

43 Wheeler RA, Twining RC, Jones JL, *et al.* Behavioral and electrophysiological indices of negative affect predict cocaine self-administration. *Neuron.* 2008; **13**: 774–85.

44 Curran GM, Booth BM, Kirchner JE, *et al.* Recognition and management of depression in a substance use disorder treatment population. *Journal of Drug and Alcohol Abuse.* 2007; **33**: 563–9.

45 Witkiewitz K, Villarroel N. Dynamic association between negative affect and alcohol lapses following alcohol treatment. *Journal of Consulting and Clinical Psychology.* 2009; **77**: 633–44.

46 Simons J, Gaher R. The Distress Tolerance Scale: development and validation of a self-report measure. *Motivation and Emotion.* 2005; **29**: 83–102.

47 Brown RA, Lejuez CW, Kahler CW, *et al.* Distress tolerance and duration of past smoking cessation attempts. *Journal of Abnormal Psychology.* 2002; **111**: 180–5.

48 Daughters SB, Lejuez CW, Bornovalova MA, *et al.* Distress tolerance as a predictor of early treatment dropout in a residential substance abuse treatment facility. *Journal of Abnormal Psychology.* 2005; **114**: 729–4.

49 Daughters SB, Lejuez CW, Kahler C, *et al.* Psychological distress tolerance and duration of most recent abstinence attempt among residential treatment seeking substance abusers. *Psychology of Addictive Behaviors.* 2005; **19**: 208–11.

50 Quinn EP, Brandon TH, Copeland AL. Is task persistence related to smoking and substance abuse? The application of learned industriousness theory to addictive behaviors. *Experimental and Clinical Psychopharmacology.* 1996; **4**: 186–90.

51 Zvolensky MJ, Baker KM, Leen-Feldner E, *et al.* Anxiety sensitivity: association with

intensity of retrospectively rated smoking-related withdrawal symptoms and motivation to quit. *Cognitive Behavior Therapy*. 2004; **33**: 114–25.

52 Douaiht A, Delay DC, Stowell KR, *et al.* Relapse prevention: clinical strategies for substance use disorders. In: Witkiewitz KA, Marlatt GA, editors. *Therapist's Guide to Evidence-based Relapse Prevention.* Amsterdam: Elsevier; 2007. pp. 37–71.

53 Verheul R, Van den Brink W, Geerlings P. A three-pathway psychobiological model of craving for alcohol. *Alcohol and Alcoholism.* 1999; **34**: 128–48.

54 Daly DC, Moss HB. *Dual Disorders: counseling clients with chemical dependency and mental illness.* 3rd ed. Center City, MN: Hazelden; 2002.

55 Westermyer JJ, Weiss RD, Zeidonis DM, editors. *Integrating Treatment for Mood and Substance Abuse.* New York: Howard Medical Publishing; 2003.

TO LEARN MORE

- A cognitive behavioural approach: treating cocaine addiction. Available at: http://archives. drugabuse.gov/TXManuals/CBT/CBT1.html
- Centre for Mindfulness in Medicine, Health Care, and Society. Available at: www.umassmed. edu/content.aspx?id=41252
- Mindfulness meditation practice CD and tapes. Available at: www.mindfulnesscds.com/
- Substance Abuse and Mental Health Services Administration publication on relapse prevention. Available at: http://store.samhsa.gov/facet/Treatment-Prevention-Recovery/term/ Relapse-Prevention?headerForList=
- Segal ZV, Williams MG, Teasdale, JD. *Mindfulness-Based Cognitive Therapy for Depression: a new approach to preventing relapse.* New York: Guilford; 2001.

CHAPTER 17

Neuropsychiatry: brain injury, mental health–substance use

John R Ashcroft

INTRODUCTION

This chapter aims to increase awareness of the prevalence of brain injury within the substance misuse population. Issues surrounding the management of substance use problems in people with established injury will be discussed, and particularly how this may differ to those without injury. Means by which to identify those with suspected brain injury will also be discussed.

A complex relationship exists between brain injury and substance use problems. Possible causes of aquired brain injury include:

➤ stroke
➤ tumours
➤ metabolic disorders
➤ infections
➤ toxins
➤ trauma.

Those with substance use problems are particularly vulnerable to traumatic brain injury,[1–3] and there is a significantly increased risk of cerebrovascular accidents in people using stimulants.[4]

SUBSTANCE USE MAY PRECEDE BRAIN INJURY

Substance use is associated with an increased risk of sustaining traumatic brain injury, with the vast majority of people testing positive for alcohol or illicit drugs at the time of hospital admission.[1]

It has been estimated that approximately one-third of (traumatic) brain injury survivors have a history of substance use prior to injury,[2] and that alcohol or other drugs are *directly* involved in more than one-third of incidents that cause traumatic brain injury[2,3] with injury typically occurring secondary to accident or assault.

Combinations of particular drugs (e.g. opiates, benzodiazepines and alcohol) can have cumulative effects on the central nervous system, further increasing the risk of injury.

Alcohol and illicit substances may interact with prescription medication or exacerbate symptoms of pre-existing medical conditions. Falls may result secondary to seizures, postural hypotension or cardiac arrythmias. Substances may also directly cause brain damage by means of neurotoxicity, cerebral ischaemia or infarction.

Stimulant use may exacerbate pre-existing hypertension and increase the risk of cerebrovascular accidents. There is evidence to suggest that amphetamines are associated with a five-fold increased risk of haemorrhagic stroke and cocaine use with a two-fold increased risk in both ischaemic and haemorrhagic stroke.[4] Combination with alcohol may further increase the risk.[5]

Brain damage may result indirectly by means of vitamin deficiency (Wernicke-Korsakoff syndrome) or hepatic impairment (hepatic encephalopathy).

Psychological disturbance may be related to intoxication or a reaction to adverse social conditions associated with substance use. Moreover, substance use may exacerbate pre-existing psychiatric disorders and interact with medication prescribed. Psychotic symptoms may be deemed *drug induced* if they persist beyond the period of acute intoxication and can be distinguished from primary psychiatric disorders. Psychiatric disorder may also be precipitated by drugs and alcohol in those predisposed.

KEY POINT 17.1

Neuropsychiatric manifestations evident following prolonged drug or alcohol use may be reflective of brain damage.

SUBSTANCE USE MAY OCCUR FOLLOWING BRAIN INJURY

Evidence suggests that there is an increased vulnerability to substance use following brain injury in those without prior substance use problems.[2,6] The use of drugs and alcohol upon an already damaged brain is particularly dangerous. Their neurotoxic effect can negatively affect recovery, in addition to enhancing the physiological effects of prescribed medication.

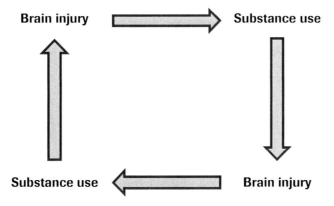

FIGURE 17.1 Substance use–brain injury cycle

Substance use may be used as a means of self-medication or simply recreationally and possibly contributes to further brain injury. In this way a **substance use–brain injury cycle** (*see* Figure 17.1) may develop, with a potentially progressive deterioration in cognitive functioning (*see* Case Study 17.1).

When further brain injury is not incurred substance use may exacerbate the residual effects of previous injury (such as coping difficulties and deficits in social skills and problem solving).

Case study 17.1

Martin (42) suffered a traumatic brain injury following a blow to the head from falling scaffold while working as a construction worker aged 26. He had suffered contusions to the left frontal and temporal lobes of the brain. Right-sided weakness and speech deficits improved with rehabilitation and speech therapy, although a number of neuropsychiatric symptoms became increasingly apparent. Following the injury Martin separated from his partner, describing how she was unable to cope with his *bad temper and mood swings.* He was unable to return to his previous job because of his physical disability and began to accrue significat debt. After separation from his partner Martin returned to live with his parents. His *aggressive and antisocial behaviour* put considerable strain on the family. Martin began to drink alcohol heavily, initially bingeing once or twice a week, although his consumption steadily increased to daily use. Since his injury he had generally *lacked motivation* in terms of performing activities of daily living, although generally with a little prompting he fared reasonably well. Since his increased alcohol consumption there was a noticeable deterioration in both his physical and mental health. He became more forgetful, was increasingly agitated and there was a significant deterioration in personal hygiene. Martin was persuaded by his parents to attend his GP in an attempt to address his excessive alcohol consumption. He agreed to a referral to the specialist alcohol sevice. History and physical examination suggested that Martin's current presentation was not simply a consequence of alcohol dependence. Rather, sustained heavy alcohol consumption had in all likelihood further damaged an already damaged and vulnerable brain, exacerbating pre-existing neuropsychiatric symptoms. Magnetic resonance imaging (MRI) of the brain displayed evidence of previous injury, in addition to cortical atrophy particularly involving the frontal lobes of the brain consistent with a diagnosis of alcohol-related dementia.

Key issues:
- The previous injury would have possibly increased Martin's vulnerability and susceptibility to futher brain damage from alcohol.
- An awareness of neurological deficits will greatly assist in the planning of future management in terms of setting realistic treatment goals.
- Intervention would aim to reduce further alcohol consumption.
- An assessment of capacity would be indicated given the potential serious consequences of continued alcohol use.

The severity of traumatic brain injury is often estimated using three domains (Table 17.1).

1 Glasgow Coma Scale (Box 17.1[7]).
2 Post traumatic amnesia – the period of dense impairment of new learning – anterograde amnesia following acute injury.[8]
3 Duration of loss of consciousness – the complete lack of responsiveness to people and other environmental stimuli.

TABLE 17.1 Severity of traumatic brain injury

	Glasgow Coma Scale Score	Post-traumatic amnesia	Loss of consciousness
Mild	13–15	Less than 1 hour	Less than 60 minutes
Moderate	9–12	60 minutes to 24 hours	1 hour to 24 hours
Severe	3–8	More than 24 hours	More than 24 hours

BOX 17.1 The Glasgow Coma Scale

Best eye response
1 Eyes fail to open
2 Eyes open in response to pain
3 Eyes open in response to speech or verbal commands
4 Eyes open spontaneously

Best verbal response
1 No verbal response
2 Incomprehensible sounds
3 Use of inappropriate words
4 Able to converse but disorientation evident
5 Able to converse and oriented to time, place and person.

Best motor response
1 No motor response
2 Extension to pain
3 Abnormal flexion to pain
4 Flexion/withdrawal from pain
5 Localises to pain
6 Able to obey commands

The distribution of severity of tramatic brain injury has been estimated as mild 80%, moderate 10–12% and severe 7–10%.[7] However, accurate estimation is complicated by the fact that many cases fail to present to the Accident and Emergency department, particularly mild injuries, or fail to be recognised at the time of assessment of head injury (*see* Case Study 17.2).

Case study 17.2

Peter (24) attended the A&E intoxicated with alcohol. He had suffered a blow to the back of the head from a bottle during a fight. His manner was verbally aggressive and he was deemed to be threatening towards others. After examination his injuries were deemed to be minor and he was asked to leave the department. Peter was later found unconscious after having collapsed ouside the department. A computerised tomograhy (CT) scan of Peter's head revealed a subdural haemorrhage.

Key issues:

- There may be clear evidence of intoxication, although it should be considered that Peter may have *also* experienced an, as yet undiagnosed, brain injury following head trauma.

Traumatic brain injury may broadly be divided into *closed* or *open*. It is possible to have head injury without brain injury and conversely brain injury may exist without evident head injury. Therefore, severity of head injury is not a reliable clinical indicator of the severity of brain injury. *Mild* head injury does not neccessarily signify *mild* brain injury.

As noted above, the vast majority of traumatic brain injuries are classified as mild (80%). However, can we really regard any brain injury as mild? Is the term *mild traumatic brain injury* an oxymoron? Although the physical and structural damage may be regarded as minor, the neuropsychiatric manifestations of the injury may be profound.

FUNCTIONAL NEUROANATOMY OF FRONTAL LOBE CIRCUITS

The location and severity of brain injury will determine the deficits incurred. The frontal lobes are particularly vulnerable to the effects of traumatic brain injury due to their size and location. They are the largest of the lobes of the brain situated at the front of the cranium. Their proximity to the sphenoid bone, an irregular wedge-shaped bone situated at the base of the skull, increases their vulnerability following trauma.

Damage to frontal lobe circuits may lead to deficits and personality change consistent with a diagnosis of *organic personality disorder*.

The World Health Organization ICD-10 classification for organic personality disorder is:

> *This disorder is characterised by a significant alteration of the habitual patterns of premorbid behaviour. The expression of emotions, needs, and impulses is particularly affected. Cognitive functions may be defective mainly or even exclusiveley in the areas of planning and anticipating the likely personal and social consequences . . .*[9]

Five major frontal-subcortical circuits have been described for this condition:[8]
1 Dorsolateral-prefrontal circuit – executive function.

2   Orbitofrontal circuit – social intelligence.
3   Anterior cingulate circuit – motivation and emotional experience.
4   Motor circuit – voluntary motor function.
5   Frontal eye fields – eye movements.

Those with brain injury typically affecting dosolateral-prefrontal circuits may have difficulties executing particular tasks. Executive dysfunction (also referred to as the dysexecutive syndrome) involves a difficulty with:

➤ planning
➤ abstract thought
➤ cognitive flexibility
➤ acquisition of rules.

In addition to traumatic injury, subcortical ischaemic vascular change has been shown to be associated with a decline in executive functioning even in individuals without dementia.[10] This is particularly relevant to people using stimulants. Therefore, it can be seen how damage to one or more of these circuits can have a profound effect on substance use management.

Difficulty with self-monitoring may lead to socially inappropriate behaviour or failure to initiate actions. Executive dysfunction may greatly affect an individual's ability to alter habitual behaviour and overcome temptation (*see* Case Study 17.3).

Case study 17.3

Sheena (37) is opiate dependent and first began to inject heroin at the age of 21. She suffered a haemorrhagic stroke at age 31 after a weekend binge of amphetamines and benzodiazepines which, although did not result in significant physical disability, led to considerable changes in her personality. Sheena is currently prescribed opiate substitution medication and although she attends regular appointments with the substance use service she continues to inject heroin. She no longer uses stimulants but will binge with alcohol occasionally at weekends. Superficially, Sheena appears motivated to refrain from heroin use but there has been minimal change in her substance use behaviour since engagement with services. During sessions, Sheena frequently displays inappropriate behaviour in the form of emotional outbursts, displays of irritability and the expression of socially inappropriate comments. She is also observed to have difficulty keeping up with the conversation and to have a tendency to lose concentration and wander off the topic. Both Sheena and the professionals involved have become increasingly frustrated at her seeming lack of progress.

Key issues:

● Brain injury is often associated with deficits in attention and concentration, information processing speed, and memory.
● Low tolerance to frustration and subsequent emotional outbursts may be directly or indirectly related to such deficits.

- Attempts should be made to minimise distractions during sessions and to take breaks or terminate sessions early if there is evidence of fatigue or frustration.
- Involvement of family and friends in the treatment programme is essential.

Poor motivation, apathy, poor memory and emotional instability may add further difficulty (*see* Case Study 17.4).

Case study 17.4

Aina (42) failed to attend a number of key worker and medical apointments and as per policy was discharged from the substance use service. She had a long history of crack cocaine and amphetamine use. Aina's lack of engagement with the service was taken to reflect a lack of desire to refrain from illicit substance use, although she had reported having not used stimulants for several weeks. For several months, Aina had consistently complained of memory and concentration difficulties associated with poor motivation and affective instability.

Key issues:
- Long-term stimulant use is associated with an increased risk of vascular changes (ischaemic and haemorrhagic) within the brain. This may result in alteration of cognitive functioning and executive dysfunction.
- Cognitive deficits directly associated with stimulant use may mimic the withdrawal state. It is important to acurately determine current substance use.
- Poor punctuality may reflect memory, attentional and concentration impairment or transportation issues.
- It may be difficult to distinguish between poor motivation associated with damage to neural circuitry or a general disinterest in the treatment programme. However, missed appointments should not be assumed to be intentional or to reflect resistance to treatment.
- Involvement of family and friends in the treatment programme is essential.

Those individuals who are more severely injured may have visible signs of head trauma such as scars and facial damage or have neurological signs such as speech and language difficulties or poor motor coordination. However, symptoms of mild traumatic brain injury are often indistiguishable from those of substance use[11] and individuals with mild brain injury and substance use problems are often unrecognised. Therefore, it is crucial to ask about previous head injury as injuries may go undetected either by the individual or services (*see* Case Study 17.5).

Case study 17.5

Richard (38) was opiate dependent and attended the substance use service to collect his prescription for methadone. His speech was deemed to be slurred and his movements slow and hesitant. Richard was advised to return later in the day when he was less intoxicated with alcohol. He became irritated and his behaviour was assumed to provide further evidence that he was drunk. He protested – an alcohol breath test was zero. He had a history of several blows to his head with associated brain injury. A past CT scan of Richard's head demonstrated damage to the left frontal and basal ganglia regions of the brain.

Key issues:

- Expressive aphasia (an impairment of spoken language characterised by non-fluent speech) and a deficit in motor coordination (associated with lesions of the basal ganglia) had been mistaken for intoxication with alcohol.
- Deficits present following brain injury can mimic intoxication with alcohol and other substances.
- People with brain injury may lack insight into deficits suffered and it is therefore important to ask about previous head injury.

Symptoms and clinical presentation may be misinterpreted as a result of poor insight into personality change or a failure to make a connection between deficit and injury. This may lead to self-medication with alcohol and substances – both prescibed and illicit.

CONCLUSION

Professionals need to understand and be openly aware of the impact of substance use problems on the brain. However, it is important to identify if the brain injury preceded the substance use or indeed is mimicking substance use. In all instances the following are pivotal to effective intervention and treatment for these individuals.

➤ Treatment providers are often trained *either* in the management of substance use or brain injury – this needs to be addressed if a good measured outcome is to be achieved.
➤ Deficits present following brain injury can mimic intoxication with alcohol and other substances.
➤ Symptoms of mild traumatic brain injury may be indistiguishable from those of substance use.
➤ Although the physical and structural damage may be minor, the neuropsychiatric manifestations of mild traumatic brain injury may be profound.
➤ People with brain injury and substance use problems may lack insight into deficits suffered or such deficits may be masked by current drug use.
➤ It is important to ask about previous head injury at the point of entry into the

substance use treatment programme as part of the comprehensive assessment process.

➤ Screening for brain injury must be an integral part of the comprehensive assessment process.

➤ Missed appointments should not be assumed to be intentional or to reflect poor motivation or resistance to treatment.

➤ Poor punctuality may reflect memory, attentional or concentration impairment.

➤ A seeming lack of motivation to engage with subtance use services, or resistance to treatment, may reflect underlying brain injury and damage to neural circuitry.

➤ Cognitive impairment may affect a person's ability to engage with any stage of a substance use programme.

➤ The diagnosis of brain injury and cognitive impairment in people experiencing substance use problems may assist in the establishment of realistic targets, outcomes and goals.

REFERENCES

1 Taylor LA, Kreutzer JS, Demm SR, *et al.* Traumatic brain injury and substance abuse: a review and analysis of the literature. *Neuropsychology Rehabilitation.* 2003; **13**: 165–88.

2 Corrigan JD, Rust E, Lamb-Heart G. The nature and extent of substance abuse problems in persons with traumatic brain injury. *Journal of Head Trauma Rehabilitation.* 1995; **10**: 29–46.

3 Boyle MJ, Vella L, Maloney E. Role of drugs and alcohol in patients with head injury. *Journal of the Royal Society of Medicine.* 1991; **84**: 608–10.

4 Westover AN, McBride S, Haley RW. Stroke in young adults who abuse amphetamines or cocaine. A population-based study of hospitalised patients. *Archives of General Psychiatry.* 2007; **64**: 495–502.

5 Green RM, Kelly KM, Gabrielsen T, *et al.* Multiple intracerebral haemorrhages after smoking 'crack' cocaine. *Stroke.* 1990; **21**: 957–62.

6 Kreutzer JS, Witol A, Sander A, *et al.* A prospective multicenter analysis of alcohol use patterns among persons with traumatic brain injury. *Journal of Head and Trauma Rehabilitation.* 1996; **11**: 58–69.

7 Teasdale G, Jennett BJ. Assessment of coma and impaired consciousness. A practical scale. *Lancet.* 1974; **2**: 81–4.

8 Arciniegas DB, Beresford TP. *Neuropsychiatry: an intoductory approach.* Cambridge: Cambridge University Press; 2001.

9 World Health Organization. The ICD-10 Classification of mental and behavioural disorders. Clinical descriptions and diagnostic guidelines. Geneva: World Health Organization; 1992. Available at: www.who.int/classifications/icd/en/GRNBOOK.pdf (accessed 19 November 2010).

10 Kramer JH, Reed BR, Mungas D, *et al.* Executive function in subcortical ischaemic vascular disease. *Journal of Neurology, Neurosurgery and Psychiatry.* 2002; **72**: 217–20.

11 Iverson GL, Lange RT, Franzen MD. Effects of mild traumatic brain injury cannot be differentiated from substance abuse. *Brain Injury.* 2005; **19**: 15–25.

TO LEARN MORE

- Corrigan JD. Substance abuse as a mediating factor in outcome from traumatic brain injury. *Archives of Physical Medicine and Rehabilitation.* 1995; **76**: 302–9.
- Kramer JH, Reed BR, Mungas D, *et al.* Executive function in subcortical ischaemic vascular disease. *Journal of Neurology, Neurosurgery and Psychiatry.* 2002; **72**: 217–20.
- Picard MM, Paluck RJ. *Traumatic Brain Injury and Substance Abuse: a reference and resource guide.* Washington: US Department of Education, Rehabilitation Service Administration; 1992.
- Taylor LA, Kreutzer JS, Demm SR, *et al.* Traumatic brain injury and substance abuse: a review and analysis of the literature. *Neuropsychological Rehabilitation.* 2003; **13**: 165–88.

Useful chapters

The *Mental Health–Substance Use* series comprises six books. To develop knowledge and understanding, chapters are interlinked, building and exploring specific areas. It is hoped the following will help readers locate relevant chapters easily.

BOOK 1: INTRODUCTION TO MENTAL HEALTH–SUBSTANCE USE

BOOK 2: DEVELOPING SERVICES IN MENTAL HEALTH–SUBSTANCE USE

Useful contacts

- Addiction Arena – www.addictionarena.com
- Addiction Medicine – http://listserv.icors.org/SCRIPTS/WA-ICORS. EXE?A0=ADD_MED
- The Addiction Project – www.theaddictionproject.com
- Addiction Rehabilitation Facilities – www.arf.org/isd/bib/mental.html
- Addiction Technology Transfer Center (ATTC) Network – www.attcnetwork.org
- Addiction Today – www.addictiontoday.org
- ADDICT-L List – http://listserv.kent.edu/archives/addict-l.html
- Alcohol and Alcohol Problems Science Database – http://etoh.niaaa.nih.gov
- Alcohol and Drug History Society – http://historyofalcoholanddrugs.typepad.com
- Alcohol Concern (64 Leman Street, London E1 8EU, UK; Tel: 020 7264 0510; Fax: 020 7488 9213; Email: contact@alcoholconcern.org.uk) – www.alcoholconcern. org.uk/servlets/home
- Alcohol Drugs and Development – www.add-resources.org
- Alcohol Focus Scotland – www.alcohol-focus-scotland.org.uk
- Alcohol Misuse (Department of Health) – www.dh.gov.uk/en/Publichealth/ Healthimprovement/Alcoholmisuse/index.htm
- Alcohol Misuse List – www.jiscmail.ac.uk/lists/ALCOHOL-MISUSE.html
- Alcohol, other Drugs and Health: current evidence – www.bu.edu/ aodhealth/index.html
- Alcohol Policy Network – www.apolnet.ca
- Alcohol Reports – www.alcoholreports.blogspot.com
- Alcoholics Anonymous – www.aa.org
- Alcoholism and Substance Abuse Providers – www.asapnys.org
- American Association of Colleges of Nursing. *Tool Kit for Cultural Competent Baccalaureate Nurses*; 2008. (This site will soon have a toolkit for graduate education as well.) – www.aacn.nche.edu/Education/pdf/toolkit.pdf
- American Psychiatric Association – www.psych.org
- American Society of Addiction Medicine – www.asam.org/CMEonline.html
- Australasian Professional Society on Alcohol and other Drugs – www.apsad.org.au
- Australian Drug Foundation – www.adf.org.au
- Australian Drug Information Network – www.adin.com.au
- Australian Government Department of Health and Ageing:
  - Alcohol – www.alcohol.gov.au

- Illicit drugs – www.health.gov.au/internet/main/publishing.nsf/content/ healthpubhlth-strateg-drugs-illicit-index.htm
- Mental health publications – www.health.gov.au/internet/main/publishing.nsf/ Content/mental-pubs
- Berman Institute of Bioethics – www.bioethicsinstitute.org
- Best Practice Portal – www.emcdda.europa.eu/best-practice
- BioMed Central – www.biomedcentral.com
- Brain Injury Australia – www.bia.net.au
- Brain Trauma Foundation – www.braintrauma.org
- Brief Addiction Science Information Source (BASIS) – www.basisonline.org
- Campaign for Effective Prevention and Treatment of Addiction – www.solutionstodrugs.com
- CASA: The National Centre on Addiction and Substance Abuse – www.casacolumbia.org
- Centre for Addiction and Mental Health – www.camh.net
- Centre for Clinical and Academic Workforce Innovation (Tel: 01623 819140; Email: ccawi@lincoln.ac.uk) – www.lincoln.ac.uk/ccawi
- Centre for Evidence-Based Mental Health (CEBMH) – www.cebmh.com
- Centre for HIV and Sexual Health, Sheffield Primary Care NHS Trust – www.sexualhealthsheffield.nhs.uk
- Centre for Independent Thought – www.centerforindependentthought.org
- Centre for Mental Health – www.centreformentalhealth.org.uk
- Clan Unity – www.clan-unity.co.uk
- Clifford Beers Foundation. *Promotion of Mental Health*, vol. 1 (1992) – www.cliffordbeersfoundation.co.uk/jcont91.htm
- Committee on Publication Ethics – http://publicationethics.org
- Communities of Practice for Local Government – www.communities.idea.gov.uk
- Community Nursing Network – www.communitynursingnetwork.org
- Co-morbid Mental Health and Substance Misuse in Scotland – www.scotland.gov.uk/ Publications/2006/06/05104841/0
- Co-occurring Centre for Excellence (US) – www.coce.samhsa.gov
- *Co-occurring Mental and Substance Abuse Disorders: a guide for mental health planning and advisory councils* (2003) – www.namhpac.org/PDFs/CO.pdf
- Creative Commons – http://creativecommons.org
- *Cultural Competency in Health: a guide for policy, partnership and participation* (2005) – www.nhmrc.gov.au/publications/synopses/hp25syn.htm
- Daily Dose: drug and alcohol news from around the world (this website is no longer in continuous service, but the archives are still available) – http://dailydose.net
- Dartmouth Psychiatric Research Centre – http://dms.dartmouth.edu/~prc
- Department of Health – www.dh.gov.uk
- Department of Primary Health Care – www.primarycare.ox.ac.uk/research/dipex
- Doctors.net.uk – www.doctors.net.uk
- Double Trouble in Recovery: http://doubletroubleinrecovery.org
  - A list of peer-reviewed journal articles on Double Trouble in Recovery: http://doubletroubleinrecovery.org/research.html
  - Citations for biomedical literature published in peer-reviewed journals. Most citations resulting from a search for Double Trouble in Recovery link to the full text article: www.ncbi.nlm.nih.gov/pubmed

- Drink and Drugs News – www.drinkanddrugs.net
- Drinks Media Wire – www.drinksmediawire.com
- Drug and Alcohol Findings – http://findings.org.uk
- Drug and Alcohol Nurses of Australia – www.danaonline.org
- Drug and Alcohol Services South Australia – www.dassa.sa.gov.au
- Drug Day Programmes list – http://health.groups.yahoo.com/group/ drug_day_programmes
- DrugInfo Clearinghouse – http://druginfo.adf.org.au
- Drug Misuse Information Scotland – www.drugmisuse.isdscotland.org
- Drug Misuse Research list – www.jiscmail.ac.uk/lists/DRUG-MISUSE-RESEARCH. html
- Drugs and Mental Health –www.thesite.org/drinkanddrugs/drugsafety/ drugsandyourbody/drugsandmentalhealth
- Drug Talk list – http://lists.sublimeip.com/mailman/listinfo/drugtalk
- Drugtext Internet Library – www.drugtext.org
- Dual Diagnosis – www.hoseahouse.org/infirmary/dualdx.html
- Dual Diagnosis: Australia and New Zealand – www.dualdiagnosis.org.au
- Dual Diagnosis Toolkit – www.rethink.org/dualdiagnosis/toolkit.html
- Dual Diagnosis Website – http://users.erols.com/ksciacca
- Enter Mental Health: www.entermentalhealth.net
- European Alcohol Policy Alliance – www.eurocare.org
- European Association for the Treatment of Addiction – www.eata.org.uk
- European Federation of Nurses Associations – www.efnweb.org
- European Monitoring Centre for Drugs and Drug Addiction – www.emcdda. europa.eu
- European Working Group on Drugs Oriented Research – www.dass.stir.ac.uk/old-site/ sections/scot-ad/ewodor.htm
- Evidence-based Practice websites – http://davisplus.fadavis.com/purnell/evidence_ based_weblinks.cfm
- Eye Movement Desensitisation and Reprocessing Training Workshops – www. emdrworkshops.com
- Faces and Voices of Recovery – www.facesandvoicesofrecovery.org
- Federation of Drug and Alcohol Professionals – www.fdap.org.uk/certification/dap. html
- Gambling International list – http://health.groups.yahoo.com/group/ GamblingIssuesInternational/join?
- Global Alcohol Harm Reduction Network – http://groups.google.com/group/ gahrnet
- Global Health Council – www.globalhealth.org
- *Guardian UK*: The most useful websites on dual diagnosis – http://society.guardian. co.uk/mentalhealth/page/0,8149,688817,00.html
- Headway – www.headway.org.uk
- Health and Safety Executive (HSE) – www.hse.gov.uk/stress
- HIT – www.hit.org.uk
- Horatio: European Psychiatric Nurses – www.horatio-web.eu
- Hub of Commissioned Alcohol Projects and Policies (HubCAPP) (this is an online resource of local alcohol initiatives throughout England and Wales) – www.hubcapp. org.uk

- Inexcess: in search of recovery – www.inexcess.tv
- International Brain Injury Association – www.internationalbrain.org
- International Centre for Alcohol Policies – www.icap.org
- International Council of Nurses – www.icn.ch
- International Council on Alcohol and Addictions – www.icaa.ch
- International Drug Policy Consortium – www.idpc.net
- International Harm Reduction Association – www.ihra.net
- International Network on Brief Interventions for Alcohol Problems (INEBRIA) – www.inebria.net
- International Nurses Society on Addictions – www.intnsa.org
- International Society for the Study of Drug Policy – www.issdp.org
- International Society of Addiction Journal Editors – www.parint.org/isajewebsite/
- Intervoice: the International Community for Hearing Voices – www.intervoiceonline.org
- IVO: scientific institute in lifestyle, addiction and related social developments – www.ivo.nl
- James Lind Alliance Guidebook – www.jlaguidebook.org
- James Lind Library – www.jameslindlibrary.org
- Join Together: advancing effective alcohol and drug policy, prevention and treatment – www.jointogether.org
- Madness and Literature Network – www.madnessandliterature.org
- Medical Council on Alcohol – www.m-c-a.org.uk
- Medline Plus – www.nlm.nih.gov/medlineplus/dualdiagnosis.html
- Mental Health (About.com) – http://mentalhealth.about.com
- Mental Health and Addiction 101 (Centre for Addiction and Mental Health, Canada) – www.camh.net/MHA101/
- Mental Health Europe – www.mhe-sme.org/en.html
- Mental Health First Aid: Australia – www.mhfa.com.au
- Mental Health First Aid: Canada – www.mentalhealthfirstaid.ca
- Mental Health First Aid: England – www.mhfaengland.org.uk
- Mental Health First Aid: Hong Kong – www.mhfa.org.hk
- Mental Health First Aid: Scotland – www.smhfa.com
- Mental Health First Aid: Singapore – www.mhfa.sg
- Mental Health First Aid: South Africa – www.mhfasa.co.za
- Mental Health First Aid: USA – www.thenationalcouncil.org/cs/program_overview
- Mental Health First Aid: Wales – www.mhfa-wales.org.uk
- Mental Health Forum – www.mentalhealthforum.net/forum
- Mental Health Foundation – www.mentalhealth.org.uk
- Mental Health in Higher Education – www.mhhe.heacademy.ac.uk/sitepages/educators/?edid=239
- Mental Health Information for All (RCPSYCH) – www.rcpsych.ac.uk/mentalhealthinfoforall.aspx
- *Mental Health Policy Implementation Guide: dual diagnosis good practice guide* (2002) – www.dh.gov.uk/en/Publicationsandstatistics/Publications/PublicationsPolicyAndGuidance/DH_4009058
- Mental Health Research Network – http://homepages.ed.ac.uk/mhrn
- The Mentor Foundation – www.mentorfoundation.org
- The Methadone Alliance Forum – www.m-alliance.org.uk/forum.html

- Middlesex University Dual Diagnosis Courses – www.mdx.ac.uk/courses/postgraduate/nursing_midwifery_health/index/aspx
- MIND: for better mental health – www.mind.org.uk
- Ministry of Justice: National Offender Management Service – www.justice.gov.uk/about/noms.htm
- Mood Disorders Association of Canada – www.mooddisorderscanada.ca
- Motivational Interventions for Drugs and Alcohol Misuse in Schizophrenia – www.midastrial.ac.uk
- Motivational Interviewing – www.motivationalinterview.org
- National Alliance on Mental Illness (US) – www.nami.org
- National Centre for Education and Training on Addiction Australia – www.nceta.flinders.edu.au
- National Comorbidity Initiative Australia – www.health.gov.au/internet/main/publishing.nsf/Content/health-pubhlth-publicat-document-metadata-comorbidity.htm
- National Consortium of Consultant Nurses in Dual Diagnosis and Substance Use – www.dualdiagnosis.co.uk
- National Drug and Alcohol Research Centre – http://ndarc.med.unsw.edu.au
- National Drug Research Institute – http://ndri.curtin.edu.au
- National Health Service – www.nhs.uk
- National Health Service Litigation Authority – www.nhsla.com
- National Institute for Health and Clinical Excellence (Midcity Place, 71 High Holborn, London, WC1V 6NA, UK; Tel: 0845 003 7780; Fax: 0845 003 7784; Email: nice@nice.org.uk) – www.nice.org.uk
- National Institute of Mental Health – www.nimh.nih.gov
- National Institute on Alcohol Abuse and Alcoholism (NIAAA) (5635 Fishers Lane, MSC 9304, Bethesda, MD 20892-9304, USA; Tel: 301-443-3860; Email: www.niaaa.nih.gov/ContactUs.htm) – www.niaaa.nih.gov
- National Institute on Drug Abuse, National Institutes of Health (6001 Executive Boulevard, Room 5213, Bethesda, MD 20892-9561, USA; Tel: 301-443-1124; Email: information@nida.nih.gov) – www.nida.nih.gov
- National Treatment Agency for Substance Misuse – www.nta.nhs.uk
- New Directions in the Study of Alcohol – www.newdirections.org.uk
- New South Wales Health Dual Disorders resources – www.druginfo.nsw.gov.au/illicit_drugs
- NHS Institute for Innovation and Improvement – www.institute.nhs.uk
- Nordic Council for Alcohol and Drug Research (NAD) – www.norden.org/en/areas-of-co-operation/alcohol-and-drugs
- O'Grady CP, Skinner WJ. *A Family Guide to Concurrent Disorders* (2007) – www.camh.net/Publications/Resources_for_Professionals/Partnering_with_families/partnering_families_famguide.pdf
- Ontario Mental Health and Addictions Knowledge Exchange Network – www.ehealthontario.ca/portal/server.pt?open=512&objID=1398&PageID=0&mode=2
- Oxford Centre for Neuroethics – www.neuroethics.ox.ac.uk
- Partnership in Coping – www.pinc-recovery.com
- Progress: National Consortium of Consultant Nurses in Dual Diagnosis and Substance Use – www.dualdiagnosis.co.uk
- Promoting Adult Learning – www.niace.org.uk/current-work/area/mental-health

- Psychiatric Nursing – www.citypsych.com/index.html
- Psychminded – www.psychminded.co.uk
- Public Access (National Institutes of Health) – http://publicaccess.nih.gov/index.htm
- Recovery Workshop – www.recoveryworkshop.com
- Rethink (UK) – www.rethink.org/dualdiagnosis
- Royal College of General Practitioners – www.rcgp.org.uk
- Royal College of Psychiatrists – www.rcpsych.ac.uk
- Royal College of Psychiatrists. *Changing Minds Campaign* – www.rcpsych.ac.uk/campaigns/previouscampaigns/changingminds.aspx
- Royal Society for the encouragement of Arts, Manufactures and Commerce (RSA) – www.thersa.org
- Sacred Space Foundation – www.sacredspace.org.uk
- SANE Australia – www.sane.org
- Schizophrenia Society of Canada – www.schizophrenia.ca
- Scholarship Society – www.scholarshipsociety.org
- Scottish Addiction Studies – www.dass.stir.ac.uk/sections/showsection.php?id=4
- Scottish Addiction Studies Library – www.drugslibrary.stir.ac.uk
- Social Care Institute for Excellence – www.scie.org.uk
- Social Care Online – www.scie-socialcareonline.org.uk
- Society for the Study of Addiction – www.addiction-ssa.org
- Spanish Peaks Mental Health Centre – www.spmhc.org
- Stigma in Mental Health and Addiction – www.cmhanl.ca/pdf/Stigma.pdf
- Substance Abuse and Mental Health Center toolkit for integrated treatment for co-occurring disorders – http://mentalhealth.samhsa.gov/cmhs/CommunitySupport/toolkits/cooccurring
- Substance Abuse and Mental Health Data Archive – www.icpsr.umich.edu/SAMHDA
- Substance Abuse and Mental Health Services Administration – www.samhsa.gov
- Substance Misuse Management in General Practice – www.smmgp.org.uk
- The International Network of Nurses (TINN) – www.tinnurses.org
- The Management Standards Consultancy – www.themsc.org
- Therapeutic Communities list – www.jiscmail.ac.uk/lists/THERAPEUTICCOMMUNITIES.html
- Think Cultural Health: bridging the healthcare gap through cultural competence continuing education. (This site, developed by the US Department of Minority Health, has continuing education modules for physicians, nurses and other healthcare providers, and the Health Care Languages Implementation Guide.) – www.thinkculturalhealth.org and https://hclsig.thinkculturalhealth.hhs.gov
- Tidal Model – www.tidal-model.com
- Tilburg University, Department of Tranzo – www.uvt.nl/tranzo
- Toc H – www.toch-uk.org.uk
- Treatment Improvement Exchange – www.treatment.org
- Trimbos Institute: Netherlands Institute on Mental Health and Addiction – www.trimbos.org
- Turning Point – www.turning-point.co.uk
- Tx Director – www.txdirector.com
- UK Database of Uncertainties about the Effects of Treatment – www.library.nhs.uk/DUETs/Default.aspx
- UK Drug Policy Commission – www.ukdpc.org.uk

- UNGASS: United Nations General Assembly Special Session on the World Drug Problem – www.ungassondrugs.org
- United Nations Office on Drugs and Crime – www.unodc.org
- University of Toronto Joint Centre for Bioethics Centre for Addiction and Mental Health Bioethics Service – www.jointcentreforbioethics.ca/partners/camh.shtml
- Update: an alcohol and other drugs information bulletin board –http://lists.sublimeip.com/mailman/listinfo/update
- US Department of Health and Human Services. *Co-occurring Mental and Substance Abuse Disorders: a guide for mental health planning and advisory councils* (2003) – www.namhpac.org/PDFs/CO.pdf
- Victorian Alcohol and Drug Association – www.vaada.org.au
- Web of Addictions: links to other websites related to addiction – www.well.com/user/woa/aodsites.htm
- Wired In to Recovery: empowering people to tackle substance use problems – http://wiredin.org.uk
- World Health Organization: Climate change and human health – www.who.int/globalchange/en
- World Health Organization: Management of substance abuse – www.who.int/substance_abuse/en
- World Health Organization: Mental health – www.who.int/mental_health/policy/en
- World Medical Association – www.wma.net/en/10home/index.html
- Youth Drug Support, Australia – www.yds.org.au
- Youth Health Talk – www.youthtalkonline.com

Index

Page numbers in **bold** indicate figures and tables.